Mastering
Advanced Assessment

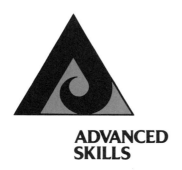

**ADVANCED
SKILLS**

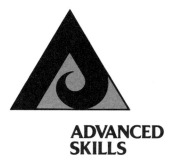

ADVANCED SKILLS

Mastering Advanced Assessment

Springhouse Corporation
Springhouse, Pennsylvania

Staff

Executive Director, Editorial
Stanley Loeb

Editorial Director
Matthew Cahill

Clinical Director
Barbara F. McVan, RN

Art Director
John Hubbard

Senior Editor
William J. Kelly

Clinical Project Director
Patricia Dwyer Schull, RN, MSN

Editors
Elizabeth Weinstein, Marylou Ambrose, Sarah Goltzer, Barbara Hodgson, Elizabeth Mauro, Barbara Trenk

Clinical Editors
Tina R. Dietrich, RN, BSN, CCRN; Carol A. Basile, RN,C, BSN, CCRN

Copy Editors
Jane V. Cray *(supervisor)*, Christina A. Price, Jennifer G. Mintzer, Nancy Papsin

Designers
Stephanie Peters *(associate art director)*, Matie Patterson *(senior designer)*, Maryanne Buschini, Darcy Feralio, Linda Franklin, Kristina Gabage, Joseph Laufer

Illustrators
Jean Gardner, Frank Grobelny, Robert Jackson, John Murphy, Robert Neumann, Judy Newhouse, George Retseck

Photographers
John Gallagher, Doug Mellor

Art Production
Robert Wieder

Typography
David Kosten *(director)*, Diane Paluba *(manager)*, Elizabeth Bergman, Joyce Rossi Biletz, Phyllis Marron, Robin Mayer, Valerie Rosenberger

Manufacturing
Deborah Meiris *(manager)*, Anna Brindisi, T.A. Landis

Production Coordination
Colleen M. Hayman

Editorial Assistants
Maree DeRosa, Beverly Lane, Mary Madden, Margaret Rastiello

Library of Congress Cataloging-in-Publication Data
Mastering advanced assessment.
    p.   cm. — (Advanced Skills™)
    Includes bibliographical references
and index.
    1. Nursing assessment.
    I. Springhouse Corporation.
    II. Series.
[DNLM: 1. Nursing Assessment.
2. Nursing Assessment — methods.
WY 100 M4224]
DNLM/DLC
                  92-49694
ISBN 0-87434-551-0   CIP

Contents

Advisory board

At the time of publication, the advisors
held the following positions.

Cecelia Gatson Grindel, RN, PhD
> Assistant Professor
> Villanova University
> College of Nursing
> Villanova, Pa.

Judith Ski Lower, RN, MSN, CCRN, CNRN
> Nurse Manager, Neurology Critical Care Unit
> Johns Hopkins Hospital
> Baltimore, Md.

Kathleen M. Malloch, RN, BSN, MBA, CNA
> Clinical Nursing Administrator
> Maryvale Samaritan Medical Center
> Phoenix, Ariz.

Marguerite K. Schlag, RN, MSN, EdD
> Director, Nursing Education and Development
> Robert Wood Johnson University Hospital
> New Brunswick, N.J.

Karen Then, RN, MN
> Assistant Professor, Faculty of Nursing
> University of Calgary, Alberta

Contributors and consultants

At the time of publication, the contributors held the following positions.

Carol A. Basile, RN,C, BSN, CCRN
Research Study Coordinator
Department of Pulmonary Medicine
Hospital of the University of Pennsylvania
Philadelphia

Vicki L. Buchda, RN, MS
Director, Special Care Unit
Maryvale Samaritan Medical Center
Phoenix, Ariz.

Tina R. Dietrich, RN, BSN, CCRN
Nurse Consultant
Bethlehem, Pa.

Margaret A. Fitzgerald, RN,C, MS, FNP
Assistant Professor, Graduate Nursing
Simmons College
Boston
Family Nurse Practitioner
Lawrence, Mass.

Jim Herbert, RN, MSN, FNP,C
Family Nurse Practitioner
Butternut Valley Health Center
Morris, N.Y.
Mary Imogene Bassett Hospital
Cooperstown, N.Y.

Margaret Massoni, RN, MSN, CS
Assistant Professor
College of Staten Island
City University of New York

Susan Russell Neary, RN,C, MS, ANP, GNP
Assistant Professor, Graduate Nursing
Simmons College
Nurse Practitioner, Home Care
Beth Israel Hospital
Boston

Catherine Paradiso, RN, MS, CCRN
Instructor
Rutgers, The State University of New Jersey
Clinical Specialist, Critical Care
St. Vincent's Medical Center
Staten Island, N.Y.

Suzanne D. Skinner, RN, MS
Former Instructor
University of Maryland School of Nursing
Baltimore

Johanna K. Stiesmeyer, RN, MS, CCRN
Critical Care Clinical Educator
El Camino Hospital
Mountain View, Calif.

At the time of publication, the consultants held the following positions.

Mary A. Mishler, RN, MSN, CNN, CS
Medical-Surgical Clinical Nurse Specialist
Our Lady of Lourdes Medical Center
Camden, N.J.

Frances W. Quinless, RN, PhD
Chairperson, Department of Nursing Education
and Services
University of Medicine and Dentistry of New Jersey
Newark

Carralee Sueppel, RN, BLS, CURN
Clinical Nursing Specialist
University of Iowa Hospitals and Clinics
Iowa City

FOREWORD

As the scope of nursing practice has continued to expand, the importance of nursing assessment has grown, too. Long gone are the days when a nurse could simply defer history taking and examination to the doctor. Now, you're expected to collect subjective and objective data in a thorough, systematic fashion, and then to formulate a diagnostic impression. Depending on where you work, you may even order diagnostic tests.

In short, nurses today are more independent—and more accountable—than ever before. Nurses working in all settings—including fast-paced hospitals, extended-care facilities, and patients' homes—have one thing in common: They must rely on themselves and on their own nursing skills. And one of the most important and sophisticated skills nurses must master is assessment.

Today, your assessment approach must be a blend of advanced clinical skills and knowledge and critical thinking. Whether you are new to nursing or have years of experience, you need a reliable guide to performing such advanced assessments.

Fortunately, *Mastering Advanced Assessment* gives you what you need—whether you're zeroing in on a patient's urgent complaint or performing a comprehensive assessment, body system by body system. This book covers everything you must know about assessment from patient interview techniques to diagnostic testing.

In the book's first two chapters, you'll find information that applies to all nursing assessments. Chapter 1 presents an overview that explains the critical role of advanced assessment in the nursing process. This chapter also covers the importance of critical-thinking skills, documentation, and collaboration. Chapter 2 explains how to take a patient's health history and how to perform a physical examination. Here you'll find a review of the four primary physical examination techniques: inspection, palpation, percussion, and auscultation.

Chapter 3 helps set *Mastering Advanced Assessment* apart from other assessment books by providing a systematic exploration of the chief complaints you're most likely to encounter. A key goal of advanced assessment is to move quickly from a patient's complaint, such as "I'm short of breath," to the appropriate history questions and examination techniques, and then to an accurate analysis of the patient's problem. This chapter will help you achieve that goal.

The next seven chapters cover assessment of the major body systems. Chapter 4 discusses the skin, hair, and nails; chapter 5, the neurologic system; chapter 6, the eyes, ears, nose, and throat; chapter 7, the respiratory system; chapter 8, the cardiovascular system; chapter 9, the gastrointestinal system; and chapter 10, the urinary and reproductive systems.

For your convenience, each of these chapters follows a format. After a brief introduction, the chapter reviews essential anatomy and physiology. Then comes a section on collecting the health history. After that, you'll find a major section explaining the physical examination. Here you'll see both illustrations and photographs that show important techniques. The next section contains a discussion of the major abnormal findings for the body system. More than just a list of abnormalities, this section is designed to help you analyze your assessment findings and reach a conclusion about what's causing your patient's problem. The last section in each body system chapter summarizes the most commonly ordered diagnostic tests.

As you use this book, you'll come upon graphic devices called logos that focus your attention on key pieces of information. The *Assessment insight* logo signals a succinct idea that deepens your understanding of a technique or principle of assessment. The *Anatomy* logo signals an illustration of a body system or structure. The *Pathophysiology* logo highlights information about disease development and progession. In chapter 8, for example, this logo accompanies a sidebar on the three causes of heart murmurs.

Throughout this book, you'll find many helpful illustrations and photographs, including color photographs. In chapter 4, for example, you'll see four pages of color photographs showing common skin abnormalities. And in chapter 7, color photographs depict important advanced assessment techniques and abnormal respiratory findings.

Following the last chapter is a listing of other books and articles on assessment recommended by the authors. Then comes the *Advanced skilltest*, a self-test containing challenging questions, some of which are based on case studies. The answers are provided along with complete rationales. This self-test will boost your confidence, as well as let you know which areas of advanced assessment you'll need to review.

I recommend *Mastering Advanced Assessment* for nurses who perform assessment in any patient-care setting. You'll appreciate the comprehensive format that covers every aspect of advanced assessment, and you'll enjoy the straightforward writing style. Once you've had the chance to use *Mastering Advanced Assessment*, you'll find yourself reaching for it again and again.

Gayle P. Andresen, RN,C, MS, ANP, GNP

Instructor, Family Medicine
University of Colorado School of Medicine
A.F. Williams Family Medical Center
Denver

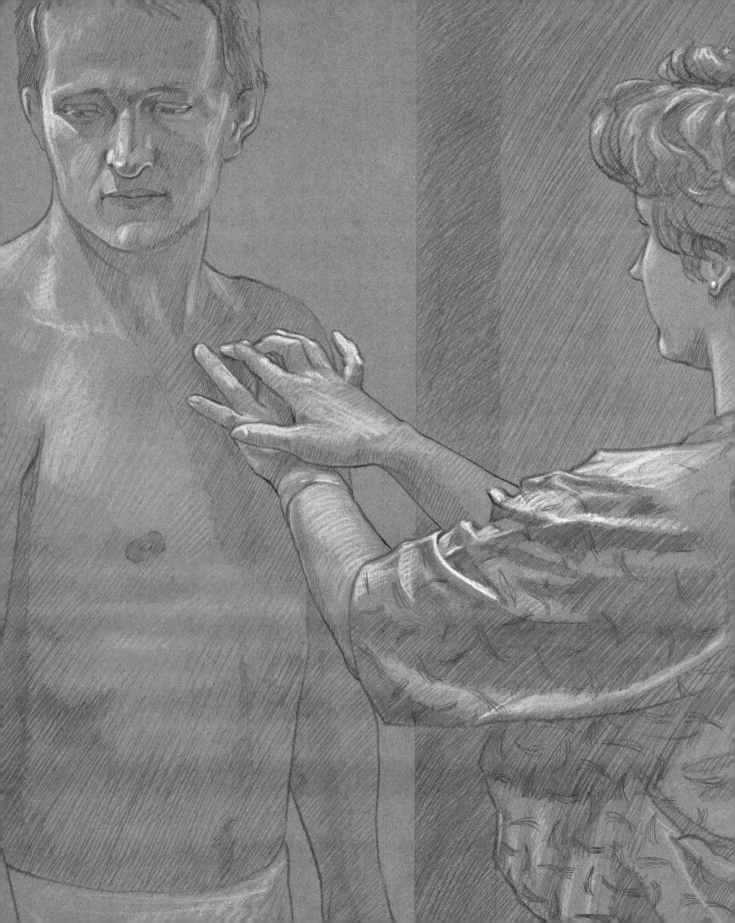

CHAPTER 1

Understanding advanced assessment

Today, you need advanced assessment skills more than ever before. Because of the trend toward admitting only the critically ill, hospitals are now populated with sicker patients. And because hospital stays have grown shorter, patients still needing sophisticated care are being discharged to extended care facilities and to their homes. So no matter where you work, you must regularly assess patients who have more complex health problems.

If you work in a hospital, standardized lengths-of-stay also make thorough, skilled assessments imperative. As you know, third-party payers have decided how long patients should be hospitalized for particular health problems. Only by recognizing and documenting a serious complication can you extend the stay of a patient who's too sick for discharge. So if your patient develops a complication—especially one with subtle signs and symptoms—the difference between proper hospital care and a dangerously early discharge may well be your

Nursing process and the scientific method

The steps of the nursing process follow the structure of the scientific method, as shown below.

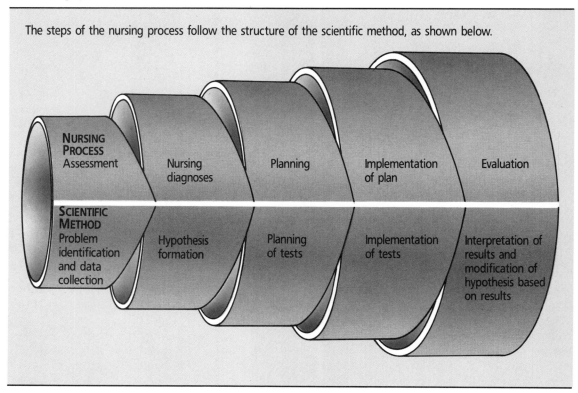

NURSING PROCESS Assessment	Nursing diagnoses	Planning	Implementation of plan	Evaluation
SCIENTIFIC METHOD Problem identification and data collection	Hypothesis formation	Planning of tests	Implementation of tests	Interpretation of results and modification of hypothesis based on results

assessment of his problem.

The aging of the population also means that more of your patients are likely to have severe, complex health problems. In our society, the percentage of people over age 65 continues to grow, and these people typically have multiple problems. As a result, you must know how one of a patient's problems affects another and how a treatment for one may affect another. For example, take a patient who suffers from both degenerative joint disease and gastritis. Administering a nonsteroidal anti-inflammatory drug may relieve symptoms of his joint disease but may exacerbate his gastritis. To monitor such patients effectively, you need both advanced knowledge and the complementary physical assessment skills.

What is advanced assessment?

Simply stated, it's a way of approaching assessment by using a full array of physical and cognitive skills. It includes the use of sophisticated assessment skills, such as auscultating carotid bruits and palpating for respiratory excursion.

But just as important as these physical skills is a focused, integrated mental approach. With this approach, your assessment truly becomes a working part of the nursing process. For example, you ask pointed questions about the patient's chief complaint to get on the right track from the start, use problem-solving techniques to uncover the cause of the problem as you assess, carefully analyze your findings to distinguish the normal from the abnormal, and interpret diagnostic test results in light of your assessment findings. This approach to assessment then leads logically to formulating appropriate nursing diagnoses and developing an effective plan of care.

Nursing process

Based on the scientific method, the nursing process is a systematic way of approaching any health problem. (See *Nursing process and the scientific method.*) To use the nursing process, you'll follow these five steps:
• Assess the patient.
• Formulate nursing diagnoses.
• Plan your care.
• Implement your plan.
• Evaluate the results.

Assessment

The first and most important step of the nursing process, assessment involves collecting all the relevant information needed to solve a health problem. All the remaining steps of this process depend heavily on the accuracy of this information, making a thorough, integrated assessment critical. Quite simply, if you don't correctly identify a patient's problem, your plan of care won't help you solve it. (See *How assessment guides diagnostic testing.*)

Keep in mind that your integrated assessment will focus not only on your patient's immediate health problem but also on his responses to it. That includes his physical, emotional, psychological, cultural, and spiritual responses.

Types of data
When your patient (or his family or friends) provides information you can't verify by observation or measurement, consider it subjective data—in short, *symptoms.* A patient's complaint of pain would be an example of a symptom. Objective data, or *signs,* can be verified. If a patient complains of a sore arm, for example, you may see a red, swollen area that feels warm. Although his complaint of pain is sub-

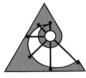

ASSESSMENT INSIGHT

How assessment guides diagnostic testing

No matter where you work, keep in mind that advanced diagnostic tests are no substitute for advanced assessment. If you detect a heart murmur on auscultation, spend a few minutes evaluating it; don't immediately recommend echocardiography.

A thorough, thoughtful assessment should always precede diagnostic tests. In fact, your assessment findings should be used to guide the choice of tests. Using this approach helps ensure that time and money won't be wasted on a battery of unnecessary diagnostic tests.

jective, the redness, warmth, and swelling that you observe are objective signs of his health problem.

During almost any assessment, you'll collect both subjective and objective data. But the amount of each will depend on the patient's problem. Consider the patient who's brought to the emergency department by a family member because he threatened suicide. You may have to rely almost exclusively on the history provided by the patient and his family member. Your only relevant observation may be that the patient seems depressed.

By contrast, another patient may have unmistakable signs of severe impetigo. With one quick observation, you'd determine his problem. You'd still collect a history to uncover the cause, but this subjective data would be secondary to your observation.

Nursing diagnoses

After collecting all the appropriate data about a patient's health problem, you'll use it to formulate your nursing diagnoses. Unlike medical diagnoses, which focus on diseases, nursing diagnoses focus on the patient's responses to his actual and potential health problems. These responses may be physical, emotional, psychological, cultural, and spiritual.

In effect, nursing diagnoses are more individualized than medical diagnoses. For instance, if you assess five different patients with the medical diagnosis of myocardial infarction, you may well devise five somewhat different sets of nursing diagnoses, each set reflecting a particular patient's response to his health problems.

Each nursing diagnosis should contain three components—the human response or problem, the related factor, and the defining characteristics. For instance, based on your assessment, you may make a nursing diagnosis of fluid volume excess related to increased sodium intake, as evidenced by edema, weight gain, shortness of breath, and S_3 heart sounds. (See *NANDA nursing diagnostic labels* and *Formulating nursing diagnoses,* page 6.)

Plan of care

Just as the nursing diagnoses grow from the assessment findings, the plan of care grows from your nursing diagnoses. Creating a useful plan takes nursing experience and awareness of the patient's individuality. This individuality, of course, should already be reflected in your nursing diagnoses.

As you formulate a plan of care, be sure to establish realistic, measurable goals and to list them in order of priority. Maslow's hierarchy of human needs can serve as a useful guide for setting priorities. This hierarchy is based on the idea that fundamental physiologic needs—for example, food and water—must be met before abstract needs—such as self-esteem. The complete Maslow hierarchy, starting with fundamental needs, is as follows: physiologic needs, safety and security, love and belonging, self-esteem, and self-actualization.

Implementation

After you've established your plan, you need to put it into action. This may require:

• *interdependent actions,* such as coordinating the contributions of other health care team members
• *dependent actions,* such as carrying out a doctor's orders
• *independent actions,* such as applying nursing interventions.

Implementation can be the most creatively demanding step of the nursing process. That's because it requires you to attain goals by applying your planned methods while still taking into account your patient's individuality and following valid scientific principles. Using critical-thinking techniques can help you apply your plan successfully.

Evaluation

In this last step of the nursing process, you evaluate the success of your plan by determining whether goals have been met. Thus, this step allows you to maintain a dynamic plan of care over time as the patient moves through the stages of illness and recovery. If you determine that a goal hasn't been met, you need to go back to the appropriate step in the nursing process and approach the problem again.

Of the five steps in the nursing process, evaluation is the most educational—if you approach it with intellectual honesty and a willingness to reassess your plan as necessary. This step can also be the most satisfying when your analysis demonstrates that the patient has met his goals.

Problem solving

One of the most fundamental nursing activities is problem solving. As we've seen, the nursing process itself serves as a system for solving a patient's health problems. But you must also solve many related problems—some large and some not so large—every day.

NANDA nursing diagnostic labels

This list contains the approved diagnostic labels of the North American Nursing Diagnosis Association (NANDA), as of 1992. The labels are arranged according to human response patterns.

Exchanging
Airway clearance, ineffective
Aspiration, high risk for
Body temperature, altered: High risk for
Bowel incontinence
Breathing pattern, ineffective
Cardiac output, decreased
Constipation
Constipation, colonic
Constipation, perceived
Diarrhea
Disuse syndrome, high risk for
Dysreflexia
Fluid volume deficit
Fluid volume deficit: High risk for
Fluid volume excess
Gas exchange, impaired
Hyperthermia
Hypothermia
Incontinence, functional
Incontinence, reflex
Incontinence, stress
Incontinence, total
Incontinence, urge
Infection, high risk for
Injury, high risk for
Nutrition, altered: Less than body requirements
Nutrition, altered: More than body requirements
Nutrition, altered: High risk for more than body requirements
Oral mucous membrane, altered
Poisoning, high risk for
Protection, altered
Skin integrity, impaired
Skin integrity, impaired: High risk for
Spontaneous ventilation, inability to sustain
Suffocating, high risk for
Thermoregulation, ineffective
Tissue integrity, impaired
Tissue perfusion, altered (renal, cerebral, cardiopulmonary, gastrointestinal, peripheral)
Trauma, high risk for
Urinary elimination, altered patterns
Urinary retention
Ventilatory weaning response, dysfunctional

Communicating
Communication, impaired verbal

Relating
Family processes, altered
Parental role conflict
Parenting, altered
Parenting, altered: High risk for
Role performance, altered
Sexual dysfunction
Sexuality patterns, altered
Social interaction, impaired
Social isolation

Valuing
Spiritual distress

Choosing
Adjustment, impaired
Coping: Defensive
Coping, family: Potential for growth
Coping, ineffective family: Compromised
Coping, ineffective family: Disabling
Coping, ineffective individual
Decisional conflict (specify)
Denial, ineffective
Health-seeking behaviors (specify)
Noncompliance (specify)
Therapeutic regimen (individual), ineffective management of

Moving
Activity intolerance
Activity intolerance: High risk for
Breast-feeding, effective
Breast-feeding, ineffective
Breast-feeding, interrupted
Diversional activity deficit
Fatigue
Growth and development, altered
Health maintenance, altered
Home maintenance management, impaired
Infant-feeding pattern, ineffective
Mobility, impaired physical
Peripheral neurovascular dysfunction, high risk for
Relocation stress syndrome
Self-care deficit: Bathing and hygiene
Self-care deficit: Dressing and grooming
Self-care deficit: Feeding
Self-care deficit: Toileting
Sleep pattern disturbance
Swallowing, impaired

Perceiving
Body image disturbance
Hopelessness
Personal identity disturbance
Powerlessness
Self-esteem, chronic low
Self-esteem disturbance
Self-esteem, situational low
Sensory-perceptual alterations (visual, auditory, kinesthetic, gustatory, tactile, olfactory)
Unilateral neglect

Knowing
Knowledge deficit (specify)
Thought processes, altered

Feeling
Anxiety
Caregiver role strain
Caregiver role strain, high risk for
Fear
Grieving, anticipatory
Grieving, dysfunctional
Pain
Pain, chronic
Post-trauma response
Rape-trauma syndrome
Rape-trauma syndrome: Compound reaction
Rape-trauma syndrome: Silent reaction
Self-mutilation, high risk for
Violence, high risk for: Self-directed or directed at others

Formulating nursing diagnoses

Each complete nursing diagnosis consists of three elements: the human response or problem statement, the related factor, and the defining characteristics. An example of each element follows its definition.

Human response or problem statement	Related factor	Defining characteristics
This statement identifies an actual or potential problem that can be affected by nursing care. When choosing a problem statement, you can use the most current list published by the North American Nursing Diagnosis Association.	A related factor may precede, contribute to, cause, or simply be associated with the human response. Identifying a related factor helps you choose the most effective interventions. Usually, the related factor is linked to the human response by the words *related to* or simply the abbreviation *R/T*.	Also called signs and symptoms, defining characteristics are the clues that lead you to your diagnosis. Like the related factor, the defining characteristics help tailor the nursing diagnosis to the particular patient. Usually, they're linked to the related factor by the words *as evidenced by* or simply the abbreviation *AEB*.
Fluid volume excess	R/T increased sodium intake	AEB edema, weight gain, shortness of breath, and S_3 heart sounds

Common methods

You can approach problem solving in a number of ways. Four of the most common ways you can use are the reflexive approach, trial and error, the intuitive approach, and the scientific method. Frequently, the approach you choose will depend on the particular problem you face.

Reflexive approach
Sometimes called the cookbook method, this approach involves using an automatic solution—that is, one that doesn't require you to make a conscious decision. Such solutions may be instinctive. For instance, if a patient says, "I feel like I'm going to vomit," you'd reflexively reach for an emesis basin.

At other times, the reflexive approach may involve applying a solution that you or someone else has decided on before the problem even arises. For example, if you're monitoring a patient's electrocardiogram, you may automatically administer lidocaine I.V. when you detect certain arrhythmias, such as ventricular tachycardia, based on standing orders.

Trial and error
Unlike the reflexive approach, the trial and error method requires thought, experimentation, and creativity. Typically, you'll use this method when no protocol exists for solving a problem. For instance, if you're using a new electronic thermometer and you don't have the manufacturer's instructions, you may experiment with the various switches before deciding on the best settings.

Because of its experimental nature, this hit-or-miss approach is related to the scientific method. But the trial and error method is considered prescientific because it's based on uncertain premises.

Intuitive approach
You've probably heard "nursing intuition" referred to as an almost magical ability, a sixth

sense that an experienced nurse possesses. Actually, this intuition is based on factual evidence. The evidence simply isn't obvious to a less experienced observer. But an experienced nurse can often detect subtle messages from patients. These messages may be expressed in body language or even silence. For example, when a nurse asks a patient with uncontrolled hypertension if he has been taking his medication regularly, she notices that he pauses before answering. Sensing that he's not telling her everything, the nurse questions him further — only to find that he has been skipping doses because he can't afford the prescription.

To use this intuitive approach, you need a certain sensitivity to and awareness of the environment. Invariably, those with nursing intuition are not only experienced and sensitive but also inclined to trust their nursing instincts.

Scientific method

To solve problems, nurses frequently turn to the scientific method, the basis of the nursing process. Using this logical approach, you proceed systematically through a series of steps:
• Identify the general problem.
• Collect relevant data from several sources.
• Formulate hypotheses (tentative assumptions made to test logical consequences).
• Plan ways to test hypotheses.
• Perform the tests.
• Interpret the results.
• Modify hypotheses, as necessary, based on the results.

When this process doesn't solve the problem, the flaw may be in your hypothesis. Or you may have failed to identify the problem properly. For example, if an alcoholic denies that he has a problem, you must address this denial in your plan of care. Addressing the alcoholism while ignoring the denial would doom your plan.

Thinking critically

When solving problems, you need to think critically. That is, you must scrutinize the premises you're using to draw your conclusions. And you must scrutinize the conclusions themselves to determine whether they're valid.

To promote critical thinking, you should question beliefs, consider face validity, and remember Occam's razor.

Question beliefs

As time passes, certain beliefs and certain ways of doing things become so strongly embedded in daily practice that their validity is taken for granted. For example, before World War II, women who had their babies in the hospital were kept in bed for as long as 2 weeks postpartum — a practice that actually increased the risk of deep vein thrombosis and subsequent pulmonary embolism. The prevailing assumption was that women needed extended bed rest to recuperate from their ordeal. But wartime surgical experience with wounded soldiers demonstrated conclusively the risks of extended bed rest.

Consider face validity

With this commonsense approach, you pose the question: Does the conclusion seem correct? That is, does it seem valid on the surface? Suppose, for instance, that you measure an infant's length and plot his growth on a chart that shows his previous measurements. If all the earlier measurements are in the 10th percentile and your new measurement is in the 90th percentile, it would lack face validity. Thus, you would remeasure the infant.

Similarly, you should question the validity of any study, laboratory finding, or assessment finding that varies markedly from the expected results. Such findings should always be rechecked.

Remember Occam's razor

Named after William of Occam, a medieval scholar, Occam's razor says that if you have several competing solutions to a problem, choose the simplest. Remembering this can protect you from overanalyzing a problem and constructing an unwieldy plan of care.

Often, your initial response to a patient's problem will be correct. Later, upon reflection, you may begin to consider the many other possibilities and feel overwhelmed. The purpose of Occam's razor is to help you focus on the most likely solution so that you can choose realistic, measurable interventions. Occam's razor can also help you rank competing solutions, placing the most practical one first.

Avoiding common errors

Several common errors can interfere with effective problem solving. Among the most common errors are false causality, suppression of the unexpected, and observer bias.

False causality
A person makes this error by assuming a causal connection between events simply because one occurs soon after the other. Consider the patient who's convinced that sniffing roses can cure a cold because he smelled a dozen roses yesterday and no longer has a cold. Though most people wouldn't believe that the fragrance of roses could cure a cold, nearly everyone makes the same basic error in logic at some point.

That's because the human mind has a strong tendency to make connections between events. Indeed, this tendency underlies much of our creativity. But our minds are so good at making connections that we often make erroneous ones that seem quite plausible. The recognition of this aspect of human thought led to the development of the scientific method as a way of examining cause and effect in a carefully controlled manner.

Suppression of the unexpected
We all have a tendency to suppress or deny evidence that doesn't fit our preconceived ideas. As a nurse, you need to guard against this basic human tendency to ignore what's not expected, especially when you're assessing a patient. Take a patient who complains of acute chest pain. If his nurse believes that the pain results from a cardiac problem, she may not consider subtle signs that point to a respi-

ratory cause as she assesses him. And this suppression of evidence can lead her to the wrong conclusion.

Remember, you may encounter a wide range of findings during a physical examination, and you need to keep your mind open. Unusual findings can threaten your sense of mastery, but you shouldn't ignore them because such findings, by their very nature, are often significant.

Observer bias
Another human tendency, observer bias can also get in the way of logical problem solving. As a educated observer, you need to guard against stereotypical thinking about patients, especially members of other cultures or classes, members of the opposite sex, and patients with health problems such as alcoholism or acquired immunodeficiency syndrome.

In some cases, observer bias can actually affect the information you collect. If during the interview a patient receives subtle messages from you about what you believe, he may tell you what he thinks you want to hear instead of telling you the truth.

Documentation

During and after your assessment, you need to document both your findings and your conclusions about the patient's problems. Documenting your assessment serves several purposes. Your notes help you organize your findings, thoughts, and conclusions, and thus help guide you through the rest of the nursing process. Using reliable assessment documentation, you can formulate nursing diagnoses and create a plan of care. Your notes also allow you to share information you've collected with other members of the health care team. And the notes act as a baseline, which you and others can use to evaluate the patient's progress.

You also need to document your assessments accurately to meet the requirements of the Joint Commission on Accreditation of Healthcare Organizations and various regulatory agencies. Good documentation can prove that quality care has been given. Peer review organizations and other quality assurance reviewers often look to the nursing assessment data for proof of quality care. Finally, in case of litigation, your record of your assessment can be used as evidence in court.

Because documentation serves these key purposes, you should always ensure that the record of your assessment is clear, concise, and accurate. In part, this means keeping current on the language of physical assessment, which continues to change. Obviously, knowing the current meanings of terms and using the terms correctly promotes effective communication among team members.

Communication is vital now more than ever because a patient's health care team may have many members, including physical therapists, occupational therapists, respiratory therapists, and registered dietitians, to name a few. Because so many people are involved, successful collaboration becomes the key to quality care. And the key to successful collaboration, in turn, is effective communication through proper documentation.

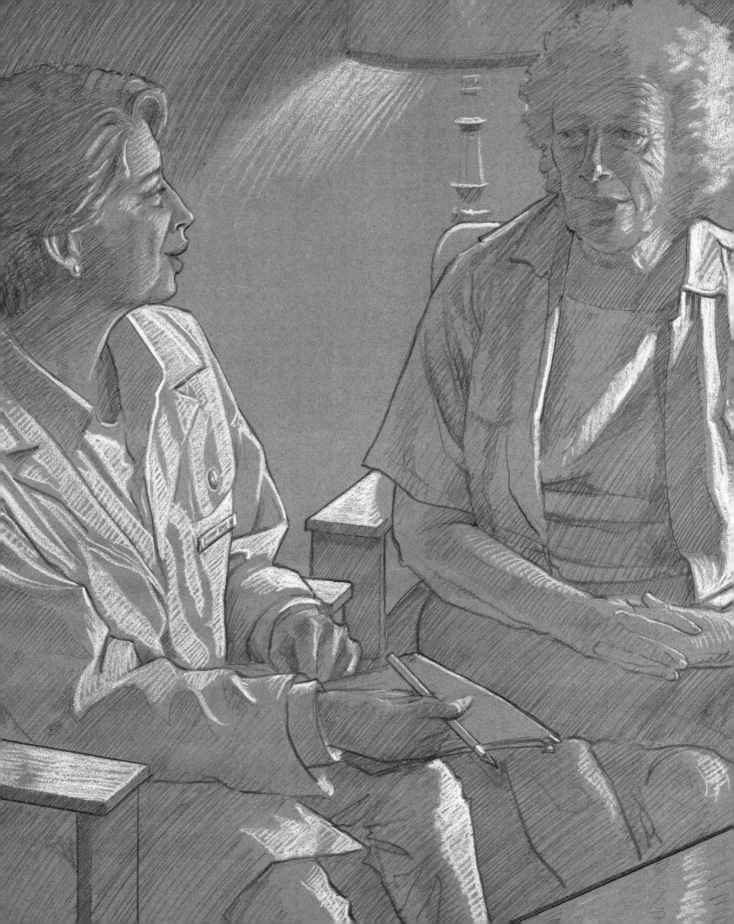

CHAPTER 2

Health history and physical examination

No matter where you work, chances are you'll be the first health care professional a patient will encounter. And during that initial meeting, you'll collect the health history and perform the physical examination that will give direction to the subsequent care he receives.

You'll use the history to explore the patient's chief complaint, learn about his past problems, and determine how he responds to his current problems. During the physical examination, you'll use the four assessment techniques to evaluate the patient's overall health and his specific problem. The information you gather and analyze during both phases of your assessment will then form the foundation of your nursing diagnoses and your plan of care.

To ensure that your information is accurate and thorough, you need to perform a skilled, systematic assessment. In this chapter, you'll find a comprehensive approach to your nursing assessment as well as guidelines and insights that will help you sharpen your skills.

Establishing the interview setting

Before taking a health history, make sure the setting is quiet and private and that the patient is comfortable. Sit facing the patient, about 3' to 4' (about 1 m) from him.

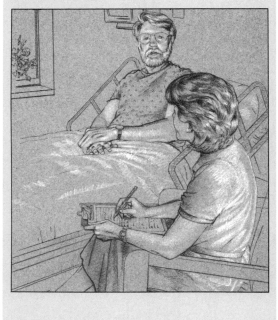

Complete health history

Unlike the medical health history, the nursing health history takes a holistic approach, focusing on the patient's illness *and* his responses to it. During the health history, you'll establish a rapport with your patient and collect important information on how the illness affects him and his family and what educational needs they have. This information then helps you direct your plan of care and initiate discharge planning. Frequently, you may find that the subjective data you collect during the health history tells you more about the patient's health status than the physical examination.

The type of health history you use will depend on whether you're gathering information about a new problem or reviewing the status of an ongoing one. You'll collect a *complete*

health history on admission when comprehensive information is needed. You'll use an *interval health history* to update information. And you'll perform a *problem-focused health history* to concentrate on a specific clinical problem.

In this chapter, the discussion will focus on the complete health history. But before reading about the specific components of such a history, review the following guidelines on interviewing your patient.

Conducting the interview

You may collect a health history in any setting—an office, the patient's hospital room, or his home. But always ensure that the immediate area is private and comfortable. Close the door to discourage interruptions and limit distractions. And make sure the room temperature is comfortable and lighting is adequate. Your patient won't provide a good history if he's shivering or looking into a bright light or glare from a window. Arrange the seating to promote eye contact and assure that you both are comfortable and relaxed. (See *Establishing the interview setting*.)

Establishing a rapport
Begin by introducing yourself to the patient and explaining that you need to take a history to identify his problem and formulate a plan of care best suited to his needs. Address the patient respectfully, using "Mr.," "Mrs.," or "Ms." and the patient's surname. Don't use the patient's first name until he gives you permission to do so.

Explaining the interview's goal will help allay the patient's fears and avoid any misconceptions. You should also discuss the duration of the first interview; the time, place, and duration of any subsequent visits; and the number of visits that will be required. Ask the patient about his expectations, and assure him of the confidentiality of all information.

To collect thorough, accurate information from the patient, you first must gain his trust. So show respect and empathy as you talk to him, and try to put him at ease and make him feel that you're interested in what he's saying. As you develop a rapport with the patient, he'll begin to share the important information you need to collect.

Throughout the interview, be alert for non-verbal communication. Body movements, gestures, touch, and voice tone convey important messages. Be aware that your own nonverbal cues can add to or relieve a patient's anxiety. Your eye movements, posture, and use of touch and space influence your interactions with a patient, especially during an initial interview, so be sure to convey your interest and concern about his problems. Your supportive attention will make him feel more relaxed and less anxious.

Listen carefully to what the patient is saying, and make eye contact with him as much as possible. If you find yourself thinking of your next question while the patient is speaking, you may need to ask him to repeat himself, thus inadvertently giving him the impression that what he's saying isn't worthwhile. (See *Interviewing the patient.*)

Communication techniques
To elicit the information you need, you may use various communication techniques. For instance, you may ask open-ended questions, closed questions, and directive questions. You'll also use common language, silence, facilitation, confirmation, restatement, reflection, clarification, confrontation, interpretation, summary, and conclusion.

Open-ended questions
Open-ended questions—such as "What brings you to the hospital today?" or "Can you tell me about your chest pain?"—tend to elicit a good deal of information. So you should use them as much as possible. Unlike closed questions, open-ended ones give the patient a chance to provide descriptive answers at his own pace. As he does, you can evaluate his alertness and his mental abilities. However, open-ended questions also allow the patient to digress and avoid discussing relevant information. So you may need to gently refocus the patient's attention.

Interviewing the patient

Depending on the situation, you may use the following tips to save interview time.
• Before starting the interview, determine whether the patient needs any immediate care. If so, provide it first so that you won't have to interrupt the interview.
• Use other sources of information, such as family members, medical history, and admission forms.
• When interviewing a newly admitted hospital patient, ask questions while you perform other tasks, such as inserting an I.V. line.
• With an acutely ill patient, collect only essential information.

Closed questions
If you need information quickly, use closed questions—such as "Has your chest pain gone away?"—because they require only one- or two-word answers. Closed questions may also cause less anxiety for patients with poor verbal skills. However, when you use these questions, you may get only a limited amount of information and may convey to the patient that you aren't interested in his plight.

Directive questions
You can help the patient focus on one subject by asking him questions, such as "When I press here, does it hurt?" and "How painful is this?" You'll use such questions when you need specific information. But you should use them cautiously because they may make the patient feel rushed, and he may not share information or fully develop his thoughts. (See *Avoid leading questions,* page 14.)

Common language
To promote clear communication, be sure to use language that the patient understands. Avoid using jargon and difficult clinical terms that create a barrier between you. If the patient uses words you don't understand, ask him to tell you what he means.

ASSESSMENT INSIGHT

Avoid leading questions

When interviewing your patient, be careful not to use leading questions that elicit "correct" answers. Such questions can seriously limit the information you receive during the health history. For example, the question "You don't use I.V. drugs, do you?" pushes the patient toward saying "No," whether he uses I.V. drugs or not. A better way to elicit this information is simply to ask, "Do you use I.V. drugs?"

Using examples from common experience can help you clarify information. For instance, to find out the size of a lesion, you might ask, "Was it as large as a dime?"

Silence
During the interview, using periods of silence encourages the patient to talk to you and allows you to observe him. These periods also allow the patient to organize his thoughts and reflect on the conversation.

Facilitation
With this technique, you use encouraging words, such as "Go on" and "I understand." Facilitation conveys empathy and encourages the patient to continue telling his story.

Confirmation
Intermittently throughout the interview, you need to make sure that you and the patient understand what's been said. To confirm that you have a clear account of what he's told you, you might say, "Just to be sure I understand, let me repeat what you said." Then repeat his account as you understand it.

Restatement
With this technique, you summarize the patient's message in your own words and then allow him to respond. You may begin your restatement by saying something like "In other words, you're saying that. . . ."

Reflection
This technique involves repeating a phrase that the patient has just used to get him to elaborate. Here's a sample of how reflection works:
   Patient: I started having pain in my foot, then I noticed the foot was cooler than my other one.
   Nurse: Your foot was cooler?
   Patient: Actually, it wasn't my entire foot, just my toes. Then, after a while, my toes started to turn blue, and I knew I had a blood clot in my leg.
   Nurse: You knew you had a blood clot in your leg?
   Patient: Yes, I had one before and the same thing happened.

Clarification
Use clarification to get a patient to clear up or elaborate on confusing or vague statements. If a patient says he's very nervous, you might say, "You feel anxious? Tell me what you mean by that."

Confrontation
Sometimes, you can help a patient gain insight into his thoughts or behavior by confronting him with inconsistencies in his narrative. Confrontation can be especially useful when a patient seems hesitant to discuss his feelings.

Interpretation
After a patient has given you information, you may interpret what he's told you. By sharing your conclusions with the patient, you allow him to confirm, deny, or offer clarification. This also allows you to offer an explanation of how the patient feels.

Summary
Briefly restating the patient's account in an orderly manner may be especially useful when his description has been detailed and rambling. A summary also signals to the patient that a segment of the interview is ending and gives him a chance to add any missing information. A summary may go something like this:
"You've told me that you've been in the hospital seven or eight times for chest pain, twice

for breathing problems, and once for a stroke. Is that correct?"

Conclusion

At the end of the interview, you might say, "I think I have all the information that I need. Do you have anything to add?" This gives the patient a last chance to supply information he believes is important.

Components of the health history

A complete health history includes a wealth of information. After collecting certain biographical data, you'll cover these topics: chief complaint, medical history, family history, psychosocial history, activities of daily living, and review of systems. If your patient is a child or an elderly person, you'll need to make some slight modifications when taking the health history.

Biographical data

Begin by asking the patient his name, address, telephone number, birth date, age, birthplace, Social Security number, race, nationality, religion, and marital status. Also find out the names of anyone living with the patient, the name and telephone number of the person to call in an emergency, and the patient's usual source of health care.

You may feel that collecting much of this data is unnecessary or too time-consuming. Yet, just by asking these simple questions, you can get a sense of the kind of person you're talking to and what his problems may be. You may also get a sense of whether the patient is a reliable historian. If he seems unable to provide accurate information, you should probably obtain the health history from a relative or friend. If you do, document who gave you the information.

Chief complaint

Ask the patient why he's seeking health care. Then record his exact words and place them in quotation marks. A properly recorded chief complaint would be "I've had a headache for 3 days." "States that he has been sick" would be

an improperly recorded chief complaint.

A description of the present illness covers details about the chief complaint, including how and when symptoms developed. While exploring the history of the present illness, you'll also ask the patient what led him to seek attention and how the illness has affected his life and ability to function.

Medical history

Ask the patient about his previous illnesses and injuries. Note the dates of significant treatments and any surgeries the patient has undergone.

Find out too if the patient has any allergies. In particular, ask him about allergies to antibiotics, such as penicillin, and to sulfa drugs.

Is the patient taking any prescription or over-the-counter drugs? Make a list of all prescribed drugs and their dosages.

Family history

Information about the general health of the patient's blood relatives helps to identify his risk of developing certain disorders. Ask the patient if any family members have a history of Alzheimer's disease, cancer, diabetes mellitus (or other endocrine or metabolic problems), hypertension, heart disease, seizures, sickle cell anemia, or kidney disease. Also ask whether any relatives have chronic conditions or unusual limitations (for instance, being bedridden because of paralysis from a cerebrovascular accident).

Psychosocial history

Try to determine how the patient feels about himself. How does he see his place in society and his relationships with others? Ask about his occupation, educational level, financial status, and responsibilities. Ask too about his sexual practices.

How has the patient coped with medical or emotional crises in the past? Has he experienced recent changes in his life or has he noticed any changes in his personality or behavior? Does he receive adequate emotional support from family and friends?

To determine the effects of change (including developmental change) on the patient's physical and psychological health, you may use one of these assessment tools: Rahe's Recent Life Changes Questionnaire or Sarason, Johnson, and Siegel's Life Experiences Survey.

With the Recent Life Changes Questionnaire, the patient checks all the events that he's experienced in the last 6 to 12 months. Each event is assigned a value based on the amount of social readjustment needed. The values are then added and a stress score is assigned. Studies have shown that a correlation exists between a high score, which indicates significant recent life changes, and the onset of health problems.

The Life Experiences Survey allows the patient to rate the desirability or undesirability of all events that have occurred in the last year. The patient uses a 7-point scale, ranging from -3 (extremely negative) to $+3$ (extremely positive). By adding all the scores, he arrives at the total change score, which may be positive or negative. Studies suggest a correlation between negative life changes and psychological problems.

Health promotion
In keeping with nursing's holistic approach, you need to understand how the patient defines health and what he does to promote his own health. Once you know this, you can determine his educational needs and evaluate whether compliance will be a problem.

Begin by asking the patient about his health beliefs. Remember that culture, religion, and personal experience heavily influence these beliefs, so be careful not to pass judgment. But do point out any obvious hazards.

Also ask the patient what he believes your role should be and what he should do to promote his own health. His answers will depend on previous experiences within the health care system, how he defines illness, and how he copes with being ill.

Socioeconomic status can influence how and when the patient seeks health care. If a patient has no insurance and has limited financial resources, he may not seek medical attention even when he's ill.

Where a patient lives and works affects his health as well. Ask him if his home and workplace have adequate heat, light, and water. Can he easily get to health care facilities, emergency services, and grocery stores?

Also find out if the patient is happy with his job. Does his employer provide protection against occupational hazards? Does he feel that his salary is adequate for the work that he does?

Activities of daily living
Ask the patient about his diet, sleep patterns, exercise patterns, and use of alcohol, drugs, and tobacco.

Diet
Nutrition plays a vital role in the way a person looks, feels, and behaves. As part of your health history, you need to collect information about which foods your patient usually eats and how he eats them. Here are some questions you might ask your patient about his dietary habits:
• Do you eat three meals a day?
• Do you prepare your own meals or does someone prepare them for you?
• Do you go to the grocery store or do you rely on someone else to do the shopping?
• Do you snack and, if so, what do you snack on?
• Do you eat foods from the four basic food groups?
• Do you have enough money to purchase the groceries that you need?

Sleep patterns
Ask about the patient's usual patterns of sleep. Is he getting enough sleep? Is his sleep disrupted? Find out when he gets most of his sleep. For example, does he work at night and sleep during the day?

Ask the patient how much sleep he needs to feel rested. Does he need to take an occasional nap during the day? Ask about any recurrent and disturbing dreams—an indication that he may be under stress or has psychological problems. Finally, ask if he has a history of narcolepsy, sleep apnea, or sleep deprivation.

Exercise patterns

Ask the patient if he exercises. If so, find out what type of exercise he does, how often, and why. Does he exercise to reduce stress? Maintain proper body weight? Lower cholesterol levels? Build muscles? This information will help you determine if the patient exercises compulsively or if he has a physical condition that could limit an exercise program.

Alcohol, drug, and tobacco use

Ask if the patient drinks alcohol or uses illicit drugs. If so, determine what kind and how much. Also find out whether he smokes. If so, ask how long he's smoked and how much he smokes.

Review of systems

During this part of the health history, you'll find out about past and present health problems in each body system. By asking questions about common symptoms, you can identify problems that the patient failed to mention earlier.

Modifications for pediatric and geriatric patients

When you assess a child or an elderly patient, you need to modify your health history somewhat. Depending on the age of your patient, you may seek slightly different information and obtain it from someone other than the patient.

Pediatric patients

Depending on how old and articulate your patient is, you may collect some or all of your data from his parents. If you're able to question the child, be sure to use language and concepts he can understand. If you're interviewing an adolescent, show your respect for his privacy by asking if he wants his parents present.

As part of your past medical history, ask about immunizations and childhood diseases. As part of the psychosocial history, you may use one of several screening tests to assess the developmental progress of infants and young children. Brazelton's Neonatal Behavioral Assessment Scale assesses the interactive behavior of the neonate. Carey and McDevitt's Infant Temperament Questionnaire measures the temperament of infants ages 4 to 8 months. And Frankenburg and Dodds's Denver Developmental Screening Test detects developmental delays in children up to age 6. Keep in mind, however, that you need special preparation before giving these tests.

Geriatric patients

An elderly patient may have sensory impairments, a decreased attention span, or an impaired memory. If you determine that your patient is confused or has difficulty communicating, you may need to rely on a family member for some or all of the health history.

Focus your interview on the patient's present illness and his current treatment regimen. Also ask about chronic illnesses and disabilities.

Assess how the patient is coping with his age, his changing role, and his relationships. As a person ages, more of his family members and friends may develop debilitating illnesses or die. Find out how your patient is coping with these changes.

Mental status examination

Depending on the patient and the circumstances, you may decide to include a mental status examination as part of your complete health history. This examination can give you insight into the patient's present psychological and physiologic functioning, his perception of his condition, and his attitude toward his current health status. During this examination, you'll assess the patient's level of consciousness, appearance, behavior, speech, cognitive functions, and emotional status.

Keep in mind that a single mental status examination won't give you definitive information about the patient's mental health. However, your skilled observations over time can yield valuable information about his mental state. For guidelines on performing a complete mental status examination, see Chapter 5.

Complete physical examination

After you've collected the appropriate health history information, you'll perform a complete physical examination of the patient. To achieve consistency and efficiency, you should always proceed in the same systematic fashion. That way, you won't skip a step or miss vital information.

Your complete examination will consist of a general survey, vital signs measurement, a nutritional assessment, and a thorough review of systems. Before reading about these elements, however, review the following guidelines on the four assessment techniques.

Techniques of assessment

To perform your physical examination, you'll use the four standard assessment techniques: inspection, palpation, percussion, and auscultation.

Inspection
The most frequently used assessment technique, inspection can reveal more than the other techniques—when it's performed correctly. An ongoing process, inspection begins when you first meet the patient and continues as you take the health history and perform the physical examination. Still, your inspection needs to be systematic. When you inspect a patient you should, for instance, proceed from head to toe, observing first for general characteristics, then for specific ones.

Palpation
Before palpating the patient, make sure your hands are clean and warm. To protect yourself, the patient, and other patients, wear gloves when you examine broken or weeping skin or mucous membranes. To establish baseline information, first examine normal areas; then assess the affected area. (See *Performing palpation.*)

You'll use four different palpation techniques, depending on the circumstances—light palpa-

tion, deep palpation, light ballottement, and deep ballottement.

Light palpation
To use light palpation, hold two or three fingers together and gently press the affected area with your fingertips to a depth of ½" to ¾" (1 to 2 cm). Feel for any masses in or directly below the skin, and determine the size and location of any deformities. Also check for tenderness and warmth. When examining the patient's breasts, move your fingertips in a circular motion.

For a respiratory examination, place the backs of your fingers and the ball of your hand over the peripheral lung fields. Then ask the patient to repeatedly say "ninety-nine" as you feel for vibrations, known as tactile fremitus, through the chest wall. If the lungs are normal, you'll feel only mild vibrations. But if the patient has pneumonia, you'll feel strong vibrations because of the increased density of the underlying lung tissue. By contrast, you'll feel decreased vibrations if the patient has pneumothorax because of the decreased density.

Deep palpation
You may use deep palpation when assessing the abdomen and pelvis. Put one hand on top of the other and press down with the fingertips of both hands to a depth of 1½" to 2" (4 to 5 cm). This technique allows you to assess organ size and to detect any masses.

Deep palpation can hurt the patient. So monitor your patient closely for pain. If necessary, stop palpating.

Light ballottement
To check for a freely movable abdominal mass, you'll use ballottement, a special palpation technique. This maneuver will also let you detect voluntary guarding.

To perform light ballottement, bounce your fingertips rapidly and lightly on the abdomen. Start low on the abdomen and move through the quadrants. This technique will cause a solid tissue mass to bounce upward toward your fingertips after you've applied light, rapid pressure.

Performing palpation

You need to be familiar with four palpation techniques: light palpation, deep palpation, light ballottement, and deep ballottement.

Light palpation
With the tips of two or three fingers held close together, press gently on the skin to a depth of ½" to ¾" (1 to 2 cm). Use the lightest touch possible; too much pressure blunts your sensitivity.

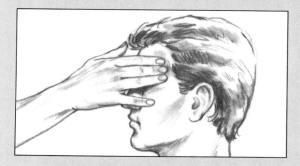

Deep palpation (bimanual palpation)
Place one hand on top of the other. Then press down about 1½" to 2" (4 to 5 cm) with the fingertips of both hands.

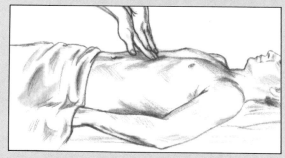

Light ballottement
Apply light, rapid pressure to the abdomen, moving from one quadrant to another. Keep your hand on the skin surface to detect tissue rebound.

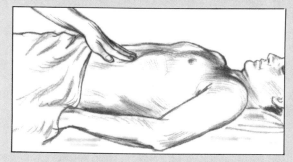

Deep ballottement
Apply abrupt, deep pressure on the patient's abdomen. Release the pressure completely, but maintain fingertip contact with the skin.

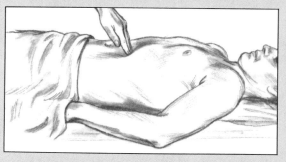

Characteristics of percussion sounds

Percussion produces sounds that vary according to the tissue being percussed. This chart lists important percussion sounds along with their characteristics and typical locations.

SOUND	INTENSITY	PITCH	DURATION	QUALITY	SOURCE
Flatness	Soft	High	Short	Flat	Muscle, bone
Dullness	Soft to moderate	High	Moderate	Thudlike	Liver, full bladder, pregnant uterus
Resonance	Moderate to loud	Low	Long	Hollow	Normal lung
Tympany	Loud	High	Moderate	Drumlike	Gastric air bubble, intestinal air
Hyperresonance	Very loud	Very low	Long	Booming	Hyperinflated lung (as in emphysema)

Deep ballottement
You can use deep ballottement to assess organ movement or mass movement. To perform deep ballottement, place your fingertips perpendicular to the patient's skin. Push your fingertips inward quickly and deeply and then quickly release the pressure without breaking contact with the abdomen. Note any rebound movement below your fingertips.

Percussion
You'll use percussion to evaluate the density of underlying tissue and to elicit tenderness. To perform this technique, you'll tap your fingers or hands against body surfaces, usually the chest and abdomen, to produce sounds and palpable vibrations.

Before percussing any area, tell the patient what you'll be doing and why. Remember, percussion can be frightening and uncomfortable for the patient.

Before percussing the abdomen, have the patient void. Otherwise, you may cause unnecessary discomfort. You also may mistake a full bladder for an abdominal mass.

When you use percussion to assess tissue density, you may hear the following percussion sounds:
• Flatness. A soft, high-pitched sound of short duration normally heard over muscles and bones.
• Dullness. A moderately soft, high-pitched sound of medium intensity normally heard over the liver. When heard over the lung, it can indicate increased density, as in pneumonia.
• Resonance. A loud, long, low-pitched sound normally heard over the lung fields.
• Tympany. A high-pitched, loud sound of medium duration usually heard over the stomach, indicating the presence of gastric air bubbles.
• Hyperresonance. A loud, low-pitched, and very long sound heard over lungs that are overinflated with air (as in emphysema).

As you percuss, always move gradually from resonant areas to dull areas and compare any sounds. For example, percuss over the abdomen and then move up to the liver. Also contrast percussion sounds from side to side and note any asymmetry in your findings. (See *Characteristics of percussion sounds.*)

Techniques of percussion
Depending on the body area you're examining and the purpose of percussion, you'll use one of three methods: indirect percussion, direct percussion, or blunt percussion. The most commonly used method, indirect percussion produces clear, crisp sounds when performed properly. Direct percussion has limited uses—

Performing percussion techniques

You should be familiar with three percussion techniques: indirect, direct, and blunt percussion.

Indirect percussion
To perform indirect percussion, place the distal phalanx of the middle finger on your nondominant hand against the patient's body surface. (This finger, known as the pleximeter, will be struck.) Then, keeping the wrist of your dominant hand loosely flexed, strike the pleximeter with the tip of your dominant middle finger (called the plexor). When you strike the pleximeter, the plexor should be perpendicular to it. Immediately after striking the pleximeter, remove the plexor; otherwise, you'll muffle the sound.

In an obese patient, percussion sounds may be muffled because of the thick subcutaneous fat layer. If so, place the lateral aspect of your nondominant thumb on the patient's body surface and sharply tap the last thumb joint with the plexor.

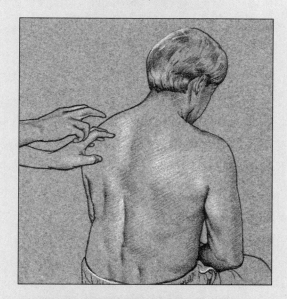

Direct percussion
This technique helps you to assess an adult's sinuses for tenderness or elicit sounds in a child's thorax. To perform direct percussion, strike the patient's body surface directly with your hand or fingertip.

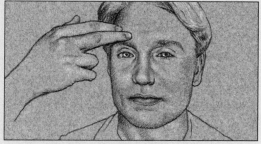

Blunt percussion
Blunt percussion can be performed in two ways. Both elicit tenderness over such organs as the kidneys, gallbladder, and liver; neither is intended to create sounds.

With the first technique, you strike the patient's body surface, using the ulnar surface of your fist. With the second technique, you place the palm of your nondominant hand over the area to be percussed. Then, strike the back of that hand with the fist of your dominant hand, as shown.

Note: Never perform blunt percussion over the thorax of an elderly patient because the ribs can fracture easily.

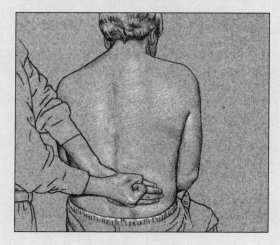

Using the stethoscope effectively

Assessing high-pitched sounds

To properly assess high-pitched sounds, such as breath sounds and S_1 and S_2 heart sounds, use the diaphragm of the stethoscope. Make sure you place the entire surface of the diaphragm firmly on the patient's skin. If the area is excessively hairy, improve diaphragm contact and reduce extraneous noise by applying water or water-soluble jelly to the skin before auscultating.

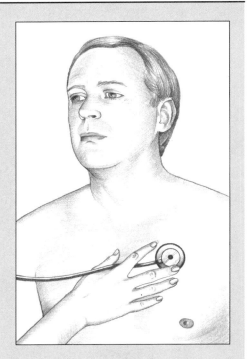

Assessing low-pitched sounds

To assess low-pitched sounds, such as heart murmurs and S_3 and S_4 heart sounds, lightly place the bell of the stethoscope on the appropriate area. Don't exert pressure. If you do, the patient's chest will act as a diaphragm, and you'll miss low-pitched sounds. If the patient is extremely thin or emaciated, use a stethoscope with a pediatric chest piece.

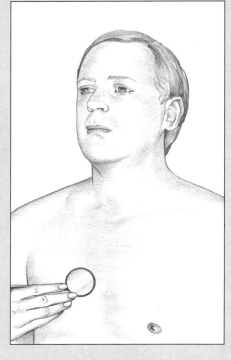

eliciting tenderness in an adult's sinuses and producing percussion sounds in a child's thorax. Blunt percussion is used only to elicit tenderness. (For more information, see *Performing percussion techniques,* page 21.)

Auscultation

This last assessment technique involves listening to body sounds—particularly those produced by the heart, lungs, blood vessels, stomach, and intestines. Although you can perform auscultation directly over a body surface using only your ears, you'll typically perform indirect auscultation with a stethoscope.

Usually, you'll auscultate last. But when you're assessing the abdomen, you should auscultate for bowel sounds before you palpate or percuss the abdomen. That's because the pressure on the abdomen may alter the bowel sounds.

Before auscultating, make sure your stethoscope tubing is no longer than 14" (35.5 cm); longer tubing may distort the sound. Also, ensure that the earpieces fit snugly and comfortably so that you don't hear any other sounds. You'll use the diaphragm of the stethoscope to hear high-pitched sounds—specifically S_1 and S_2 heart sounds, friction rubs, breath sounds, and bowel sounds. To hear low-pitched sounds—such as heart murmurs and S_3 and S_4 heart sounds—you'll use the bell of the stethoscope. (See *Using the stethoscope effectively.*)

Components of the physical examination

You'll begin your physical examination with a general survey of the patient's appearance; then obtain his vital signs. For a complete examination, you should also perform a nutritional assessment before moving on to a thorough review of the body systems.

General survey

As the first step in the physical examination, the general survey provides important information about the patient's health and overall status. This survey requires skilled, focused observations and a confident, professional approach.

During your survey, be sure to note the following: any signs of physical or emotional distress, the patient's facial characteristics, body type, posture, movements, voice, speech, dress, grooming, hygiene, and psychological state. If you performed a mental status examination as part of your health history, you will have already evaluated some of this information. After you perform your general survey, record your findings in a one-paragraph summary.

Physical or emotional distress
Note whether the patient appears ill and in need of immediate attention. What's his state of consciousness? Does he appear to be in pain? Is he dyspneic? Is he wringing his hands, speaking rapidly, or having difficulty listening to you?

Facial characteristics
Note the patient's facial expression. Is he showing signs of tension? Is his expression appropriate for the situation? Also, does he look his stated age?

Body type, posture, and movements
Classify the patient's body build as stocky, average, or slender. Is he cachectic or obese? Does he have a barrel chest? Do you note finger clubbing, edema, or joint contractures?

Note whether the patient's body is symmetrical. Are structures on one side similar to those on the other side? Minor variations, such as differences in breast size, are normal.

When he walks, note his coordination and the symmetry and smoothness of his gait. If he's in bed, is he able to turn, sit up, and reposition himself? Is he slumping? Does he lean forward to breathe?

Voice and speech
Listen to the tone and clarity of the patient's voice. Also note his vocal strength. Is he hoarse? Note too the patient's vocabulary and word usage.

Dress, grooming, and hygiene
What's the general condition of the patient's clothes? Are they appropriate? Do you smell any obvious odors, such as alcohol, urine, or excessive cologne? Does the patient seem indifferent about his appearance? Does he seem able to care for himself?

Psychological state
Assess the patient's level of consciousness, awareness, attentiveness, attention span, and orientation. Determine if he's able to follow simple instructions. Does he appear relaxed and comfortable, nervous, fidgety, or anxious? Does he have any bizarre mannerisms?

Vital signs
Taking vital signs may be considered a routine nursing function, but remember that it provides extremely important information. During your initial examination, you'll record baseline values. Then you'll take vital signs at regular intervals. With a hospitalized patient, you'll usually take vital signs every 4 to 6 hours. With a patient in a critical care area, you'll take them every 1 to 2 hours. When a patient first returns from surgery or any invasive procedure, you may take vital signs as often as every 15 minutes.

Your initial measurements can alert you to a problem that needs immediate attention. But, usually, a series of readings will provide much more valuable information than any single set of vital signs. Always analyze vital signs together, not separately, because two or more abnormal vital signs can provide important clues to a patient's problem. A rapid, thready pulse and low blood pressure, for instance, can suggest shock.

Before you take a patient's vital signs, try to help him relax. Physical or emotional stress can alter your measurements. If you obtain an abnormal value, take the vital sign again.

Temperature
Body temperature is the difference between the amount of heat the body produces and the amount of heat it loses. Recorded either in degrees Fahrenheit (° F) or degrees Celsius (° C), normal body temperature ranges from

How body temperature differs by route

Normal body temperature varies, depending on the route you use to measure it. This chart gives you the normal ranges for oral, rectal, axillary, and tympanic temperatures.

ROUTE	NORMAL RANGES
Oral	97.7° to 99.5° F (36.5° to 37.5° C)
Rectal	98.7° to 100.5° F (37° to 38° C)
Axillary	96.7° to 98.5° F (36° to 36.9° C)
Tympanic	98.2° to 100° F (36.7° to 37.7° C)

96.7° to 100.5° F (36° to 38° C), depending on the route used to measure it. (See *How body temperature differs by route.*)

Body temperature varies with age, sex, physical activity, and environmental conditions. Plus, temperature changes may occur with metabolic diseases (such as hyperthyroidism), severe infection, myocardial infarction, and surgery.

Pyrexia (fever) is an abnormally elevated temperature. Hyperthermia is defined as a temperature above 105° F (40.6° C). Hypothermia is a body temperature below 93° F (33.9° C), taken rectally.

If you need to convert a Celsius measurement to Fahrenheit, multiply the Celsius temperature by 1.8 and add 32. To convert from Fahrenheit to Celsius, subtract 32 from the Fahrenheit temperature and divide by 1.8.

Oral temperature. You can use the oral route on adults who are awake, alert, oriented, and cooperative. To measure temperature orally, you'll use either a glass or an electronic thermometer. A glass thermometer takes 3 to 5 minutes to record body temperature; an electronic thermometer takes 10 to 30 seconds.

Rectal temperature. You may take a rectal temperature on infants, young children, and confused or unconscious patients. As with the oral route, you can use either a glass or an electronic thermometer. First lubricate it; then

insert it into the anal canal, pointing it toward the umbilicus.

Axillary temperature. Axillary measurements are less accurate and take about 11 minutes to obtain. Although used infrequently, this noninvasive method may be preferred when the patient's immune system is impaired—for example, from chemotherapy—to prevent the spread of infection.

Tympanic temperature. You may also use an electronic tympanic thermometer to measure temperature. With this method, the reading is unaffected by mouth breathing or other patient activity, and the thermometer responds quickly to subtle thermal changes.

Pulse
When you take a patient's pulse, you're assessing the pressure of blood being ejected with each heartbeat. You can assess a patient's pulse by palpating or auscultating over different arterial pulse points and noting the rate, rhythm, and amplitude.

The most easily accessible pulse is the radial pulse. To palpate it, use the pads of your index and middle fingers. Don't use your thumb because it has a pulse of its own. In cardiovascular emergencies, you may palpate femoral and carotid pulses. These arteries are larger and closer to the heart and reflect more directly the heart's activity. (See *Identifying pulse sites.*)

Pulse rate. To assess the radial pulse rate, press the area over the artery until you can feel a pulse. If it has a regular rhythm, count the pulse for 15 seconds and then multiply by 4 to get the rate per minute. If the rhythm is irregular, count the pulse for a full 60 seconds.

Age has an effect on the normal heart rate. Infants have a pulse rate of about 125 beats/minute; by age 4, the rate is about 100 beats/minute. By adolescence, the rate falls to between 60 and 100 beats/minute. Tachycardia is a pulse rate above 100 beats/minute; bradycardia, a pulse rate less than 60 beats/minute.

Healthy persons can have normal changes in pulse rate. Fear, anger, and pain stimulate the sympathetic nervous system and can increase the pulse rate, whereas stimulation of the vagus nerve during sleep, vomiting, or suctioning can decrease the rate.

Pulse rhythm. When assessing pulse rhythm, you're indirectly assessing the heart's electrical conduction. Normally, the pulse should be regular. If you detect an irregularity, evaluate whether it follows a pattern. Is the rate regular with a few early, sporadic beats? Is it irregular in response to respirations? Is there no pattern at all? Pulses that fade on inspiration and strengthen on expiration are called paradoxical pulses and can occur with deep breathing or with cardiac tamponade.

When you note an irregularity, auscultate the apical pulse and palpate the radial pulse at the same time. You should palpate a heartbeat every time you hear one. If you don't, document the difference between the apical pulse rate and the radial pulse rate. The difference, known as the pulse deficit, provides an indirect evaluation of the ability of every heart contraction to eject enough blood into the peripheral circulation. Ultimately, an electrocardiogram may be needed to diagnose pulse irregularities.

Pulse amplitude. You'll also assess the amplitude (or force) of the patient's pulse. To document your findings, you may use a numerical scale that ranges from +3 (for a bounding pulse) to 0 (for an unpalpable pulse). As an alternative, you may simply describe the force of the patient's pulse. (See *Documenting pulse amplitude,* page 26.)

Respiration
When you observe a patient breathing, you're evaluating the lungs' ability to take in oxygen and expel carbon dioxide. As you watch, focus on the rate, depth, and rhythm of each breath.

Determine respiratory rate by counting the patient's respirations for 60 seconds. You should do this while still holding his wrist after taking his pulse, so he doesn't know you're counting his respirations. If he realizes what you're doing, he may alter his respiratory pattern. The normal adult respiratory rate is 12 to

Identifying pulse sites

This illustration shows the locations of the major peripheral arterial pulses and the apical pulse.

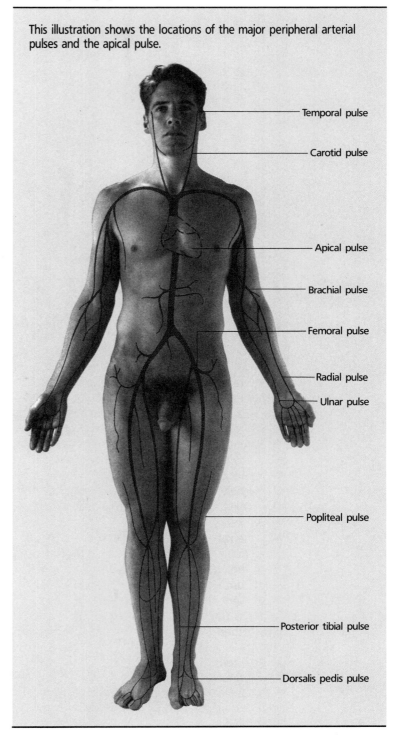

Temporal pulse

Carotid pulse

Apical pulse

Brachial pulse

Femoral pulse

Radial pulse

Ulnar pulse

Popliteal pulse

Posterior tibial pulse

Dorsalis pedis pulse

Documenting pulse amplitude

To document pulse amplitude, you may use a numerical scale or a descriptive term. Numerical scales differ slightly from facility to facility, but the one shown here is among the most commonly used.

+3 = **bounding pulse** (readily palpable, forceful, not easily obliterated by finger pressure)

+2 = **normal pulse** (easily palpable and obliterated only by strong finger pressure)

+1 = **weak or thready pulse** (hard to feel and easily obliterated by slight finger pressure)

  0 = **absent pulse** (not palpable)

20 breaths/minute; the normal rate for children is higher. Respiratory rate increases with emotional stress, metabolic disorders (such as diabetes mellitus), and lung diseases (such as emphysema). Respiratory rate decreases with depression of the central nervous system—for instance, when a patient receives anesthesia.

Also observe respiratory depth as the chest rises and falls, and describe breaths as shallow, moderate, or deep. Shallow respirations may indicate a chest injury; deep respirations, neurologic dysfunction. Note any abnormal sounds, such as wheezing or stridor. Normal respirations should be quiet and easy.

Observe the rhythm and symmetry of the chest wall as it expands during inspiration. Skeletal deformity, broken ribs, and collapsed lung tissue can cause unequal chest expansion. A patient with chronic obstructive pulmonary disease or respiratory distress may use the accessory muscles of respiration. Normally, the respiratory pattern should be regular. Irregular breathing patterns, such as Biot's or Cheyne-Stokes respirations, occur with neurologic disorders.

Blood pressure

When you take a patient's blood pressure, you're indirectly measuring the pressure exerted on the arterial walls with each heart contraction. Blood pressure measurements help you evaluate cardiac output, fluid and circulatory status, and arterial resistance.

As you know, a blood pressure measurement consists of a diastolic and a systolic reading. The systolic reading reflects the maximum pressure exerted on the arterial wall at the peak of left ventricular contraction. The diastolic reading reflects the minimum systemic arterial pressure that occurs during left ventricular relaxation. The diastolic reading is more significant because it evaluates the arterial pressure with the heart at rest.

Normal systolic blood pressure ranges from 100 to 140 mm Hg; normal diastolic pressure, from 60 to 90 mm Hg. A systolic pressure of less than 95 mm Hg and a diastolic pressure of less than 60 mm Hg indicates hypotension. Such readings may result from any condition that reduces the total blood volume or decreases cardiac output. A systolic blood pressure of greater than 140 mm Hg and a diastolic pressure of greater than 90 mm Hg indicates hypertension. These elevations may be idiopathic or result from an underlying disease. Remember that factors—such as physical activity, emotional stress, body position, and age—affect arterial pressure.

Measuring blood pressure. Usually, you'll use a stethoscope and a sphygmomanometer to obtain a patient's blood pressure. But if you have difficulty obtaining an audible blood pressure, you can use a Doppler probe or measure blood pressure by palpation.

Typically, you'll check blood pressure at the brachial or popliteal arterial site. If you use the popliteal artery, the systolic measurement may be higher and the diastolic may be lower than measurements taken at the brachial artery.

Take initial blood pressure readings in both arms. A pressure difference of 5 to 10 mm Hg between arms is normal. A difference of greater than 15 mm Hg can indicate cardiac disease, aortic coarctation, or arterial obstruction. Also note any wide difference between systolic and diastolic pressures, known as abnormal pulse pressure. (See *Measuring blood pressure.*)

Measuring blood pressure

To assess a patient's blood pressure accurately, follow this procedure.

• Have the patient lie supine or sit erect, and tell him what you're going to do. His arm should be extended at heart level and well supported. If the artery is below heart level, a false-high reading may result. Be sure the patient is relaxed and comfortable when you take his blood pressure so that the reading is accurate.

• Wrap the cuff snugly around the upper arm above the antecubital area. For an adult, place the lower border of the cuff about 1″ (2.5 cm) above the antecubital space. The center of the bladder should rest directly over the medial aspect of the arm. Most cuffs have an arrow for you to position over the brachial artery.

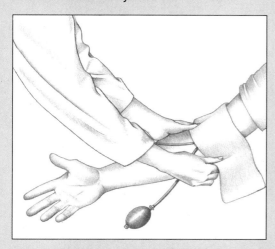

• If necessary, connect the appropriate tube to the rubber bulb of the air pump and the other tube to the manometer. Then insert the stethoscope's earpieces into your ears.

• Locate the brachial artery by palpation. Center the bell of the stethoscope over the part of the artery where you detect the strongest beats, and hold it in place with one hand. Using the bell will help you to hear Korotkoff's sounds, which are low-pitched.

• Using the thumb and index finger of your other hand, turn the thumbscrew on the rubber bulb of the air pump clockwise to close the valve.

• Then, while auscultating the sound over the bra-

chial artery, pump air into the cuff to compress and eventually occlude arterial blood flow. Pump air until the mercury column or aneroid gauge registers 160 mm Hg or at least 10 mm Hg above the last audible sound.

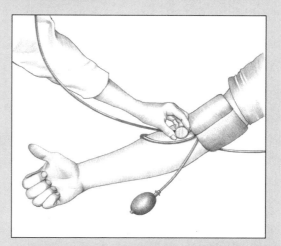

• Carefully open the valve of the air pump and slowly deflate the cuff—no faster than 5 mm Hg/second. While releasing air, watch the mercury column drop or the aneroid gauge descend and auscultate the sound over the artery.

• When you hear the first beat or a clear tapping sound, note the pressure on the column or gauge. This is the systolic pressure. The beat or tapping is the first of the five Korotkoff sounds. The second sound resembles a murmur or swish; the third sound, a crisp tapping; the fourth sound, a soft, muffled tone; and the fifth sound is the last sound heard.

• Continue to release air gradually while auscultating the sound over the artery.

• Note the diastolic pressure—the fourth Korotkoff sound. If you continue to hear sounds as the column or gauge falls to zero (common in children) record the pressure at the beginning of the fourth sound. This is important because a distinct fifth sound is absent in some patients.

• Rapidly deflate the cuff. Record the pressure, wait 15 to 30 seconds, then repeat the procedure and record the pressure to confirm your original findings. After doing so, remove and fold the cuff.

Nutritional status

As part of a complete assessment, you should also evaluate your patient's nutritional status. To do so, you'll determine his height, weight, and skin-fold thickness. You'll then compare these measurements with those on standard comparison charts. Depending on the circumstances, biochemical measurements may also be needed.

Height

Measure and record the patient's height in centimeters or inches. Have adults or older children take off their shoes and stand erect against a flat, vertical measuring surface with a right-angle head scale. You can measure height in a patient who isn't ambulatory by using a length board. This board is designed specifically for measuring the recumbent patient.

Weight

Weigh the patient, preferably using a standard platform scale with a balance beam. If your patient can't stand, you may use an electronic platform scale or a bed scale. (See *Suggested weights for adults.*)

Skin-fold thickness

You can measure the patient's body fat by determining skin-fold thickness, which is an indirect indication of subcutaneous fat and caloric status. These measurements are more useful for patients who are malnourished, of normal weight, or only moderately overweight than they are for obese patients.

To measure skin-fold thickness, you'll use calipers. The most common site is the nondominant triceps. First, determine the midpoint between the acromion and the olecranon processes. Then, relax the arm, and grasp a fold of bare skin between your left thumb and forefinger and pull it away from the muscle. Place the calipers on either side of the skin fold, directly at the midpoint. When the calipers stop moving, read the measurement to the nearest 0.5 mm. Repeat the measurement once or twice to ensure accuracy.

Biochemical measurements

Certain tests can also be used to determine the level of malnutrition or the presence of other nutritional deficits. Commonly used tests include total lymphocyte count, serum albumin level, total iron-binding capacity, serum transferrin level, creatinine-height index, hemoglobin level, hematocrit, nitrogen balance, and skin antigen tests.

Review of systems

You need to conduct your review of systems in a methodical manner. You can select a body systems approach, a body regions approach, or a head-to-toe approach. But once you find an approach that works for you — one that is thorough, minimizes changes in patient position, and aids your documentation — you should stick with it. (See *Patient positioning and draping guidelines,* page 30.) The approach presented below can serve as a general guideline for performing your systematic examination.

Skin

Stand in front of the patient and look at the exposed areas of his hands, face, and forearms. As you continue assessing the other regions of the body, look for any lesions, and note their type, color, location, and distribution. Take note of any changes in skin temperature or texture, cyanosis, or finger clubbing. Ask the patient if he's had any itching, rashes, sores, or lumps. Also examine and palpate the nails.

Head

Examine the hair, scalp, skull, and face. As you do, ask the patient if he's experienced recent headaches, syncope, dizziness, or trauma.

Eyes. Note the position and alignment of the eyes. Then inspect the eyelids, sclerae, and conjunctivae. Also check the patient's visual acuity and assess his pupillary reaction and accommodation to light and his visual fields. Ask if he's had pain, itching, swelling, discharge, or difficulty seeing.

Ears. Assess the auricles, canals, and eardrums. Then check for auditory acuity, using your watch. If you think the patient's hearing is diminished, perform the Rinne and Weber tests. Ask if he's had vertigo, tinnitus, pain, discharge, or difficulty hearing.

Nose and sinuses. Examine the exterior of the nose; then inspect the nasal mucosa, septum, and turbinates, using a light and nasal speculum. Palpate the frontal and maxillary sinuses for tenderness. Determine whether the patient has had discharge, epistaxis, pain, or difficulty smelling.

Mouth and pharynx. Examine the patient's lips, buccal mucosa, gums, teeth, hard palate, tongue, and pharynx. Ask if he's had tongue or gum soreness, bleeding gums, taste or voice changes, a sore throat, or difficulty chewing or swallowing.

Neck
Inspect and palpate the cervical lymph nodes and note any masses or unusual pulsations in the neck. Look for tracheal deviation; then palpate the thyroid gland. Ask if the patient has had neck stiffness or pain.

Back
Inspect and palpate the spine and muscles of the back; then assess for costovertebral tenderness. Determine whether the patient has had back pain or spasms.

Posterior thorax and lungs
Inspect, palpate, and percuss the posterior thorax and determine the level of diaphragmatic dullness on each side. As you auscultate the lungs, identify any abnormal sounds. Ask if the patient has experienced difficulty breathing, coughing, or hemoptysis.

Breasts and axillae
Standing in front of the patient, examine her breasts—first with her arms relaxed, then with her arms elevated and, finally, with her hands on her hips. With the patient lying down, palpate her breasts. Inspect the axillae and palpate the axillary nodes. Has the patient had pain, swelling, lumps, breast tenderness, nipple changes, or discharge?

Suggested weights for adults

This chart provides a guideline for determining appropriate weights. Higher weights in each category typically apply to men, who tend to have more muscle and bone; lower weights usually apply to women, who have less muscle and bone. Suggested weights for people age 35 and over are higher than those for younger adults because recent research shows that older people can carry somewhat more weight without impairing their health. Height is measured without shoes; weight is measured without clothes.

HEIGHT	WEIGHT (LB)	
	Ages 19 to 34	Age 35 and over
5'0"	97 to 128	108 to 138
5'1"	101 to 132	111 to 143
5'2"	104 to 137	115 to 148
5'3"	107 to 141	119 to 152
5'4"	111 to 146	122 to 157
5'5"	114 to 150	126 to 162
5'6"	118 to 155	130 to 167
5'7"	121 to 160	134 to 172
5'8"	125 to 164	138 to 178
5'9"	129 to 169	142 to 183
5'10"	132 to 174	146 to 188
5'11"	136 to 179	151 to 194
6'0"	140 to 184	155 to 199
6'1"	144 to 189	159 to 205
6'2"	148 to 195	164 to 210
6'3"	152 to 200	168 to 216
6'4"	156 to 205	173 to 222
6'5"	160 to 211	177 to 228
6'6"	164 to 216	182 to 234

Source: U.S. Department of Agriculture, U.S. Department of Health and Human Services. *Nutrition and Your Health: Dietary Guidelines for Americans*, 3rd ed. Washington, D.C., 1990.

Patient positioning and draping guidelines

Requirements for patient positioning and draping vary with the body system or region you're assessing. These illustrations show the primary positioning and draping arrangements to use during a routine assessment.

Head, neck, and chest examinations
To examine the patient's head, neck, anterior and posterior chest, and lungs, have him sit on the edge of the examination table.

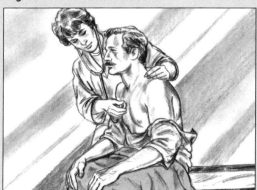

Breast examination
To begin examining a woman's breasts, have her sit. For the second part of the examination, ask her to lie down. When she does, place a small pillow or folded towel beneath her shoulder on the side being examined. To spread the breast more evenly over the chest, ask her to place her arm over her head.

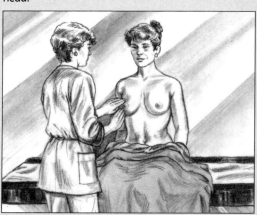

Abdominal examination
To examine the abdomen, place the patient supine. If the patient is a woman, ensure her privacy during abdominal assessment by placing a towel over her breasts and upper thorax. Pull the sheet down as far as the symphysis pubis, but don't expose this area.

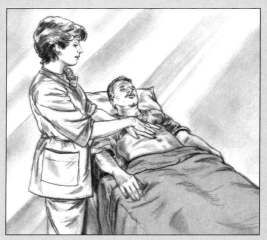

Gynecologic examination
To assess a woman's reproductive system, place her in the lithotomy position. Drape a sheet over her chest and knees and between her legs. Her buttocks should be at or just beyond the edge of the table and her feet in the stirrups. The rectal examination may also be performed with the patient in this position.

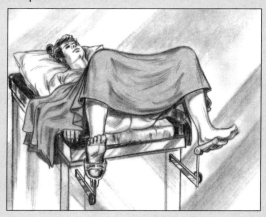

Anterior thorax and lungs
Inspect, palpate, and percuss the thorax. Then auscultate the anterior lung fields.

Cardiovascular system
Inspect and palpate carotid pulsations, and auscultate for carotid bruits. Then elevate the head of the bed about 30 degrees, observe jugular venous pulsations, and measure jugular venous pressure. Inspect and palpate the precordium, and assess the apical impulse. Then, auscultate with the bell of the stethoscope at the apex and lower sternal border. With the diaphragm of the stethoscope, auscultate the aortic, pulmonic, tricuspid, and mitral areas. Also auscultate for physiologic splitting of S_2, any abnormal heart sounds, or murmurs. Ask if the patient has had chest pain or palpitations.

Abdomen
With the patient supine and the head of the bed flat, inspect, auscultate, palpate, and percuss the abdomen. Palpate, first lightly, then deeply, to assess the liver, spleen, kidneys, and aorta. Ask about pain, dysphagia, nausea, vomiting, diarrhea, and hematemesis.

Male genitalia and rectum
With the patient lying on his left side, inspect the sacrococcygeal and perianal areas. Then palpate the anal canal, rectum, and prostate. With the patient standing, examine his penis and scrotum, and check for hernias. Ask about penile discharge, odor, pain, burning, itching, and sexual difficulties.

Female genitalia and rectum
With the patient in the lithotomy position, examine the external genitalia, vagina, and cervix. After performing a Papanicolaou (Pap) smear, palpate the uterus and adnexa. Then perform a rectovaginal and rectal exam. Ask the patient about discharge, odor, pain, burning, itching, and sexual difficulties.

Legs
Observe the muscle mass of the legs. Observe also for varicose veins and ask the patient if he's experienced coldness, numbness, edema, intermittent claudication, or discoloration. Then inspect for swelling, discoloration, ulcers, and pitting edema. Look too for enlarged joints or deformities. With the patient standing, examine the alignment of the legs. Palpate all pulses and inguinal lymph nodes. Finally, test the range of motion. Ask about pain, cramping, stiffness, and twitching.

Neurologic system
Observe as the patient walks normally, walks heel-to-heel, walks on his toes, hops in place, and does shallow knee bends. After checking for pronator drift, assess the strength of his grip and of his vertically raised arms.

Assess the patient's deep tendon reflexes. Then test sensory function in his hands, feet, arms, and legs. If necessary, also assess the cranial nerves by testing the sense of smell, temporal and masseter muscle strength, corneal reflexes, facial movements, and gag reflex.

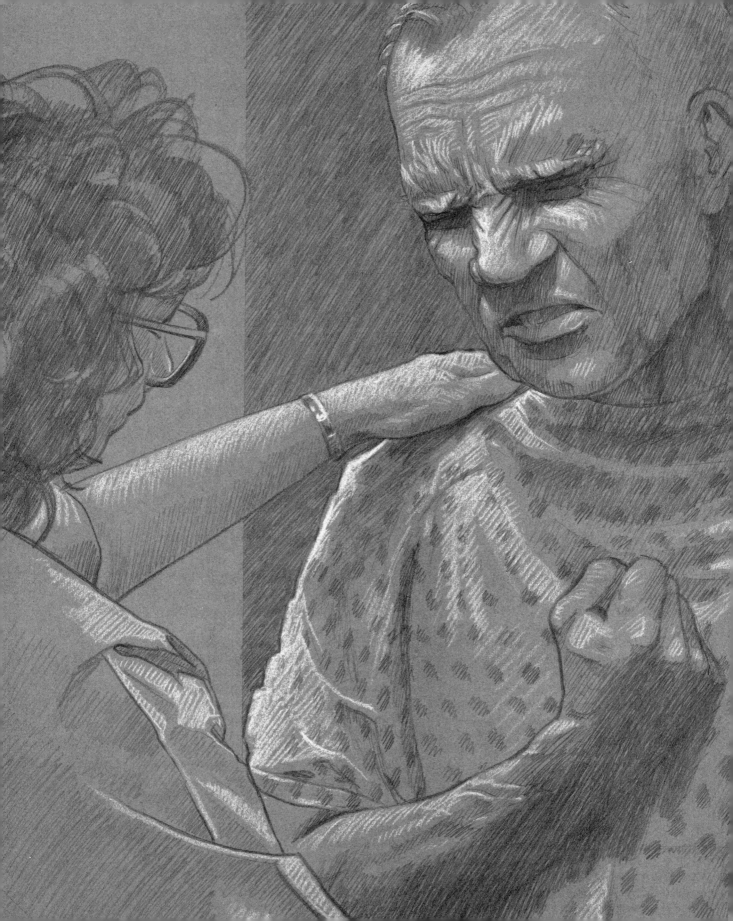

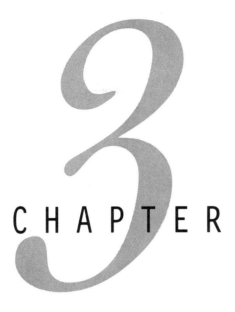

CHAPTER

Exploring the chief complaint

Almost every initial assessment you perform begins with a patient's chief complaint. To ensure that it ends with definitive, useful information, you must take a focused, systematic approach to exploring the chief complaint. That means asking the right health history questions, conducting a physical examination based on the history data you collect, and analyzing the possible causes of the patient's problem.

One aid to asking the right questions about any chief complaint is the PQRST mnemonic device. This aid will help you to explore complaints systematically and collect the specific information you need. (See *Using the PQRST mnemonic device*, page 34.)

In this chapter, you'll get guidance on exploring 25 of the most common chief complaints. For each one, you'll find a concise description, detailed questions to ask during the history, areas to focus on during the physical examination, and several common causes to consider.

Using the PQRST mnemonic device

To fully explore any chief complaint, use the PQRST mnemonic device as a guide. When you ask the questions listed here, you'll encourage the patient to describe his symptoms in greater detail. Only when you have such clarification can you correctly interpret this subjective information.

P Q R S T

Provocative or palliative	**Quality or quantity**	**Region or radiation**	**Severity scale**	**Timing**
• What were you doing when you first noticed the symptom? • What seems to trigger it? Stress? Certain positions or activities? Certain foods? • What makes the symptom worse? • What relieves the symptom? Changing your diet? A different position? Taking medication? Being active?	• How would you describe the symptom? How does it feel, look, or sound? • How severe is the symptom now? • Is the symptom so severe that it prevents you from performing any activities? • Is it more or less severe than at any other time?	• Where does the symptom occur? • Does the symptom spread? In the case of pain, does it travel down your back or arms? Does it radiate up your neck? Does it travel down your legs?	• How would you rate the symptom at its worst on a scale of 1 to 10, with 10 being the most extreme? • Does the symptom force you to lie down, sit down, or slow down? • Does the symptom seem to be getting better, worse, or staying about the same?	• On what date did the symptom first occur? • Did it start suddenly or gradually? • How often do you have the symptom? Hourly? Daily? Weekly? Monthly? Seasonally? • When do you usually have the symptom? During the day? At night? In the early morning? Does it awaken you? • Do you have the symptom before, during, or after meals? • How long does an episode last?

Fever

An abnormal elevation of body temperature above 98.6° F (37° C), fever (or pyrexia) is a common sign arising from disorders that affect virtually every body system. As a result, fever alone has little diagnostic value. However, persistently high fever is a medical emergency.

Fever can be classified as low (oral reading of 99° to 100.4° F [37.2° to 38° C]), moderate (100.5° to 104° F [38° to 40° C]), or high (above 104° F). Fever above 108° F (42.2° C) causes unconsciousness and, if prolonged, brain damage.

Fever can also be classified as intermittent or sustained. Intermittent fever, the most common type, refers to the daily fluctuations between normal and above-normal temperatures. Sustained fever refers to a persistent elevation with little fluctuation.

Health history

If your patient complains of fever, ask him appropriate questions from the following list.
• When did the fever begin? How high did it reach? Is the fever constant, or does it disappear and then reappear later?
• Ask if the patient also has chills, fatigue, or pain.
• Has the patient had any immunodeficiency disorders or treatments, infections, recent trauma or surgery, or diagnostic tests? Has he traveled recently?
• Which medications is the patient taking? Has he recently had anesthesia?

Physical examination

Based on your history findings, use the appropriate physical examination techniques to further explore the chief complaint. Because fever can accompany many disorders, your physical examination may range from a brief evaluation of one body system to a comprehensive review of all systems.

Causes

Your assessment may lead you to suspect one or more of the following causes.

Infectious and inflammatory disorders. Fever may be low, as in Crohn's disease and ulcerative colitis, or extremely high, as in bacterial pneumonia. It may be remittent, as in infectious mononucleosis; sustained, as in meningitis; or relapsing, as in malaria. Fever may arise abruptly, as in Rocky Mountain spotted fever, or insidiously, as in mycoplasmal pneumonia. Typically, it accompanies a self-limiting disorder, such as the common cold.

Medications. Fever and rash commonly result from hypersensitivity to quinidine, methyldopa (Aldomet), procainamide hydrochloride (Pronestyl), phenytoin (Dilantin), anti-infectives, barbiturates, iodides, and some antitoxins. Fever can also result from the use of chemotherapeutic agents and medications that decrease sweating, such as anticholinergics. Plus, toxic doses of salicylates, amphetamines, and tricyclic antidepressants can cause fever.

Other causes. Fever may also result from an injection of contrast media used in diagnostic tests, from surgery, and from blood transfusion reactions.

Fatigue

A common symptom, fatigue is a feeling of excessive tiredness, lack of energy, or exhaustion, accompanied by a strong desire to rest or sleep. Fatigue differs from weakness, which involves the muscles, but may accompany it.

A normal response to physical overexertion, emotional stress, and sleep deprivation, fatigue can also result from psychological and physiologic disorders, especially viral infections and endocrine, cardiovascular, or neurologic disorders.

Health history

If your patient complains of fatigue, ask him appropriate questions from the following list.
• When did the fatigue begin? Is it constant or intermittent? If it's intermittent, when does it occur? Does the fatigue worsen with activity and improve with rest, or vice versa? (The former usually signals a physiologic disorder; the latter, a psychological disorder.)
• Has the patient experienced any recent stressful changes at home or at work?
• Has he changed his eating habits? Has he recently lost or gained weight?
• Ask if the patient or anyone in his family has a history of cardiovascular, endocrine, or neurologic disorders, viral infections, or psychological disorders.
• Which medications is the patient taking?

Physical examination

Observe the patient's general appearance for signs of depression or organic illness. Is he unkempt? Expressionless? Tired or unhealthy looking? Is he slumped over? Assess his mental status, noting especially any agitation, attention deficits, mental clouding, or psychomotor impairment.

Causes

Your assessment may lead you to suspect one or more of the following causes.

Anemia. Fatigue after mild activity is often the first symptom of anemia. Other signs and symptoms vary but typically include dyspnea, pallor, and tachycardia.

Cancer. Unexplained fatigue is often the earliest indication of cancer. Related signs and symptoms reflect the type, location, and stage of the tumor, and usually include abnormal bleeding, anorexia, nausea, pain, a palpable mass, vomiting, and weight loss.

Chronic infection. In a patient with a chronic infection, fatigue is usually the most prominent symptom—and sometimes the only one.

Congestive heart failure. Persistent fatigue and lethargy are characteristic symptoms of congestive heart failure. Left ventricular failure produces exertional and paroxysmal nocturnal dyspnea, orthopnea, and tachycardia. Right ventricular failure causes neck vein distention and, sometimes, a slight but persistent nonproductive cough.

Depression. Chronic depression is almost always accompanied by persistent fatigue that's unrelated to exertion. The patient may also complain of anorexia, constipation, headache, and sexual dysfunction.

Diabetes mellitus. The most common symptom in this disorder, fatigue may begin insidiously or abruptly. Related findings include polydipsia, polyphagia, polyuria, and weight loss.

Myasthenia gravis. The cardinal symptoms of this disorder are easy fatigability and muscle weakness that worsen with exertion and abate with rest. These symptoms are related to the specific muscle groups affected.

Other causes. Fatigue can be caused by anxiety, myocardial infarction, rheumatoid arthritis, systemic lupus erythematosus, and malnutrition. Certain drugs—notably antihypertensives and sedatives—and most types of surgery also cause fatigue.

Dizziness

A common symptom, dizziness is a sensation of imbalance or faintness sometimes associated with blurred or double vision, confusion, and weakness. Dizziness may be mild or severe, have an abrupt or gradual onset, and be aggravated by standing up quickly and alleviated by lying down. Episodes are usually brief.

Dizziness typically results from inadequate blood flow and oxygen supply to the cerebrum and spinal cord. It may occur with anxiety, respiratory and cardiovascular disorders, and postconcussion syndrome. What's more, it's a key symptom of certain serious disorders, such as hypertension and vertebrobasilar artery insufficiency.

Health history

If your patient complains of dizziness, ask him appropriate questions from the following list.
• When did the dizziness start? How severe is it? How often does it occur, and how long does each episode last? Does the dizziness abate spontaneously? Is it triggered by standing up suddenly or bending over?
• Ask if the patient has blurred vision, chest pain, a chronic cough, diaphoresis, a headache, or shortness of breath.
• Does he have a history of hypertension or another cardiovascular disorder? Also ask about diabetes mellitus, anemia, respiratory or anxiety disorders, and head injury.
• Which medications is the patient taking?

Physical examination

Assess the patient's level of consciousness, respirations, and body temperature. As you observe his breathing, look for accessory muscle use or barrel chest. Look also for finger clubbing, cyanosis, dry mucous membranes, and poor skin turgor. Then, evaluate the patient's motor and sensory functions and reflexes.

Palpate the extremities for peripheral edema and capillary refill. Then, auscultate the patient's heart rate and rhythm and his breath sounds. Take his blood pressure while he's lying down, sitting, and standing. If the diastolic pressure exceeds 100 mm Hg, notify the doctor immediately and have the patient lie down.

Causes

Your assessment may lead you to suspect one or more of the following causes.

Cardiac arrhythmias. Dizziness lasts for several minutes or longer and may precede fainting. Other signs and symptoms include blurred vision; confusion; hypotension; palpitations; paresthesia; weakness; and an irregular, rapid, or thready pulse.

Hypertension. Dizziness may precede fainting but may be relieved by rest. Other findings include blurred vision; elevated blood pressure; headache; and retinal changes, such as hemorrhage, exudate discharge, and papilledema.

Transient ischemic attack. Dizziness of varying severity occurs during a transient ischemic attack. Lasting from a few seconds to 24 hours, an attack may be triggered by turning the head to the side and typically signals an impending cerebrovascular accident. During an attack, blindness or visual field deficits, diplopia, hearing loss, numbness, paresis, ptosis, and tinnitus may also occur.

Other causes. Dizziness may result from anemia, generalized anxiety disorder, orthostatic hypotension, panic disorder, and postconcussion syndrome. Also, dizziness may be an adverse reaction to certain drugs, including antianxiety agents, central nervous system depressants, narcotic analgesics, decongestants, antihistamines, antihypertensives, and vasodilators.

Papular rash

Consisting of small, raised, circumscribed and, possibly, discolored lesions, a papular rash can erupt anywhere on the body and in various configurations. A characteristic sign of many cutaneous disorders, a papular rash may also result from allergies or from infectious, neoplastic, or systemic disorders.

Health history

If your patient reports a papular rash, ask him appropriate questions from the following list.
• When and where did the rash erupt? What did it look like? Has it spread or changed in any way? If so, when and how did it spread?
• Does the rash itch or burn? Is it painful or tender?
• Ask if the patient has had a fever, GI distress, or a headache. Does he have any allergies? Has he had any previous skin disorders, infections, sexually transmitted diseases, or tumors? What childhood diseases has he had?
• Has he recently been bitten by an insect or a rodent or exposed to anyone with an infectious disease?
• Which drugs is he taking? Has he applied any topical agents to the rash and, if so, when was the last application?

Physical examination

Observe the color, configuration, and location of the rash.

Causes

Your assessment may lead you to suspect one or more of the following causes.

Acne vulgaris. The rupture of enlarged comedones produces inflamed and, possibly, painful and pruritic papules, pustules, nodules, or cysts. They may appear on the face and, occasionally, on the shoulders, chest, and back.

Insect bites. Venom from insect bites—especially those of ticks, lice, flies, and mosquitoes—may cause an allergic reaction that produces a papular, macular, or petechial rash. Associated findings include fever, headache, lymphadenopathy, myalgia, nausea, and vomiting.

Kaposi's sarcoma. A neoplastic disorder most commonly found in patients with acquired immunodeficiency syndrome, Kaposi's sarcoma produces purple or blue papules or macules on the extremities, ears, and nose. Firm pressure causes these lesions to decrease in size, but they return to their original size within 10 to 15 seconds. The lesions may become scaly, ulcerate, and bleed.

Psoriasis. In this disorder, small, erythematous, pruritic papules appear on the scalp, chest, elbows, knees, back, buttocks, and genitalia. The papules may be painful. They enlarge and coalesce, forming elevated, red, scaly plaques covered by silver scales, except in moist areas, such as the genitalia. The scales may flake off easily or thicken, covering the plaque. Other common findings include pitted fingernails and arthralgia.

Other causes. Infectious mononucleosis or sarcoidosis may produce a papular rash. Such a rash may also be caused by antibiotics, sulfonamides, benzodiazepines, lithium (Lithane), gold salts, allopurinol (Zyloprim), isoniazid (Laniazid), and salicylates.

Pustular rash

Crops of pustules (small, elevated, circumscribed lesions), vesicles (small blisters), and bullae (large blisters) filled with purulent exudate make up a pustular rash. The lesions vary in size and shape and may be generalized or localized (limited to the hair follicles or sweat glands).

Pustules may result from skin disorders, systemic disorders, ingestion of certain drugs, and exposure to skin irritants. Although many pustular lesions are sterile, a pustular rash usually indicates infection.

Health history
If your patient reports a pustular rash, ask him appropriate questions from the following list.
• When and where did the rash erupt? Did another type of skin lesion precede the pustules?
• What does the rash look like? Has it spread or changed in any way? If so, how and where did it spread?
• Determine whether the patient has a history of skin disorders or allergies. What about family members?

• Which medications is the patient taking? Has he applied any topical medication to the rash and, if so, when did he last apply it?

Physical examination
Examine the entire skin surface, noting if it's dry, oily, moist, or greasy. Record the exact location, distribution, color, shape, and size of the lesions.

Causes
Your assessment may lead you to suspect one or more of the following causes.

Folliculitis. A bacterial infection of the hair follicles, folliculitis produces individual pustules, each pierced by a hair. The patient may also suffer from pruritus. Hot-tub folliculitis is characterized by pustules on the area covered by a bathing suit.

Scabies. Threadlike channels or burrows under the skin characterize scabies, a disorder that can also produce pustules, vesicles, and excoriations. The lesions are 1 to 10 cm long, with a swollen nodule or red papule containing the itch mite. In men, crusted lesions often develop on the glans and shaft of the penis and on the scrotum. In women, lesions may form on the nipples. Other common sites include the wrists, elbows, axillae, and waist.

Other causes. A pustular rash may result from blastomycosis, furunculosis, and pustular psoriasis. Also, certain drugs—such as bromides, iodides, corticotropin, corticosteroids, lithium (Lithane), phenytoin (Dilantin), phenobarbital (Luminal), isoniazid (Laniazid), and oral contraceptives—can cause a pustular rash.

Vesicular rash

The lesions in a vesicular rash are scattered or linear vesicles that are sharply circumscribed and usually less than 0.5 cm in diameter. They may be filled with clear, cloudy, or bloody fluid. Lesions larger than 0.5 cm in diameter are called bullae. A vesicular rash may be mild or severe, transient or permanent.

Health history

If your patient complains of a vesicular rash, ask him appropriate questions from the following list.

• When and where did the rash erupt? Did other skin lesions precede the vesicles?

• What does the rash look like? Has it spread or changed in any way? If so, how and where did it spread?

• Does the patient have a history of allergies or skin disorders? Does anyone else in his family?

• Has the patient recently had an infection or been bitten by an insect?

Physical examination

Examine the patient's skin and note the location, general distribution, color, shape, and size of the lesions. Check for crusts, macules, papules, scales, scars, and wheals. Note whether the outer layer of epidermis separates easily from the basal layer.

Palpate the vesicles or bullae to determine whether they're flaccid or tense.

Causes

Your assessment may lead you to suspect one or more of the following causes.

Burns. Thermal burns that affect the epidermis and part of the dermis often cause vesicles and bullae, along with erythema, moistness, pain, and swelling.

Herpes zoster. First, fever and malaise occur. Then, the vesicular rash appears along a dermatome. This is accompanied by pruritus, deep pain, and paresthesia or hyperesthesia, usually of the trunk and sometimes of the arms and legs. The vesicles erupt, dry up, and form scabs in about 10 days. Occasionally, herpes zoster involves the cranial nerves; such involvement produces dizziness, eye pain, facial palsy, hearing loss, impaired vision, and loss of taste.

Other causes. Other causes of vesicular rashes include dermatitis, herpes simplex, insect bites, pemphigus, scabies, tinea pedis, and toxic epidermal necrolysis.

Headache

The most common neurologic symptom, a headache may be mild to severe, localized or generalized, constant or intermittent. About 90% of all headaches are benign and can be described as vascular, muscle-contraction, or a combination of both.

Occasionally, this symptom indicates a severe neurologic disorder. A generalized, pathologic headache may result from disorders associated with intracranial inflammation, increased intracranial pressure (ICP), meningeal irritation, or a vascular disturbance. A headache may also result from eye and sinus disorders and from the effects of drugs, tests, and treatments. (See *What causes headache?* pages 40 and 41.)

Health history

If your patient complains of a headache, ask him appropriate questions from the following list.

• When did the headache first occur? Is the pain mild, moderate, or severe? Is it localized or generalized? If it's localized, where does it occur? Is it constant or intermittent? If it's intermittent, what's the duration? How would the patient describe the pain; for example, is it stabbing, dull, throbbing, or viselike? Does anything seem to trigger it, exacerbate it, or relieve it?

• Has the patient also experienced confusion, dizziness, drowsiness, eye pain, fever, muscle twitching, nausea, photophobia, seizures, speaking or walking difficulties, neck stiffness, visual disturbances, vomiting, or weakness?

• Has the patient been under unusual stress at home or at work? Has his family noticed any changes in his behavior or personality?

• Does he have a history of blood dyscrasia, cardiovascular disease, glaucoma, hemorrhagic disorders, hypertension, poor vision, seizures, or smoking? Has he had any recent traumatic injuries; dental work; or sinus, ear, or systemic infections?

• Which medications is the patient taking?

PATHOPHYSIOLOGY

What causes headache?

Headache pain can be extracranial or intracranial. Like other types of pain, headache depends on the stimulation of specialized pain receptors. However, most cranial structures, including the brain parenchyma, choroid plexus, pia arachnoid membrane, parts of the dura mater, ventricular linings, and the skull itself, don't contain pain receptors. Extracranial structures sensitive to pain include the skin, scalp, and mucosa. Intracranial structures responsive to pain include the blood vessels, venous sinuses and their tributaries, sensory cranial nerves, dural arteries, and the arteries and dura at the base of the brain.

Extracranial pain
Three cranial nerves transmit pain sensations. The trigeminal nerve (CN V) contains the pain fibers above the tentorium cerebelli; pain is referred to the frontal and temporal areas as far back as above the ears. The glossopharyngeal and vagus nerves (CN IX and CN X) contain the pain fibers for structures below the tentorium cerebelli. Usually, these nerves transmit pain impulses from the occipital and upper cervical areas.

Pain stemming from the sinuses, ears, eyes, or teeth results from inflammation of the ostia or turbinates or from displacement of the cranial nerves, causing referred pain to the head.

Intracranial pain
The pain of meningitis is thought to be caused by a chemical irritation of the meningeal nerve endings. Ruptured cerebral aneurysm, acute epidural hemorrhage, subarachnoid hemorrhage, and subdural hematoma all stimulate meningeal nerve endings, causing chemical meningitis.

Headache can be caused by displaced pain-sensitive structures. Displacement may result from a space-occupying lesion and enlargement of brain tissue, as occurs with brain abscess, brain tumor, hematoma, or brain edema. Displacement may also result from dilation of the cranial arteries by such disorders as hypertension, acute cerebrovascular insufficiency, hypercapnia, hypoxia, or toxic systemic reactions, as well as the use of vasodilators.

Physical examination
Observe the rate and depth of the patient's respirations, noting any breathing difficulty or abnormal patterns. Then inspect his head for bruising, swelling, and sinus bleeding. Check also for Battle's sign, neck stiffness, otorrhea, and rhinorrhea.

Assess the patient's level of consciousness (LOC): Is he drowsy, lethargic, or comatose? Examine his eyes, noting pupillary size, equality, and response to light. With the patient both at rest and active, note any tremors.

Gently palpate the skull and sinuses for tenderness. Unless head trauma has occurred, slowly move the neck to check for nuchal rigidity or pain. Then assess the patient's motor strength. Palpate his peripheral pulses, noting their rate, rhythm, and intensity.

Check for a positive Babinski's reflex. As you percuss for other reflexes, note any hyper-reflexia. Then auscultate over the temporal artery, listening for bruits. Be sure to monitor the patient's blood pressure and pulse pressure.

Causes
Your assessment may lead you to suspect one or more of the following causes.

Brain abscess. A headache stemming from a brain abscess typically intensifies over a few days, localizes to a particular spot, and is aggravated by straining. The headache may be accompanied by a decreased LOC (drowsiness to deep stupor), focal or generalized seizures, nausea, and vomiting. Depending on the abscess site, the patient may also have aphasia, ataxia, impaired visual acuity, hemiparesis, personality changes, or tremors. Signs of an infection may or may not appear. The patient's history may include systemic, chronic middle

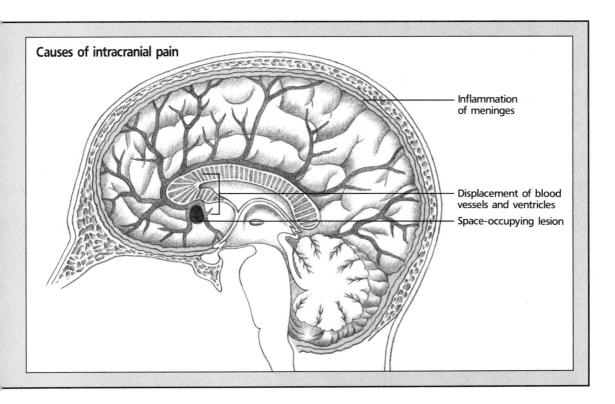

Causes of intracranial pain

Inflammation of meninges

Displacement of blood vessels and ventricles

Space-occupying lesion

ear, mastoid, or sinus infection; osteomyelitis of the skull or a compound fracture; or a penetrating head wound.

Brain tumor. Initially, the headache develops near the tumor site and becomes generalized as the tumor grows. Pain is usually intermittent, deep-seated, dull, and most intense in the morning. It's aggravated by coughing, stooping, Valsalva's maneuver, and changes in head position.

Cerebral aneurysm (ruptured). This headache is sudden and excruciating. It may be unilateral and usually peaks within minutes of the rupture. The headache may be accompanied by nausea, vomiting, and signs of meningeal irritation. The patient may lose consciousness. His history may include hypertension or other cardiovascular disorders, a stressful life-style, or smoking.

Encephalitis. The patient has a severe, generalized headache accompanied by a deteriorating LOC over a 48-hour period. Fever, focal neurologic deficits, irritability, nausea, nuchal rigidity, photophobia, seizures, and vomiting may also develop. His history may reveal exposure to the viruses that commonly cause encephalitis, such as mumps or herpes simplex.

Epidural hemorrhage (acute). A progressively severe headache immediately follows a brief loss of consciousness. Then the patient's LOC rapidly and steadily declines. Accompanying signs and symptoms include increasing ICP, ipsilateral pupil dilation, nausea, and vomiting. The patient's history usually reveals head trauma within the past 24 hours.

Glaucoma (acute angle-closure). An ophthalmic emergency, glaucoma may cause an excruciating headache. Other signs and symptoms include blurred vision, cloudy cornea, halo vision, moderately dilated and fixed pupil, photophobia, nausea, and vomiting.

Hypertension. Patients with hypertension may have a slightly throbbing occipital headache on awakening. Then, during the day, the severity may decrease. But if the patient's diastolic blood pressure exceeds 120 mm Hg, the headache remains constant.

Meningitis. The patient experiences a severe, constant, generalized headache that starts suddenly and worsens with movement. He may also have chills, fever, hyperreflexia, nuchal rigidity, and positive Kernig's and Brudzinski's signs. His history may include recent systemic or sinus infection, dental work, or exposure to bacteria or viruses that commonly cause meningitis, such as *Haemophilus influenzae, Streptococcus pneumoniae*, enteroviruses, and mumps.

Migraine. A severe, throbbing headache, migraine may follow a 5-to-15-minute prodrome of dizziness; tingling of the face, lips, or hands; unsteady gait; and visual disturbances. Other signs and symptoms include anorexia, nausea, photophobia, and vomiting.

Sinusitis (acute). Patients with sinusitis have a dull, periorbital headache that's typically aggravated by bending over or touching the face. They may also have fever, malaise, nasal discharge, nasal turbinate edema, sinus tenderness, and sore throat. Sinusitis is relieved by sinus drainage.

Subarachnoid hemorrhage. The hallmarks of this disorder are a sudden, violent headache along with dizziness, hypertension, ipsilateral pupil dilation, nausea, nuchal rigidity, seizures, vomiting, and an altered LOC that may rapidly progress to coma. The patient's history may include congenital vascular defects, arteriovenous malformation, cardiovascular disease, smoking, or excessive stress.

Subdural hematoma. A severe, localized headache usually follows head trauma that causes an immediate loss of consciousness, a latent period of drowsiness, confusion or personality changes, and agitation. Later, signs of increased ICP may develop. If the head trauma occurred within 3 days of the onset of signs and symptoms, the hematoma is acute; within 3 weeks, subacute; after more than 3 weeks, chronic. About 50% of patients with this disorder have no history of head trauma.

Other causes. Cervical traction, lumbar puncture, myelography, use of vasodilators, and withdrawal from vasopressors or sympathomimetic drugs can also cause headache. So can indomethacin (Indocin); digoxin (Lanoxin); aspirin (Ecotrin); and anticoagulants, such as warfarin sodium (Coumadin).

Paresthesia

Paresthesia is an abnormal sensation, commonly described as a numbness, prickling, or tingling, that's felt along peripheral nerve pathways. It may develop suddenly or gradually and be transient or permanent. A common symptom of many neurologic disorders, paresthesia may also occur in certain systemic disorders and.with the use of certain drugs.

Health history
If your patient complains of paresthesia, ask him appropriate questions from this list.
• When did the paresthesia begin? What does it feel like? Where does it occur? Is it transient or constant?
• Has the patient had recent trauma, surgery, or an invasive procedure that may have injured peripheral nerves? Has he been exposed to industrial solvents or heavy metals? Ask if he's had long-term radiation therapy. What about neurologic, cardiovascular, metabolic, renal, or chronic inflammatory disorders, such as arthritis or lupus erythematosus?
• Which medications is the patient taking?

Physical examination

Focus on the patient's neurologic status, assessing his level of consciousness and cranial nerve function. Also note his skin color and temperature.

Test muscle strength and deep tendon reflexes in the extremities affected by paresthesia. Systematically evaluate light touch, pain, temperature, vibration, and position sensation. Then palpate his pulses.

Causes

Your assessment may lead you to suspect one or more of the following causes.

Arterial occlusion (acute). A patient with a saddle embolism may complain of sudden paresthesia and coldness in one or both legs. Aching pain at rest, intermittent claudication, and paresis are also characteristic. The leg becomes mottled, and a line of temperature and color demarcation develops at the level of the occlusion. Pulses are absent below the occlusion and capillary refill is diminished.

Brain tumor. Tumors that affect the parietal lobe may cause progressive contralateral paresthesia accompanied by agnosia, agraphia, apraxia, homonymous hemianopia, and loss of proprioception.

Herniated disk. Herniation of a lumbar or cervical disk may cause acute or gradual paresthesia along the distribution pathways of the affected spinal nerves. Other neuromuscular effects include muscle spasms, severe pain, and weakness.

Herpes zoster. Paresthesia, an early symptom of herpes zoster, occurs in the dermatome supplied by the affected spinal nerve. Within several days, this dermatome is marked by a pruritic, erythematous, vesicular rash accompanied by sharp, shooting pain.

Spinal cord injury. Paresthesia may occur in a partial spinal cord transection after spinal shock resolves. The paresthesia may be unilateral or bilateral and occur at or below the level of the lesion.

Other causes. Paresthesia may result from arthritis, a cerebrovascular accident, a migraine headache, multiple sclerosis, peripheral neuropathies, vitamin B_{12} deficiency, hypocalcemia, and heavy metal or solvent poisoning. Also, long-term radiation therapy, parenteral gold therapy, and certain drugs—such as phenytoin (Dilantin), chemotherapeutic agents, D-penicillamine (Depen), and isoniazid (Laniazid)—may cause paresthesia.

Diplopia

Also called double vision, diplopia occurs when the extraocular muscles fail to work together, causing images to fall on noncorresponding parts of the retina. Diplopia can result from orbital lesions, eye surgery, or impaired function of the cranial nerves that supply the extraocular muscles.

Classified as binocular or monocular, diplopia is usually intermittent at first or affects near or far vision exclusively. *Binocular diplopia* usually results from ocular deviation or displacement or retinal surgery. *Monocular diplopia* may result from an early cataract, retinal edema or scarring, or poorly fitting contact lenses. Diplopia may also occur with hysteria or malingering.

Health history

If your patient complains of diplopia, ask him appropriate questions from the following list.
• Determine when the patient first noticed the diplopia. Are the images side by side (horizontal), one above the other (vertical), or both? Is the diplopia intermittent or constant? Find out if both eyes are affected or just one. Is near or far vision affected? Does the diplopia occur only when he gazes in certain directions? Has the problem worsened, remained the same, or subsided? Does it worsen as the day progresses? Can the patient correct the problem by tilting his head? If so, ask him to show you, and note the direction of the tilt.
• Does the patient have eye pain?
• Has he had recent eye surgery? Does he wear contact lenses?
• Does he have a history of vision problems?

Does anyone in his family?
• Which medications is the patient taking?

Physical examination
Observe the patient for conjunctival infection, exophthalmos, lid edema, ocular deviation, and ptosis. Have him occlude one eye at a time; if he sees double with only one eye, he has monocular diplopia. Test his visual acuity and extraocular muscle function.

Causes
Your assessment may lead you to suspect one or more of these causes.

Botulism. Hallmark signs and symptoms of botulism are diplopia, dysarthria, dysphagia, and ptosis. Early findings include diarrhea, dry mouth, sore throat, and vomiting. Later, descending weakness or paralysis of extremity and trunk muscles causes dyspnea and hyporeflexia.

Intracranial aneurysm. A life-threatening disorder, intracranial aneurysm initially produces diplopia and eye deviation, perhaps accompanied by a dilated pupil on the affected side and ptosis. Other findings include a decreased level of consciousness; dizziness; neck and spinal pain and rigidity; a severe, unilateral, frontal headache, which becomes violent after rupture of the aneurysm; tinnitus; unilateral muscle weakness or paralysis; and vomiting.

Other causes. Alcohol intoxication, diabetes mellitus, encephalitis, eye surgery, head injury, migraine, and orbital tumors may also cause diplopia.

Visual floaters

Particles of blood or cellular debris that move about in the vitreous humor appear as spots or dots when they enter the visual field. Chronic floaters commonly occur in elderly or myopic patients. But the sudden onset of visual floaters often signals retinal detachment, an ocular emergency.

Health history
If your patient complains of visual floaters, ask him appropriate questions from this list.
• When did the floaters first appear? What do they look like? Did they appear suddenly or gradually? If they appeared suddenly, did the patient also see flashing lights and have a curtainlike loss of vision?
• Is the patient nearsighted, and does he wear corrective lenses?
• Does the patient have a history of eye trauma or other eye disorders, allergies, granulomatous disease, diabetes mellitus, or hypertension?
• Which medications is the patient taking?

Physical examination
Inspect the eyes for signs of injury, such as bruising or edema. Then assess the patient's visual acuity, using the Snellen alphabet or "E" chart.

Causes
Your assessment may lead you to suspect one or more of the following causes.

Retinal detachment. Floaters and light flashes appear suddenly in the portion of the visual field where the retina has detached. As retinal detachment progresses (a painless process), gradual vision loss occurs, with the patient seeing a "curtain" falling in front of his eyes. Ophthalmoscopic examination reveals a gray, opaque, detached retina with an indefinite margin. Retinal vessels appear almost black.

Vitreous hemorrhage. Rupture of retinal vessels produces a shower of red or black dots or a red haze across the visual field. Vision blurs suddenly in the affected eye, and visual acuity may be greatly reduced.

Other causes. Visual floaters may also result from posterior uveitis.

Vision loss

Vision loss can occur suddenly or gradually, be temporary or permanent, and may range from

PATHOPHYSIOLOGY

How glaucoma causes vision loss

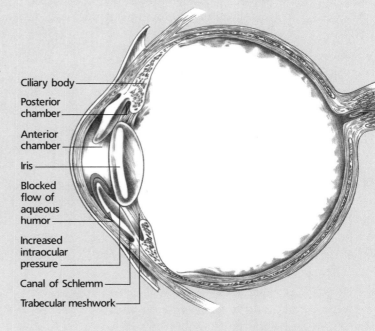

In a normally functioning eye, the ciliary body produces aqueous humor, which flows from the posterior chamber to the anterior chamber and then through the trabecular meshwork to the canal of Schlemm (outflow channel). From there, the aqueous humor travels into the venous circulation.

When the iris comes in contact with the trabecular meshwork, this flow is blocked, causing a sudden increase in intraocular pressure—acute angle-closure glaucoma. The resulting compromise in the optic nerve's blood supply can lead to blindness.

Ciliary body

Posterior chamber

Anterior chamber

Iris

Blocked flow of aqueous humor

Increased intraocular pressure

Canal of Schlemm

Trabecular meshwork

---

a slight impairment to total blindness. It may result from eye, neurologic, and systemic disorders, as well as from trauma and reactions to certain drugs.

Health history
If your patient complains of vision loss, ask him appropriate questions from the following list.
• When did the loss first occur? Did it occur suddenly or gradually? Does it affect one or both eyes? Does it affect all or part of the visual field?
• Is the patient experiencing blurred vision, halo vision, nausea, pain, photosensitivity, or vomiting with the vision loss?
• Has the patient had a recent facial or eye injury?
• Does the patient have a history of cardiovascular or endocrine disorders, infections, or allergies? Does anyone in his family have a history of vision loss or other eye problems?

• Which medications is the patient taking?

Physical examination
Observe the patient's eyes for conjunctival or scleral redness, drainage, edema, foreign bodies, and signs of trauma. With a flashlight, examine the cornea and iris. Observe the size, shape, and color of the pupils. Then test direct and consensual light reflexes and visual accommodation, extraocular muscle function, and visual acuity. Gently palpate each eye, noting any hardness. Then auscultate over the neck and temple for carotid bruits.

Causes
Your assessment may lead you to suspect one of the following causes.

Glaucoma. Acute angle-closure glaucoma may cause rapid blindness. (See *How glaucoma causes vision loss*.) Findings include halo vision, nonreactive pupillary response, photophobia, rapid onset of unilateral inflammation and pain, and reduced visual acuity. By contrast, chronic open-angle glaucoma progresses slowly. Usually bilateral, it causes aching eyes, halo vision, peripheral vision loss, and reduced visual acuity.

Eye trauma. Sudden unilateral or bilateral vision loss may occur after an eye injury. The loss may be total or partial, permanent or temporary. The eyelids may be reddened, edematous, and lacerated.

Other causes. Vision loss may also be caused by congenital rubella or syphilis, herpes zoster, Marfan's syndrome, a pituitary tumor, retrolental fibroplasia, and drugs such as digitalis glycosides, indomethacin (Indocin), ethambutol (Myambutol), quinine sulfate (Strema), and methanol.

Dyspnea

Patients typically describe dyspnea as shortness of breath, but this symptom also refers to difficult or uncomfortable breathing. Its severity varies greatly and is often unrelated to the seriousness of the underlying cause. Dyspnea may arise suddenly or slowly and may subside rapidly or persist for years.

Health history
If your patient complains of dyspnea, ask him appropriate questions from the following list.
• When did the dyspnea first occur? Did it begin suddenly or gradually? Is it constant or intermittent? Does it occur during activity or while he's resting? Does anything seem to trigger, exacerbate, or relieve it? Has he ever had dyspnea before?
• Ask the patient if he also has a productive or nonproductive cough or chest pain.
• Has the patient recently had an upper respiratory tract infection or experienced trauma? Does he smoke? If so, how much and for how long? Has he been exposed to any allergens? Does he have any known allergies?
• Which medications is he taking?

Physical examination
Observe the patient's respirations, noting their rate and depth, and any breathing difficulties or abnormal respiratory patterns. Check too for flaring nostrils, grunting respirations, inspiratory stridor, intercostal retractions during inspiration, and pursed-lip expirations.

Also examine the patient for barrel chest, diaphoresis, neck vein distention, finger clubbing, and peripheral edema. Note the color, consistency, and odor of any sputum.

Palpate his chest for asymmetrical expansion, decreased diaphragmatic excursion, tactile fremitus, and subcutaneous crepitation. Also check the rate, rhythm, and intensity of his peripheral pulses.

As you percuss the lung fields, note dull, hyperresonant, or tympanic percussion sounds. Auscultate the lungs for bronchophony, crackles, decreased or absent unilateral breath sounds, egophony, pleural friction rubs, rhonchi, whispered pectoriloquy, and wheezing. Then auscultate the heart for abnormal sounds or rhythms, such as ventricular or atrial gallop, and for pericardial friction rubs and tachycardia. Be sure to monitor the patient's blood pressure and pulse pressure.

Causes
Your assessment may lead you to suspect one or more of the following causes.

Adult respiratory distress syndrome. In adult respiratory distress syndrome (ARDS), acute dyspnea is followed by accessory muscle use, crackles, grunting respirations, progressive respiratory distress, rhonchi, and wheezes. In the late stages, anxiety, cyanosis, decreased mental acuity, and tachycardia occur. Severe ARDS can produce signs of shock, such as cool, clammy skin and hypotension. The typical patient has no history of underlying cardiac or pulmonary disease but has sustained a recent pulmonary or systemic insult.

Airway obstruction (partial). Inspiratory stridor and acute dyspnea occur as the patient tries to overcome the obstruction. Related findings include accessory muscle use, anxiety, asymmetrical chest expansion, cyanosis, decreased or absent breath sounds, diaphoresis, hypotension, and tachypnea. The patient may have aspirated vomitus or a foreign body or been exposed to an allergen.

Asthma. Acute dyspneic attacks occur along with accessory muscle use, apprehension, dry cough, flushing or cyanosis, intercostal retractions, tachypnea, and tachycardia. On palpation, you'll detect decreased tactile fremitus. Hyperresonance occurs on chest percussion. On auscultation, you'll note wheezing and rhonchi or, during a severe episode, decreased breath sounds.

Congestive heart failure. Dyspnea usually develops gradually or occurs as chronic paroxysmal nocturnal dyspnea. In ventricular failure, dyspnea occurs with basilar crackles, dependent peripheral edema, distended neck veins, fatigue, orthopnea, tachycardia, ventricular or atrial gallop, and weight gain. The patient may have a history of cardiovascular disease or may be taking drugs that can precipitate congestive heart failure (CHF), such as amiodarone (Cordarone), certain beta blockers, or corticosteroids.

Myocardial infarction. Sudden dyspnea occurs with crushing substernal chest pain that may radiate to the back, neck, jaw, and arms. The patient's history may include heart disease, hypertension, hypercholesterolemia, or use of drugs that can precipitate a myocardial infarction (MI), such as cocaine, dextrothyroxine sodium (Choloxin), estramustine phosphate sodium (Emcyt), or recombinant interleukin-2.

Pneumonia. Dyspnea occurs suddenly, usually accompanied by fever, pleuritic chest pain that worsens with deep inspiration, and shaking chills. The patient also has a dry or productive cough, depending on the stage and type of pneumonia. Sputum may be discolored and foul-smelling. Crackles, decreased breath sounds, dullness on percussion, and rhonchi may also be present. The history may include exposure to a contagious organism, hazardous fumes, or air pollution.

Pulmonary edema. In this disorder, severe dyspnea is often preceded by signs of CHF, such as crackles in both lung fields, cyanosis, tachycardia, tachypnea, and marked anxiety. The patient may have a dry cough or one that produces copious amounts of pink, frothy sputum. The history may reveal cardiovascular disease, cyanosis, fatigue, and pallor.

Pulmonary embolism. Severe dyspnea occurs with intense angina-like or pleuritic pain aggravated by deep breathing and thoracic movement. Other findings include crackles, cyanosis, diffuse wheezing, dull percussion sounds, low-grade fever, nonproductive cough, pleural friction rubs, restlessness, tachypnea, and tachycardia. The patient's history may include acute MI, CHF, hip or leg fractures, oral contraceptive use, pregnancy, thrombophlebitis, or varicose veins.

Other causes. Dyspnea may also result from anemia, anxiety, cardiac arrhythmias, cor pulmonale, inhalation injury, lung cancer, pleural effusion, and sepsis.

Dysphagia

Difficulty swallowing, or dysphagia, is the most common—and sometimes the only—symptom of esophageal disorders. This symptom may also result from oropharyngeal, respiratory, neurologic, and collagen disorders, and from exposure to toxins. Patients with dysphagia have an increased risk of aspiration and choking, and of malnutrition and dehydration. (See *Classifying dysphagia*, pages 48 and 49.)

Health history

If your patient complains of dysphagia, ask him appropriate questions from the following list.
• When did the dysphagia start? Is swallowing painful? If so, is the pain constant or intermittent? Can the patient point to the spot where the dysphagia is most intense? Does eating alleviate or aggravate the dysphagia? Does he have more trouble swallowing solids or liquids? Does the dysphagia disappear after he tries to

Classifying dysphagia

Swallowing occurs in three distinct phases, and dysphagia can be classified by the phase affected. Determining the phase of a patient's dysphagia can help to identify the symptom's cause.

Phase 1
Swallowing begins in the *transfer phase* with the chewing and moistening of food with saliva. The tongue presses against the hard palate to transfer the chewed food to the back of the throat; the trigeminal nerve (CN V) then stimulates the swallowing reflex. Phase 1 dysphagia typically results from a neuromuscular disorder.

Phase 2
In the *transport phase,* the soft palate closes against the pharyngeal wall to prevent nasal regurgitation. At the same time, the larynx rises and the vocal cords close to keep the food out of the lungs; breathing stops momentarily as the throat muscles constrict to move food into the esophagus. Phase 2 dysphagia usually indicates spasm or carcinoma.

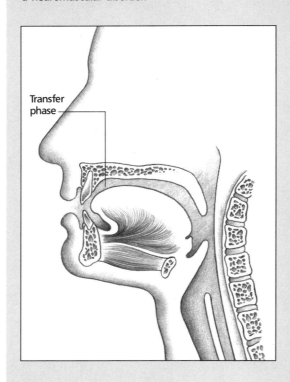

Transfer phase

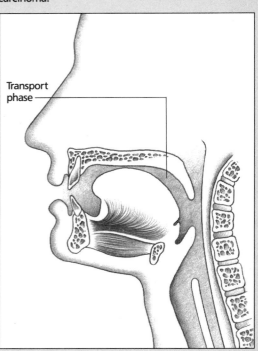

Transport phase

swallow a few times? Is swallowing easier if he changes position?
• Ask if the patient or anyone in his family has a history of esophageal, oropharyngeal, respiratory, neurologic, or collagen disorders. Has he recently had a tracheotomy or been exposed to a toxin?

Physical examination
Evaluate the patient's swallowing and his cough and gag reflexes. As you listen to his speech, note any signs of muscle weakness. Does he have aphasia or dysarthria? Is his voice nasal or hoarse? Check his mouth for dry mucous membranes and thick secretions. Then observe for tongue and facial weakness.

Esophageal carcinoma. Typically, painless dysphagia accompanies rapid weight loss. As the carcinoma advances, dysphagia becomes painful and constant. The patient complains of a cough with hemoptysis, hoarseness, sore throat, and steady chest pain.

Esophagitis. A patient with corrosive esophagitis will have dysphagia accompanied by excessive salivation, fever, hematemesis, intense pain in the mouth and anterior chest, and tachypnea. Monilial esophagitis will produce dysphagia and sore throat. In reflux esophagitis, dysphagia is a late symptom that usually accompanies stricture.

Hiatal hernia. The patient with a hiatal hernia may complain of belching, dysphagia, dyspepsia, flatulence, heartburn, regurgitation, and retrosternal or substernal chest pain that are aggravated by lying down or bending over.

Other causes. Dysphagia results from botulism, esophageal diverticulum, external esophageal compression, hypocalcemia, laryngeal nerve damage, and Parkinson's disease. Radiation therapy and a tracheotomy may also cause dysphagia.

Hoarseness

A rough or harsh-sounding voice, hoarseness can be acute or chronic. It may result from infections or inflammatory lesions or exudates in the larynx, from laryngeal edema, from compression or disruption of the vocal cords or recurrent laryngeal nerve damage, or from irritating polyps on the vocal cords. Hoarseness can also occur with aging because the laryngeal muscles and mucosa atrophy, leading to diminished control of the vocal cords. Hoarseness may be exacerbated by excessive alcohol intake, smoking, inhalation of noxious fumes, excessive talking, and shouting.

Health history
If your patient complains of hoarseness, ask him appropriate questions from the following list.

Phase 3
Peristalsis and gravity work together in the *entrance phase* to move food through the esophageal sphincter and into the stomach. Phase 3 dysphagia results from lower esophageal narrowing by diverticulitis, esophagitis, and other disorders.

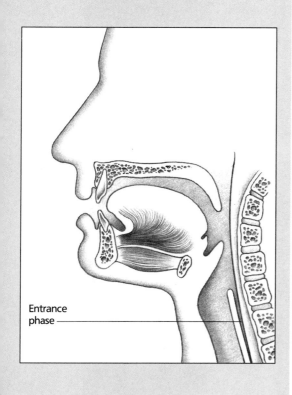

Entrance phase

Causes
Your assessment may lead you to suspect one or more of the following causes.

Airway obstruction. A life-threatening condition, upper airway obstruction is marked by respiratory distress. Dysphagia occurs along with gagging and dysphonia.

• When did the hoarseness start? Is it constant or intermittent? Does anything relieve or exacerbate it? Has the patient been overusing his voice?

• Ask if the patient has also had a cough, a dry mouth, difficulty swallowing dry food, shortness of breath, or a sore throat.

• Does the patient have a history of cancer or other disorders? Does he regularly drink alcohol or smoke? If so, how much?

Physical examination

Inspect the patient's mouth and throat for redness or exudate, possibly indicating an upper respiratory tract infection. Ask him to stick out his tongue: If he can't, the hypoglossal nerve (CN XII) may be impaired.

As the patient breathes, observe for asymmetrical chest expansion, intercostal retractions, nasal flaring, stridor, and other signs of respiratory distress.

Palpate the patient's neck for masses and the cervical lymph nodes and thyroid gland for enlargement. Then palpate the trachea to assess for deviation.

As you percuss the chest wall, note any dullness. Then, auscultate the lungs for crackles, rhonchi, tubular sounds, or wheezes. To detect bradycardia, auscultate the heart.

Causes

Your assessment may lead you to suspect one or more of the following causes.

Inhalation injury. Exposure to a fire or an explosion can cause an inhalation injury, which produces coughing, hoarseness, orofacial burns, singed nasal hair, and soot-stained sputum. Subsequent signs and symptoms include crackles, rhonchi, wheezes, and rapid deterioration to respiratory distress.

Reviewing the cough mechanism

Coughing, a necessary protective mechanism, clears the airways. The cough reflex occurs when mechanical, chemical, thermal, inflammatory, or psychogenic stimuli activate the cough receptors, which are thought to be located in the nose, sinuses, auditory canals, nasopharynx, larynx, trachea, bronchi, pleurae, diaphragm and, possibly, the pericardium and GI tract. Once a cough receptor is stimulated, the glossopharyngeal and vagus nerves (CN IX and CN X) transmit the impulse to the cough center in the medulla. From there, the impulse is transmitted to the larynx and to the intercostal and abdominal muscles.

Deep inspiration (shown in the first illustration) is followed by a closure of the glottis (shown in the second illustration), relaxation of the diaphragm, and contraction of the abdominal and intercostal muscles. The resulting increased pressure in the lungs opens the glottis to release the forceful, noisy expiration known as a cough (shown in the third illustration).

Deep inspiration

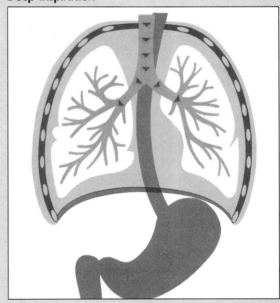

Laryngitis. Persistent hoarseness may be the only sign of chronic laryngitis. In acute laryngitis, hoarseness or a complete loss of voice develops suddenly. Related findings include cough, fever, pain (especially during swallowing or speaking), profuse diaphoresis, rhinorrhea, and sore throat.

Vocal cord polyps. With this disorder, a raspy hoarseness will be the chief complaint. The patient may also have a chronic cough and a crackling voice.

Other causes. Hoarseness may result from hypothyroidism, pulmonary tuberculosis, rheumatoid arthritis, and laryngeal cancer (most common in men ages 50 to 70). Prolonged intubation, surgical severing of the recurrent laryngeal nerve, and a tracheostomy may also produce hoarseness.

Nonproductive cough

A nonproductive cough is a noisy, forceful expulsion of air from the lungs that doesn't yield sputum or blood. One of the most common symptoms of a respiratory disorder, a nonproductive cough can be ineffective and cause damage, such as airway collapse, rupture of the alveoli, or blebs.

A nonproductive cough that later becomes productive is a classic sign of a progressive respiratory disease. An acute nonproductive cough has a sudden onset and may be self-limiting. A nonproductive cough that persists beyond 1 month is considered chronic; often, such a cough results from cigarette smoking. (See *Reviewing the cough mechanism.*)

Health history
If your patient complains of a nonproductive cough, ask him appropriate questions from the following list.

Effect of closed glottis

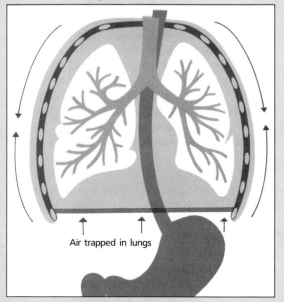

Air trapped in lungs

Release of cough

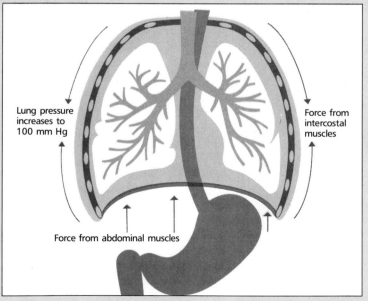

Lung pressure increases to 100 mm Hg

Force from intercostal muscles

Force from abdominal muscles

• When did the cough begin? Does any body position or specific activity relieve or exacerbate it? Does it get better or worse at certain times of the day? How does the cough sound? Does it occur often? Is it paroxysmal?

• Is the cough accompanied by pain?

• Has the patient had recent changes in appetite, energy level, exercise tolerance, or weight? Has he had surgery recently? Does he have any allergies? Does the patient smoke? Has he been exposed recently to fumes or chemicals?

• Which medications is the patient taking?

Physical examination

Note whether the patient appears agitated, anxious, confused, diaphoretic, flushed, lethargic, nervous, pale, or restless. Is his skin cold or warm, clammy or dry?

Observe the rate and depth of his respirations, noting any abnormal patterns. Then examine his chest configuration and chest wall motion.

Check the patient's nose and mouth for congestion, drainage, inflammation, and signs of infection. Then inspect his neck for vein distention and tracheal deviation.

As you palpate the patient's neck, note any enlarged lymph nodes or masses. Next, percuss his chest while listening for dullness, flatness, and tympany. Finally, auscultate his lungs for crackles, decreased or absent breath sounds, pleural friction rubs, rhonchi, and wheezes.

Causes

Your assessment may lead you to suspect one or more of the following causes.

Asthma. Typically, an asthma attack occurs at night, starting with a nonproductive cough and mild wheezing. Then, it progresses to audible wheezing, chest tightness, a cough that produces thick mucus, and severe dyspnea. Other signs include accessory muscle use, cyanosis, diaphoresis, flaring nostrils, flushing, intercostal and supraclavicular retractions on inspiration, prolonged expirations, tachycardia, and tachypnea.

Interstitial lung disease. With this disorder,

the patient has a nonproductive cough and progressive dyspnea. He may also be cyanotic and fatigued, and have fine crackles, finger clubbing, chest pain, and a recent weight loss.

Other causes. Nonproductive coughing may be caused by an airway occlusion, atelectasis, hypersensitivity pneumonitis, pericardial effusion, pleural effusion, pulmonary embolism, and sinusitis. Also, incentive spirometry, intermittent positive-pressure breathing, and suctioning can bring on a nonproductive cough.

Productive cough

With productive coughing, the airway passages are cleared of accumulated secretions that normal mucociliary action doesn't remove. The sudden, forceful, noisy expulsion contains sputum, blood, or both.

Usually caused by a cardiopulmonary disorder, productive coughing typically stems from an acute or chronic infection that causes inflammation, edema, and increased mucus production in the airways. Such coughing can also result from inhaling antigenic or irritating substances; in fact, its most common cause is cigarette smoking.

Health history

If your patient complains of a productive cough, ask him appropriate questions from the following list.

• When did the cough begin? How much sputum does the patient cough up daily? Is sputum production associated with the time of day, meals, activities, or the environment? Has it increased since coughing began? What are the color, odor, and consistency of the sputum? How does the cough sound and feel? Has the patient ever had a productive cough before?

• Ask if the patient also has changes in appetite or weight.

• Does the patient have a history of recent surgery or allergies? Does he smoke or drink alcohol? If so, how much? Does he work around chemicals or respiratory irritants?

• Which medications is the patient taking?

Physical examination

As you examine the patient's mouth and nose for congestion, drainage, and inflammation, note his breath odor. Then inspect his neck for vein distention. As he breathes, observe the chest for accessory muscle use, intercostal and supraclavicular retractions, and uneven expansion.

Palpate his neck for enlarged lymph nodes, masses, and tenderness. Next, percuss his chest, listening for dullness, flatness, and tympany. Finally, auscultate for abnormal breath sounds, crackles, pleural friction rubs, rhonchi, and wheezes.

Causes

Your assessment may lead you to suspect one or more of the following causes.

Bacterial pneumonia. With this disorder, an initially dry cough becomes productive. Rust-colored sputum appears in pneumococcal pneumonia; brick red or currant jelly sputum, in *Klebsiella* pneumonia; salmon-colored sputum, in staphylococcal pneumonia; and mucopurulent sputum, in streptococcal pneumonia.

Lung abscess. The cardinal sign of a ruptured lung abscess is coughing that produces copious amounts of purulent, foul-smelling and, possibly, blood-tinged sputum. A ruptured abscess can also cause anorexia, diaphoresis, dyspnea, fatigue, fever with chills, halitosis, headache, inspiratory crackles, pleuritic chest pain, tubular or amphoric breath sounds, and weight loss.

Other causes. Productive coughing can result from acute bronchiolitis, aspiration and chemical pneumonitis, bronchiectasis, cystic fibrosis, pertussis, pulmonary embolism, pulmonary edema, and tracheobronchitis. Also, expectorants, incentive spirometry, and intermittent positive-pressure breathing can cause productive coughing.

Hemoptysis

The expectoration of blood or bloody sputum from the lungs or tracheobronchial tree is

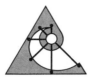

Hemoptysis or hematemesis?

If your patient begins bleeding from his mouth, determine if he's experiencing *hemoptysis* (coughing blood from the lungs) or *hematemesis* (vomiting blood from the stomach). Here's how the two conditions compare.

Hemoptysis
• Bright red or pink; frothy
• Mixed with sputum
• Produces negative litmus paper test (paper remains blue)

Hematemesis
• Dark red; may have a coffee-ground appearance
• Mixed with food
• Produces positive litmus paper test (paper turns pink)

known as hemoptysis. Usually resulting from a tracheobronchial tree abnormality, hemoptysis is associated with inflammatory conditions or lesions that cause erosion and necrosis of bronchial tissues and blood vessels.

Sometimes, hemoptysis is confused with bleeding from the mouth, throat, nasopharynx, or GI tract. (See *Hemoptysis or hematemesis?*) Severe hemoptysis requires emergency endotracheal intubation and suctioning.

Health history

If your patient complains of hemoptysis, ask him appropriate questions from the following list.
• When did the hemoptysis begin? How much blood or sputum is the patient expectorating? How often?
• Did the patient recently have a flulike syndrome? Has he had any recent invasive pulmonary procedures or chest trauma?
• Ask the patient if he smokes, or if he ever smoked. If so, how much? Does he have a history of cardiac, respiratory, or bleeding disorders?

• Which medications is the patient taking? Is he taking anticoagulants?

Physical examination

After assessing the patient's level of consciousness, examine his nose, mouth, and pharynx for sources of bleeding. Observe the rate and depth of his respirations, noting any breathing difficulty or abnormal breathing patterns. Also, as he breathes, look for abnormal chest movement, accessory muscle use, and retractions. Inspect the skin for central and peripheral cyanosis, diaphoresis, lesions, and pallor.

Palpate the rate, rhythm, and intensity of the peripheral pulses. Then feel the chest, noting abnormal pulsations, diaphragmatic tenderness, and fremitus. Check the level of the patient's diaphragm and assess respiratory excursion. If the patient has a history of trauma, carefully check the position of the trachea and note any edema.

As you percuss over the lung fields, note any dullness, flatness, hyperresonance, or tympany. Then auscultate the lungs for crackles, rhonchi, and wheezes, and the heart for bruits, gallops, murmurs, and pleural friction rubs. Be sure to monitor the patient's blood pressure and pulse pressure.

Causes

Your assessment may lead you to suspect one or more of the following causes.

Bronchitis (chronic). With this disorder, the patient usually has a productive cough that lasts at least 3 months and leads to expectoration of blood-streaked sputum. Other respiratory signs include dyspnea, prolonged expiration, scattered rhonchi, and wheezing.

Lung abscess. A patient with a lung abscess expectorates copious amounts of bloody, purulent, foul-smelling sputum. He also has anorexia, chills, diaphoresis, fever, headache, and pleuritic or dull chest pain. Lung auscultation may reveal tubular breath sounds or crackles. Percussion reveals dullness on the affected side. The patient may have a history of a recent pulmonary infection or evidence of poor oral hygiene with dental or gingival disease.

Lung cancer. Ulceration of the bronchus commonly causes recurring hemoptysis (an early sign), which can vary from blood-streaked sputum to blood. Related findings include anorexia, chest pain, dyspnea, fever, a productive cough, weight loss, and wheezing.

Pulmonary edema. A patient with pulmonary edema may expectorate copious amounts of frothy, blood-tinged, pink sputum. He may also complain of dyspnea and orthopnea. On examination, you may detect diffuse crackles in both lung fields and a ventricular gallop.

Tracheal trauma. With tracheal trauma, the bleeding appears to come from the back of the throat. Accompanying signs and symptoms include airway occlusion, dysphagia, hoarseness, neck pain, and respiratory distress.

Other causes. Hemoptysis may also result from bronchiectasis, coagulation disorders, cystic fibrosis, lung or airway injuries from diagnostic procedures, and primary pulmonary hypertension.

Back pain

Back pain may be acute, chronic, constant, or intermittent. It also may remain localized in the back or radiate along the spine or down one or both legs. A patient's pain may be exacerbated by activity (most commonly, stooping or lifting) and alleviated by rest. Or it may be unaffected by both.

Intrinsic back pain results from muscle spasm, nerve root irritation, fracture, or a combination of these causes. It usually occurs in the lower back or lumbosacral area. Back pain may also be referred from the abdomen, possibly signaling a life-threatening disorder.

Health history

If your patient complains of back pain, ask him appropriate questions from the following list.
• When did the pain first occur? What does it feel like? Is it mild, moderate, or severe? Is it constant or intermittent? Where exactly is it? Is it associated with activity? If the patient is a

woman, does the pain occur before or during her menses? What relieves or exacerbates it?
• Ask if the patient has had recent episodes of abdominal tenderness or rigidity, fever, nausea, or vomiting. Does he feel any unusual sensations in his legs? Has he had urinary frequency or urgency or painful urination?
• Does the patient have a history of trauma, back surgery, or urinary tract surgery, procedures, obstructions, or infections?
• Which medications is the patient taking?

Physical examination

Observe the rate and depth of the patient's respirations, noting any breathing difficulty or abnormal breathing patterns. Check his skin for diaphoresis, discoloration, edema, mottling, and pallor. Then inspect his back, legs, and abdomen for signs of trauma. After checking for abdominal distention, take a baseline abdominal girth measurement.

Because palpation and percussion can affect the frequency and intensity of bowel sounds, you should auscultate the abdomen first. Listen for bowel sounds in each quadrant. Then listen over the abdominal aorta for bruits and over the lungs for crackles. Be sure to monitor the patient's blood pressure and pulse pressure.

Palpate the abdominal, epigastric, and pelvic areas for abdominal rigidity, enlarged organs, masses, and tenderness. If you feel any pulsations, don't palpate deeply. Check the peripheral pulses for rate, rhythm, and intensity. Then gently palpate the painful area, noting contractions, excessive muscle tone, or spasm.

Finally, percuss each abdominal quadrant, noting any abnormal sounds, increased pain, or tenderness.

Causes

Your assessment may lead you to suspect one or more of the following causes.

Abdominal aortic aneurysm (dissecting).
Low back pain and dull upper abdominal pain often accompany a rapidly enlarging aneurysm and may indicate the early stages of rupture. On palpation, you may detect tenderness over the aneurysmal area and a pulsating epigastric

mass. Other signs include absent femoral and pedal pulses, mottling of the skin below the waist, and signs of hypovolemic shock.

Pancreatitis. Fulminating, continuous abdominal pain that may radiate to the back and both flanks characterizes pancreatitis. You may also note abdominal tenderness, rigidity, and distention; fever; hypoactive bowel sounds; pallor; tachycardia; and vomiting. The patient's history may include alcohol abuse, use of thiazide diuretics, gallbladder disease, or trauma.

Pyelonephritis (acute). The patient with acute pyelonephritis has progressive back pain or tenderness in the flank area, accompanied by costovertebral angle and abdominal pain in one or two quadrants. Associated signs and symptoms include dysuria, high fever, hematuria, nocturia, shaking chills, vomiting, and urinary frequency and urgency. The history may reveal a recent urinary tract procedure, urinary tract infection or obstruction, compromised renal function, or neurogenic bladder.

Other causes. Back pain may also result from appendicitis, cholecystitis, a lumbosacral sprain, osteoporosis, a perforated ulcer, renal calculi, tumors, and vertebral osteomyelitis.

Chest pain

Patients describe chest pain in many ways. They may report a dull ache, a sensation of heaviness or fullness, a feeling of indigestion, or a sharp, shooting pain. The pain may be constant or intermittent; it may radiate to other body parts; and it may arise suddenly or gradually. Patients may say that stress, anxiety, exertion, deep breathing, or certain foods seem to trigger the pain.

Chest pain may indicate several acute and life-threatening cardiopulmonary and GI conditions. But it can also result from musculoskeletal and hematologic disorders, anxiety, and certain drugs.

Health history

If your patient complains of chest pain, ask him appropriate questions from the following list.
• When did the chest pain begin? Did it develop suddenly or gradually? Is the pain localized or diffuse? Does it radiate to the neck, jaw, arms, or back? Is the pain sharp and stabbing or dull and aching? Is it constant or intermittent? Does breathing, changing positions, or eating certain foods exacerbate or relieve the pain?
• Find out if the patient has had related complaints, such as coughing, dyspnea, headache, nausea, palpitations, vomiting, or weakness.
• Does the patient have a history of cardiac or respiratory disease, cardiac surgery, chest trauma, or intestinal disease? Does he have a family history of cardiac disease?
• Does the patient drink alcohol or use any illicit drugs? Which medications is he taking?

Physical examination

Assess the patient's skin temperature, color, and general appearance, noting coolness, cyanosis, diaphoresis, mottling below the waist, pallor, peripheral edema, and prolonged capillary refill time. Look too for facial edema, jugular vein distention, and tracheal deviation. And note any signs of altered level of consciousness, anxiety, dizziness, or restlessness.

Then observe the rate and depth of the patient's respirations, noting any abnormal patterns or breathing difficulty. If the patient has a productive cough, examine the sputum.

Palpate the patient's neck, chest, and abdomen. Note any asymmetrical chest expansion, masses, subcutaneous crepitation, tender areas, tracheal deviation, or tactile fremitus. Also, palpate his peripheral pulses, and record their rate, rhythm, and intensity.

As you percuss over an affected lung, note any dullness. Then auscultate the lungs to identify crackles, diminished or absent breath sounds, pleural friction rubs, rhonchi, or wheezes. Auscultate the heart for clicks, gallops, murmurs, and pericardial friction rub. To check for abdominal bruits, apply the bell of the stethoscope over the abdominal aorta. Be sure to monitor the patient's blood pressure closely.

Causes

Your assessment may lead you to suspect one or more of the following causes.

Angina. Anginal pain usually begins gradually, builds to a peak, and then slowly subsides. The pain can last from 2 to 10 minutes. It occurs in the retrosternal region and radiates to the neck, jaw, and arms. Associated signs and symptoms include diaphoresis, dyspnea, nausea, vomiting, palpitations, and tachycardia. On auscultation, you may detect an atrial gallop (or S_4) or a murmur. Attacks may occur at rest or be provoked by exertion, emotional stress, or a heavy meal.

Aortic aneurysm (dissecting). A patient with a dissecting aortic aneurysm complains of sudden, excruciating, tearing pain in the chest and neck, radiating to the upper back, lower back, and abdomen. Other signs and symptoms include abdominal tenderness; heart murmurs; jugular vein distention; systolic bruits; tachycardia; weak or absent femoral or pedal pulses; and pale, cool, diaphoretic, mottled skin below the waist.

Cholecystitis. With this disorder, the patient has sudden epigastric or right upper quadrant (RUQ) pain, which may be steady or intermittent, radiate to the back, and be sharp or intense. Other signs and symptoms include chills, diaphoresis, nausea, and vomiting. Palpation of the RUQ may reveal distention, rigidity, tenderness, and a mass.

Myocardial infarction. Usually, the patient has severe, crushing substernal pain that radiates to the left arm, jaw, or neck. The pain may be accompanied by anxiety, clammy skin, diaphoresis, dyspnea, a feeling of impending doom, nausea, vomiting, pallor, and restlessness. The patient may have an atrial gallop, crackles, hypotension or hypertension, murmurs, and a pericardial friction rub. A history of heart disease, hypertension, hypercholesterolemia, or cocaine abuse is common.

Peptic ulcer. A sharp, burning pain arising in the epigastric region, usually hours after eating, characterizes peptic ulcer. Other signs and symptoms include epigastric tenderness, nausea, and vomiting. Food or antacids usually relieve the pain.

Pneumothorax. A collapsed lung produces a sudden, sharp, severe chest pain that's often unilateral and increases with chest movement. You may detect decreased breath sounds, hyperresonant or tympanic percussion sounds, and subcutaneous crepitation. Other signs and symptoms include accessory muscle use, anxiety, asymmetrical chest expansion, nonproductive cough, tachycardia, and tachypnea. The history may include chronic obstructive pulmonary disease, lung cancer, diagnostic or therapeutic procedures involving the thorax, or thoracic trauma.

Pulmonary embolism. Typically, the patient experiences sudden dyspnea with an intense angina-like or pleuritic ischemic pain aggravated by deep breathing and thoracic movement. Other findings include anxiety, cough with blood-tinged sputum, crackles, dull percussion sounds, restlessness, and tachycardia. If the embolism is large, the cardiovascular, pulmonary, and neurologic systems may be compromised. The patient's history may reveal thrombophlebitis, a hip or leg fracture, acute myocardial infarction, congestive heart failure, pregnancy, or the use of oral contraceptives.

Other causes. Chest pain may also result from abrupt withdrawal of beta blockers, acute bronchitis, anxiety, esophageal spasm, lung abscess, muscle strain, pancreatitis, pneumonia, a rib fracture, or tuberculosis.

Palpitations

Defined as a person's conscious awareness of his own heartbeat, palpitations are usually felt over the precordium or in the throat or neck. The patient may describe his heart as pounding, jumping, turning, fluttering, flopping, or missing or skipping beats. Palpitations may be regular or irregular, fast or slow, and paroxysmal or sustained. Beside cardiac causes, palpi-

tations may stem from anxiety, drug reactions, hypertension, thyroid hormone deficiency, and several other problems.

Health history
If your patient complains of palpitations, ask him appropriate questions from the following list.
• When did the palpitations start? Where does the patient feel them? How would he describe them? What was he doing when they started? How long did they last? Has he ever had palpitations before?
• Does the patient have chest pain, dizziness, or weakness along with the palpitations?
• Is the patient under unusual stress at home or at work? Has he recently undergone multiple blood transfusions or an infusion of phosphate?
• Does the patient have a history of thyroid disease, calcium or vitamin D deficiency, malabsorption syndrome, bone cancer, renal disease, hypoglycemia, or cardiovascular or pulmonary disorders that may produce arrhythmias or hypertension?
• Which medications is the patient taking? Is he taking an over-the-counter drug that contains caffeine or a sympathomimetic, such as a cough, cold, or allergy preparation? Does he smoke or drink alcohol? If so, how much?

Physical examination
Assess the patient's level of consciousness, noting any anxiety, confusion, or irrational behavior. Check his skin for pallor and diaphoresis. Then observe the eyes for exophthalmos.

Note the rate and depth of his respirations, checking for abnormal patterns and breathing difficulty. Also, inspect the fingertips for capillary nail bed pulsations.

To check for thyroid gland enlargement, gently palpate the patient's neck. Then palpate his muscles for weakness and twitching. Evaluate his peripheral pulses, noting the rate, rhythm, and intensity. And assess his reflexes for hyperreflexia.

Auscultate the heart for gallops and murmurs, and the lungs for abnormal breath sounds. Be sure to monitor blood pressure and pulse pressure.

Causes

Your assessment may lead you to suspect one or more of the following causes.

Acute anxiety attack. Palpitations may be accompanied by diaphoresis, facial flushing, and trembling. The patient usually hyperventilates, which may lead to dizziness, syncope, and weakness.

Cardiac arrhythmias. Paroxysmal or sustained palpitations may occur with dizziness, fatigue, and weakness. Other signs and symptoms include chest pain; confusion; decreased blood pressure; diaphoresis; pallor; and an irregular, rapid, or slow pulse rate. The patient may be using drugs that can cause cardiac arrhythmias—for instance, digitalis glycosides, sympathomimetics, ganglionic blockers, anticholinergics, or methylxanthines.

Thyrotoxicosis. In this disorder, sustained palpitations may accompany diaphoresis, diarrhea, dyspnea, heat intolerance, nervousness, tachycardia, tremors, and weight loss despite increased appetite. Exophthalmos and an enlarged thyroid gland may also develop.

Other causes. Palpitations may also arise from anemia, aortic insufficiency, hypocalcemia, hypertension, hypoglycemia, mitral valve stenosis or prolapse, and pheochromocytoma.

Abdominal pain

Usually, abdominal pain results from GI disorders, but it can also stem from reproductive, genitourinary, musculoskeletal, or vascular disorders, from drug use, or from the effects of toxins. Abdominal pain may originate in the abdominopelvic viscera, the parietal peritoneum, or the capsules of the liver, kidneys, or spleen. The pain may be acute or chronic, diffuse or localized.

Visceral pain develops slowly into a dull ache that's poorly localized in the epigastric, periumbilical, or lower midabdominal region. By contrast, somatic pain develops quickly after an insult and is sharp and well-localized. Mov-

ing or coughing aggravates it. Abdominal pain may also be referred from another site with the same or a similar nerve supply. (See *Recognizing types of abdominal pain.*)

Health history

If your patient complains of abdominal pain, ask him appropriate questions from the following list.
• When did the pain begin? What does it feel like? How long does it last? Where exactly is it? Does it radiate to other areas, such as the chest or back? Does it get better or worse when the patient changes position, moves, exerts himself, coughs, eats, or has a bowel movement?
• Find out if the patient had a fever during episodes of pain. Does he have appetite changes, constipation, diarrhea, nausea, pain with urination, pink or cloudy urine, vomiting, or urinary frequency or urgency?
• Does the patient have a history of adrenal disease, heart disease, recent infection, or recent blunt trauma to the abdomen, flank, or chest? Has he had any condition that could predispose him to emboli or that could narrow an arterial lumen? Has he recently undergone a urinary tract procedure or surgery? Has he traveled to a foreign country recently?
• Is the patient a woman of childbearing age? If so, what was the date of her last menses? Has her menstrual pattern changed? Could she be pregnant?
• Does the patient have a history of I.V. drug or alcohol abuse? Which prescription and over-the-counter drugs is he taking?

Physical examination

After assessing the patient's level of consciousness, observe his skin for diaphoresis, jaundice, and turgor. Then check for coolness, discoloration, and edema of the arms and legs. Inspect the abdomen and chest for signs of trauma: A bluish discoloration around the umbilicus (Cullen's sign) and around the flank area (Turner's sign) can indicate blunt trauma. Obtain and record a baseline measurement of abdominal girth at the umbilicus.

After inspecting for neck vein distention, observe the rate and depth of respirations,

Recognizing types of abdominal pain

AFFECTED ORGAN	VISCERAL PAIN	PARIETAL PAIN	REFERRED PAIN
Stomach	Midepigastrium	Midepigastrium and left upper quadrant	Shoulders
Small intestine	Periumbilical area	Over affected site	Midback (rare)
Appendix	Periumbilical area	Right lower quadrant	Right lower quadrant
Proximal colon	Periumbilical area and right flank for ascending colon	Over affected site	Right lower quadrant and back (rare)
Distal colon	Hypogastrium and left flank for descending colon	Over affected site	Left lower quadrant and back (rare)
Gallbladder	Midepigastrium	Right upper quadrant	Right subscapular area
Ureters	Costovertebral angle	Over affected site	Groin; scrotum in men, labia in women (rare)
Pancreas	Midepigastrium and left upper quadrant	Midepigastrium and left upper quadrant	Back and left shoulder
Ovaries, fallopian tubes, and uterus	Hypogastrium and groin	Over affected site	Inner thighs

noting any abnormal patterns. Observe the color and odor of the patient's urine.

Because palpation and percussion can affect the frequency and intensity of bowel sounds, you should auscultate the abdomen first. Listen for bowel sounds in each quadrant, noting whether the sounds are high-pitched and tinkling, hyperactive, or absent.

Then, listen to the patient's heart and breath sounds for abnormalities. Be sure to monitor his blood pressure and pulse pressure.

As you systematically palpate the abdominal, pelvic, flank, and epigastric areas, note any enlarged organs, masses, rigidity, tenderness, rebound tenderness, or tenderness with guarding. Check the patient's peripheral pulses for rate, rhythm, and intensity.

Percuss each abdominal quadrant, noting tenderness, increased pain, and percussion sounds. Dull percussion sounds indicate free fluid; hollow sounds, air.

Causes
Your assessment may lead you to suspect one or more of the following causes.

Abdominal aortic aneurysm (dissecting). Constant, dull upper abdominal pain radiating to the lower back typically accompanies rapid aneurysmal enlargement and may herald a rupture. Palpation may reveal an epigastric mass that pulsates before rupture. On auscultation, you may detect a systolic bruit over the aneurysm. You may also note abdominal rigidity, increasing abdominal girth, and signs of hypovolemic shock.

Abdominal trauma. The patient may have generalized or localized abdominal pain along with abdominal ecchymosis, abdominal tenderness, or vomiting. If he is hemorrhaging into the peritoneal cavity, you may note abdominal rigidity, dullness on percussion, and increasing abdominal girth. You may hear hollow bowel sounds if an abdominal organ has been perforated, or bowel sounds may be absent. Bowel sounds heard in the chest cavity usually signal a diaphragmatic tear.

Appendicitis. The patient with appendicitis may have sudden pain in the epigastric or umbilical region that increases over a few hours or days, along with flulike symptoms. Anorexia, constipation or diarrhea, nausea, and vomiting precede the pain, which may be dull or severe. Pain localizes at McBurney's point in the right lower quadrant. Abdominal rigidity and rebound tenderness may also occur.

Ectopic pregnancy. Lower abdominal pain may be sharp, dull, or cramping, and either constant or intermittent. The pain may be accompanied by breast tenderness, nausea, vaginal bleeding, vomiting, and urinary frequency. The patient typically has a 1- to 2-month history of amenorrhea after sexual intercourse. Rupture of the fallopian tube produces sharp lower abdominal pain, which may radiate to the shoulders and neck and become extreme on cervical or adnexal palpation.

Hepatitis. Liver enlargement from any type of hepatitis causes discomfort or dull pain and tenderness in the right upper quadrant. Associated signs and symptoms include anorexia, clay-colored stools, dark urine, jaundice, nausea, pruritus, and vomiting.

Intestinal obstruction. With an intestinal obstruction, short episodes of intense, colicky, cramping pain alternate with pain-free periods. Accompanying signs and symptoms include obstipation, pain-induced agitation, tympany, visible peristaltic waves, and abdominal distention, tenderness, and guarding. You may note high-pitched, tinkling, or hyperactive bowel sounds proximal to the obstruction and lower-pitched, hypoactive, or absent bowel sounds distal to the obstruction.

Pancreatitis. The characteristic symptom of pancreatitis is fulminating, continuous upper abdominal pain that may radiate to both flanks and to the back. Abdominal tenderness, fever, nausea, pallor, tachycardia, and vomiting may also occur. Some patients have abdominal distention and rigidity, hypoactive bowel sounds, and rebound tenderness. The patient's history may include alcohol abuse, gallbladder disease, trauma, a scorpion bite, or ingestion of a drug

that can cause pancreatitis—such as a thiazide diuretic.

Renal calculi. Depending on the location of the calculi, the patient may feel severe abdominal or back pain. However, the classic symptom of renal calculi is colicky pain that travels from the costovertebral angle to the flank, the suprapubic region, and the external genitalia. The pain may be dull or excruciating. Abdominal distention, agitation, chills, fever, nausea, urinary urgency, and vomiting may also occur.

Other causes. Abdominal pain may result from adrenal crisis, cholecystitis, congestive heart failure, diabetic ketoacidosis, diverticulitis, hepatic abscess, mesenteric artery ischemia, myocardial infarction, an ovarian cyst, a perforated ulcer, peritonitis, pneumonia, pneumothorax, pyelonephritis, renal infarction, and splenic infarction. Also, salicylates and nonsteroidal anti-inflammatory drugs can produce abdominal pain.

Pyrosis

A substernal burning sensation that rises in the chest and may radiate to the neck or throat, pyrosis results from the reflux of gastric contents into the esophagus. Usually, it is accompanied by regurgitation. Because increased intra-abdominal pressure contributes to reflux, pyrosis commonly occurs with pregnancy, ascites, or obesity, but it may also be caused by GI disorders, connective tissue disease, and certain drugs. (See *How pyrosis develops.*)

In most cases, pyrosis develops after meals or when a person lies down, bends over, lifts heavy objects, or exercises vigorously. It generally worsens with swallowing and improves when the person sits upright or takes antacids. Some patients confuse pyrosis with a myocardial infarction (MI), but a patient who is having an MI typically has other symptoms besides a burning sensation.

When a patient complains of pyrosis, you'll obtain a health history, but you won't perform a physical examination.

How pyrosis develops

A barrier to reflux, the lower esophageal sphincter (LES) normally relaxes only to allow food to pass from the esophagus into the stomach. But hormonal fluctuations, mechanical stress, and the effects of certain foods and drugs can lower LES pressure. When LES pressure falls and intra-abdominal or intragastric pressure rises, the normally con-tracted LES relaxes inappropriately and allows reflux of gastric acid or bile secretions into the lower esophagus. There, the reflux irritates and inflames the esophageal mucosa, producing pyrosis.

Persistent inflammation can cause LES pressure to decrease even more and may trigger a recurrent cycle of reflux and pyrosis.

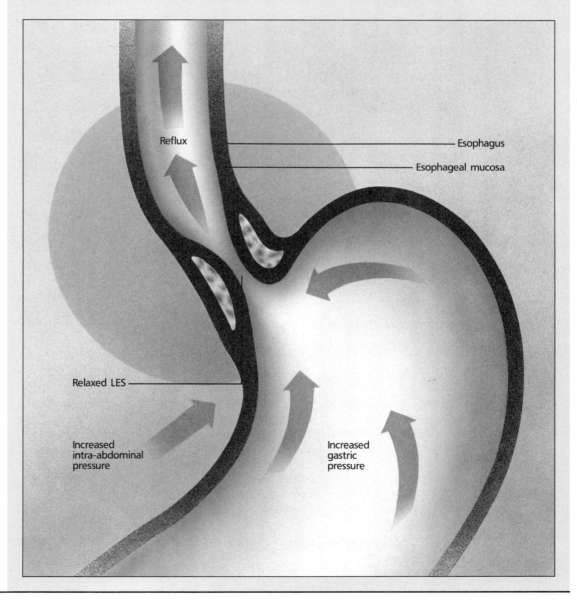

Reflux

Esophagus

Esophageal mucosa

Relaxed LES

Increased
intra-abdominal
pressure

Increased
gastric
pressure

Health history

If your patient complains of pyrosis, ask him appropriate questions from the following list.
• When did the pyrosis start? Do certain foods or beverages seem to trigger it? Does stress or fatigue seem to aggravate it? Do movement, certain body positions, or very hot or cold liquids worsen or relieve it? Where exactly is the burning sensation? Does it radiate to other areas? Does it cause the patient to regurgitate sour or bitter-tasting fluids? Has he ever had pyrosis before?
• Does the patient have a history of GI problems or connective tissue disease? If the patient is a woman, is she pregnant?
• Which medications is the patient taking?

Causes

Your assessment may lead you to suspect one or more of the following causes.

Esophageal cancer. Pyrosis may be a sign of esophageal cancer, depending on the tumor's size and location. The first symptom is usually painless dysphagia that progressively worsens. Eventually, partial obstruction and rapid weight loss occur. The patient may complain of a feeling of substernal fullness, hoarseness, nausea, sore throat, steady pain in the posterior and anterior chest, and vomiting.

Gastroesophageal reflux. Severe, chronic pyrosis is the most common symptom of this disorder. The pyrosis usually occurs within 30 minutes to 1 hour after eating and may be triggered by certain foods or beverages. It worsens when the person lies down or bends over and abates when he sits, stands, or ingests antacids. Other findings include a dull retrosternal pain that may radiate, dysphagia, flatulent dyspepsia, and postural regurgitation.

Peptic ulcer. Pyrosis and indigestion usually signal the onset of a peptic ulcer attack. Most patients experience a gnawing, burning pain in the left epigastrium, although some report sharp pain. The pain typically occurs when the stomach is empty and is often relieved by eating or by taking antacids. The pain may also occur after the patient ingests coffee, aspirin, or alcohol.

Scleroderma. A connective tissue disease, scleroderma may cause esophageal dysfunction resulting in pyrosis, bloating after meals, odynophagia, the sensation of food sticking behind the sternum, and weight loss. Other GI effects include abdominal distention, constipation or diarrhea, and malodorous, floating stools.

Other causes. Pyrosis may also be caused by esophageal diverticula, obesity, and several drugs, including acetohexamide (Dymelor), tolbutamide (Orinase), lypressin (Diapid), aspirin, anticholinergic agents, and drugs having anticholinergic effects.

Nausea

A profound feeling of revulsion to food, or a signal of impending vomiting, nausea is usually accompanied by anorexia, diaphoresis, hypersalivation, pallor, tachycardia, tachypnea, and vomiting. A common symptom of GI disorders, nausea may also result from electrolyte imbalances; infections; metabolic, endocrine, and cardiac disorders; early pregnancy; drug therapy; surgery; and radiation therapy. Also, severe pain, anxiety, alcohol intoxication, overeating, and ingestion of something distasteful can trigger nausea.

Health history

If your patient complains of nausea, ask him appropriate questions from the following list.
• When did the nausea begin? Is it intermittent or constant? How severe is it?
• Ask about related signs and symptoms, such as abdominal pain, anorexia, changes in bowel habits, excessive belching or flatus, weight loss, or vomiting.
• If the patient is a woman, is she pregnant or could she be? Does the patient have a history of GI, endocrine, or metabolic disorders; recent infections; cancer; or radiation therapy or chemotherapy?
• Which medications is the patient taking? Does he drink alcohol and, if so, how much?

Physical examination

Examine the patient's skin for bruises, jaundice, poor turgor, and spider angiomas. Then inspect his abdomen for distention.

Because palpation and percussion can affect the frequency and intensity of bowel sounds, you should auscultate the abdomen first. Listen for bowel sounds in each quadrant. Then, using the bell of the stethoscope, listen for abdominal bruits.

As you palpate the abdomen, note any rigidity, tenderness, or rebound tenderness. Next, palpate the size of the liver. Finally, percuss the abdomen and liver for any abnormalities.

Causes

Your assessment may lead you to suspect one or more of the following causes.

Appendicitis. The patient with appendicitis will feel nauseated and may vomit. He'll also have vague epigastric or periumbilical discomfort that localizes in the right lower quadrant.

Cholecystitis (acute). In this disorder, nausea commonly follows severe right upper quadrant pain that may radiate to the back or shoulders. Associated findings include abdominal tenderness, vomiting and, possibly, abdominal rigidity and distention, diaphoresis, and fever with chills.

Gastritis. Patients with gastritis often have nausea, especially after ingestion of alcohol, aspirin, spicy foods, or caffeine. Belching, epigastric pain, fever, malaise, and vomiting of mucus or blood may also occur.

Other causes. Nausea may result from cirrhosis, electrolyte imbalances, labyrinthitis, metabolic acidosis, myocardial infarction, renal and urologic disorders, and ulcerative colitis. Use of anesthetics, antibiotics, antineoplastics, ferrous sulfate, oral potassium, and quinidine, and overdoses of digitalis and theophylline may also trigger nausea, as may radiation therapy and surgery—especially abdominal surgery.

Weight loss

Weight loss can reflect decreased food intake, increased metabolic requirements, or a combination of the two. Its causes include endocrine, neoplastic, GI, and psychological disorders; nutritional deficiencies; infections; and neurologic lesions that cause paralysis and dysphagia. Weight loss may also accompany conditions that prevent sufficient food intake, such as painful oral lesions, ill-fitting dentures, and the loss of teeth. Weight loss may stem from poverty, adherence to fad diets, excessive exercise, or drug use.

Health history

If your patient complains of weight loss, ask him appropriate questions from the following list.
• When did the patient first notice he was losing weight? How much weight has he lost? Was the loss intentional? If not, can he think of any reason for it?
• Ask what the patient usually eats in a day. Have his eating habits changed recently? Why?
• Have the patient's stools changed recently? For instance, has he noticed bulky, floating stools or has he had diarrhea? What about abdominal pain, excessive thirst, excessive urination, heat intolerance, nausea, or vomiting?
• Has the patient felt anxious or depressed? If so, why?
• Which medications is he taking? Does he take diet pills or laxatives to lose weight?

Physical examination

Record the patient's height and weight. As you take his vital signs, note his general appearance. Does he appear well-nourished? Do his clothes fit? Is muscle wasting evident?

Next, examine his skin for turgor and abnormal pigmentation, especially around the joints. Does he have jaundice or pallor? Examine his mouth, including the condition of his teeth or dentures. Also check his eyes for exophthalmos and his neck for swelling.

Finally, palpate the patient's abdomen for liver enlargement, masses, and tenderness.

Causes

Your assessment may lead you to suspect one or more of the following causes.

Anorexia nervosa. A psychogenic disorder, anorexia nervosa is most common in young women and is characterized by a severe, self-imposed weight loss. This may be accompanied by amenorrhea, blotchy or sallow skin, cold intolerance, constipation, frequent infections, loss of fatty tissue, loss of scalp hair, and skeletal muscle atrophy.

Cancer. Weight loss is frequently a sign of cancer. Associated signs and symptoms reflect the type, location, and stage of the tumor, and typically include abnormal bleeding, anorexia, fatigue, nausea, pain, a palpable mass, and vomiting.

Crohn's disease. Weight loss occurs with abdominal pain, anorexia, and chronic cramping. Other findings include abdominal distention, tenderness, and guarding; diarrhea; hyperactive bowel sounds; pain; and tachycardia.

Depression. In severe depression, weight loss may occur along with anorexia, apathy, fatigue, feelings of worthlessness, and insomnia or hypersomnia. Other signs and symptoms include incoherence, indecisiveness, and suicidal thoughts or behavior.

Leukemia. Acute leukemia causes a progressive weight loss accompanied by bleeding tendencies, high fever, and severe prostration. Chronic leukemia causes a progressive weight loss with anemia, anorexia, bleeding tendencies, an enlarged spleen, fatigue, fever, pallor, and skin eruptions.

Other causes. Weight loss may result from adrenal insufficiency, diabetes mellitus, gastroenteritis, lymphoma, ulcerative colitis, and thyrotoxicosis. Drugs such as amphetamines, chemotherapeutic agents, laxatives, and thyroid preparations can also cause weight loss.

Hematuria

A cardinal sign of renal and urinary tract disorders, hematuria is the presence of blood in the urine. Hematuria may be evident or confirmed by a urine test for occult blood.

The bleeding may be continuous or intermittent, is often accompanied by pain, and may be aggravated by prolonged standing or walking. Dark or brownish blood indicates renal or upper urinary tract bleeding; bright red blood, lower urinary tract bleeding.

Health history

If your patient complains of hematuria, ask him appropriate questions from the following list.
• Ask when the patient first noticed the hematuria. Does it occur every time he urinates? Is he passing any clots? Has he ever had hematuria before?
• Does the patient have any pain? If so, does the pain occur only when he urinates, or is it continuous?
• Does the patient have bleeding hemorrhoids? Has he had any recent trauma or performed any strenuous exercise? Does he have a history of renal, urinary, prostatic, or coagulation disorders? If the patient is a woman, is she menstruating?
• Which medications is the patient taking?

Physical examination

Check the urinary meatus for any bleeding or abnormalities. Then, palpate the abdomen and flanks, noting any pain or tenderness. Finally, percuss the abdomen and flanks, especially the costovertebral angle, to elicit any tenderness.

Causes

Your assessment may lead you to suspect one or more of the following causes.

Bladder cancer. A primary cause of gross hematuria in men, bladder cancer may produce pain in the bladder, rectum, pelvis, flank, back, or leg. You may also note signs and symptoms of urinary tract infection.

Calculi. Both bladder and renal calculi produce hematuria, which may be accompanied by signs and symptoms of urinary tract infection. Bladder calculi usually produce gross hematuria, pain referred to the penile or vulvar area and, in some patients, bladder distention. Renal calculi may produce either microscopic or gross hematuria.

Glomerulonephritis. Usually, acute glomerulonephritis begins with gross hematuria. It may also produce anuria or oliguria, flank and abdominal pain, and increased blood pressure. Chronic glomerulonephritis typically causes microscopic hematuria accompanied by generalized edema, increased blood pressure, and proteinuria.

Nephritis. Acute nephritis causes fever, a maculopapular rash, and microscopic hematuria. In chronic interstitial nephritis, the patient may have dilute, almost colorless urine along with polyuria.

Pyelonephritis (acute). A typical sign of pyelonephritis is microscopic or macroscopic hematuria that progresses to grossly bloody hematuria. After the infection resolves, microscopic hematuria may persist for a few months. Other related findings include flank pain, high fever, and signs and symptoms of a urinary tract infection.

Renal infarction. Patients with renal infarction usually have gross hematuria. Other signs and symptoms include anorexia; costovertebral angle tenderness; and constant, severe flank and upper abdominal pain.

Other causes. Hematuria may result from benign prostatic hyperplasia, bladder trauma, obstructive nephropathy, polycystic kidney disease, renal trauma, and urethral trauma. Also, diagnostic tests—such as cystoscopy and renal biopsy—and drugs—such as anticoagulants, oxyphenbutazone (Oxalid), and thiabendazole (Mintezol)—may cause hematuria.

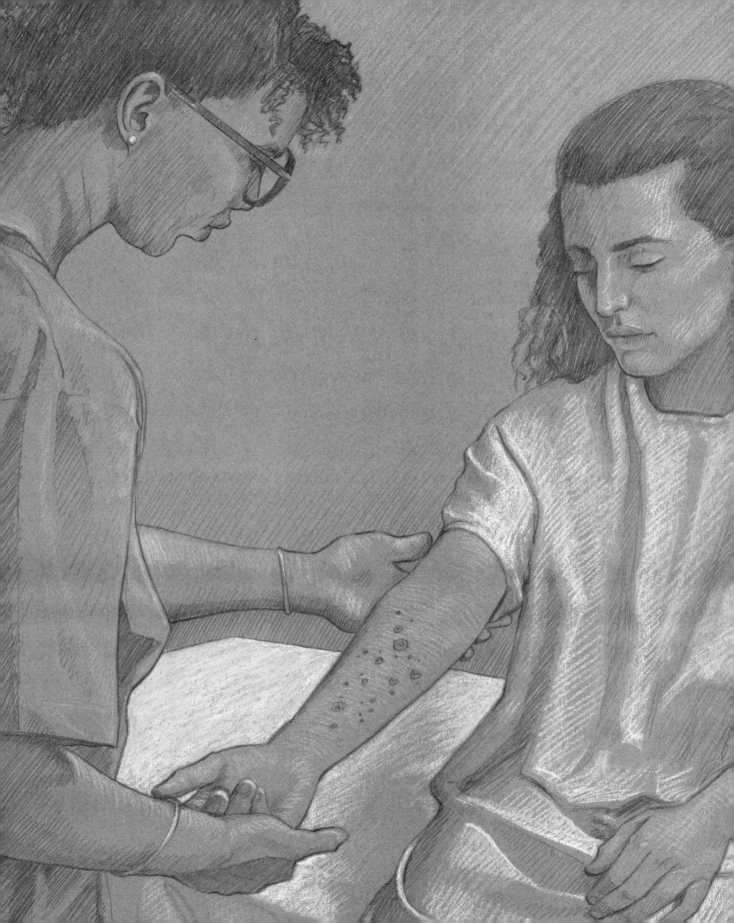

CHAPTER 4

Skin, hair, and nails

Your patient's skin protects him from the external world. Along with the hair and nails, the skin also acts as a visible barometer of changes within the body.

As a nurse, you observe your patient's skin regularly during routine care, so you're often the first to detect an abnormality. In a more formal assessment, you should always include the skin, hair, and nails—even if your patient's chief complaint is associated with a different body system. Your evaluation will provide a reliable picture of his overall health.

In this chapter, you'll first review the anatomy and physiology of the skin, hair, and nails. Next, you'll find guidelines for taking a health history of a patient with a skin, hair, or nail problem. The third section describes techniques you'll use during the physical examination. Then comes a section that will help you use the information you've gathered to identify the major disorders of the skin, hair, and nails. The final section covers pertinent diagnostic tests.

Anatomy and physiology

To assess your patient's skin, hair, and nails, you'll need to understand their structure and function. You should be familiar with the appearance of the skin, hair, and nails in both healthy and diseased states and understand how they change as a patient ages.

Skin

Also called the integumentary system, the skin is the body's largest organ. It makes up about 15% of the total body weight and contains cells, hair follicles, glands, and blood vessels.

As a system, the skin has several important functions in helping the body maintain homeostasis. Primarily, the skin protects the underlying tissues from trauma and provides a barrier against bacteria and any other harmful agents that come in contact with it. The skin also senses temperature, pain, touch, and pressure, which are transmitted to the central nervous system through sensory nerve fibers.

The skin helps regulate body temperature by means of sweat production and evaporation. Blood vessels in the skin dilate or constrict in response to temperature to further assist thermoregulation. Synthesis of vitamin D, another function of the skin, occurs as a result of exposure to ultraviolet rays.

Structure

The skin consists of two distinct layers: the outer epidermis and the deeper, thicker dermis. The subcutaneous tissue lies beneath these layers. (See *Reviewing skin structure.*)

Epidermis

The outermost layer of the skin, the epidermis is about 0.04 mm thick and made of avascular, stratified squamous epithelial tissue. Two layers can be distinguished in the epidermis epithelium: the stratum corneum, or superficial layer, and the deeper basal cell layer.

The stratum corneum is formed from epithelial cells in the deeper layer that migrate to the outer surface of the skin. The epidermal cells die as they reach the surface, and epidermal regeneration is continuous. Equilibrium between cell production and cell destruction or loss is essential to protect the integrity of the skin surface. During the migration of epidermal cells, which lasts about 14 days, some of the intracellular contents are transformed into keratin, a tough protein substance. The remaining cell membranes along with the keratinized cells make up the superficial layer, which is continuously shed or worn away as the deeper basal cell layer produces new cells.

The basal cell layer also contains melanocytes, which produce melanin and are responsible for skin color. Although the actual number of melanocytes is about the same in everyone, these cells are more productive in some people than in others, causing variations in skin color.

Melanin production intensifies when the skin is exposed to ultraviolet rays. Some ultraviolet ray exposure is necessary for vitamin D synthesis, but melanin protects the skin from the sun's most damaging rays. The epidermis has no blood supply, so nutrient distribution and waste removal take place through diffusion.

Dermis

Beneath the epidermis lies a thicker layer—the dermis, or corium—of about 0.5 cm. This layer consists of connective tissue and an extracellular material called matrix. Collagen, elastin, and reticular fibers are all part of this matrix and contribute to the strength and pliability of the skin. Blood and lymphatic vessels, nerves, and hair follicles are located in the dermis, as are the sebaceous, apocrine, and eccrine glands.

Wound healing and control of infection take place in the two distinct layers of the dermis: the papillary dermis and the reticular dermis. The papillary dermis has projections, or papillae, which nourish the avascular epidermis. The reticular dermis lies under the superficial papillary dermis and covers the subcutaneous tissue.

Sebaceous glands. Part of the same structure that contains the hair follicles and arrector pili muscles, these glands consist of a single short duct that originates from a group of lobules in

Reviewing skin structure

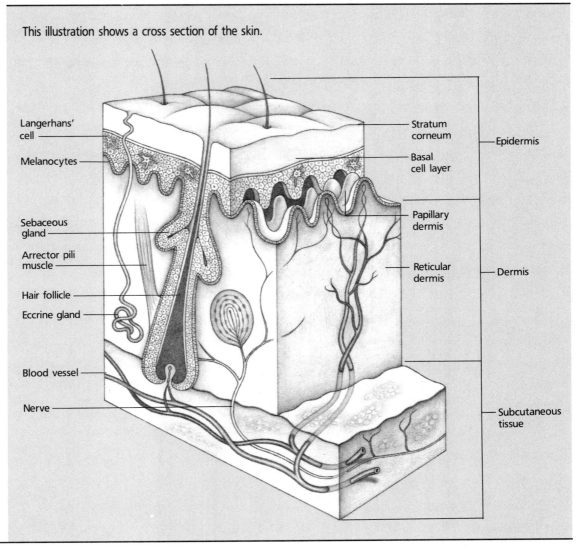

This illustration shows a cross section of the skin.

Langerhans'
cell

Melanocytes

Sebaceous
gland

Arrector pili
muscle

Hair follicle

Eccrine gland

Blood vessel

Nerve

Stratum
corneum

Basal
cell layer

Papillary
dermis

Reticular
dermis

Epidermis

Dermis

Subcutaneous
tissue

the dermis. Their main function is to produce sebum, which is secreted onto the skin or into the hair follicle. The fats, cholesterol, and salts contained in the sebum help make the skin and hair pliant. Sebaceous glands are found primarily in the skin of the scalp, face, upper body, and anogenital region.

Apocrine and eccrine glands. Commonly known as the sweat glands, the apocrine and eccrine glands lie in the dermis. The apocrine glands are located primarily in the axillae and anogenital areas, whereas the eccrine glands are distributed over most of the body. Both types of glands have secretory coils with ducts throughout the dermis. The eccrine gland ducts open on the skin surface, and the apocrine gland ducts lead to the hair follicles. Both glands secrete a watery fluid, which is initially odorless but can develop an odor as a result of bacterial decomposition. This release of sweat helps regulate body temperature.

Subcutaneous tissue

Located beneath the dermis, subcutaneous tissue is composed of fat cells, loose connective tissue, nerve fibers, and blood vessels. The thickness and consistency of subcutaneous tissue varies, depending on its location. It provides insulation against heat and cold and cushioning against shock.

Normal changes

Aging produces many normal skin changes. You should be familiar with these normal changes so that you can distinguish them from pathologic ones. Not only illness but also hormonal fluctuation and emotional stress can cause skin changes needing treatment.

Skin appearance

Skin changes are probably the signs of aging you'll notice most. The thinner, wrinkled skin of your elderly patients results from the thinning of the subcutaneous fat layer, especially in the extremities. You'll notice creases and lines, which form as a result of decreased elastin and collagen fibers. Wrinkles appear when the skin becomes lax and skin turgor decreases. Dry skin is common because of diminished sebum production. White patients often look paler as they age, and their skin becomes more opaque, owing to the reduced vascularity of the dermis. When exposed to the sun, the skin thickens, yellows, and develops deep creases and lines.

Not all elderly people develop spots and lesions, but many of them do. Brown spots, commonly known as liver spots, form on the backs of the hands and the forearms. Purple lesions called senile purpura can develop as a result of weakened, leaky capillaries. You'll often notice seborrheic keratoses and actinic keratoses on exposed areas. Probably the most common and harmless skin marks you'll see on elderly patients are cherry angiomas, usually found on the trunk.

Susceptibility to disease

With aging, all skin functions and processes decline. These include the response to injury, barrier protection, cell renewal, immune response, thermoregulation, sensation, sweat and sebum production, and vitamin D synthesis.

As a result of depressed immune responses, elderly patients are more prone to disease, including skin diseases. Diminished cell renewal also places them at greater risk for infection, poor wound healing, and tissue atrophy. They also develop carcinomas of the skin, especially squamous cell and basal cell carcinomas, at a higher rate than younger people.

Hair

The hair covers most of the body surface, with the exception of the palms and soles. Adults have two types of hair covering the body—vellus and terminal. Vellus hair is short, very fine, and unpigmented. Terminal hair, the normally pigmented hair visible on the scalp and eyebrows, is much coarser and thicker.

Structure

The hair is formed from keratin by matrix cells. At the lower end of the hair shaft is the hair bulb, which contains melanocytes and determines hair color. Each hair lies in a hair follicle and is attached to a smooth arrector pili muscle at its base. Sebaceous glands secrete sebum into the hair follicle. (See *Reviewing hair structure.*)

Normal variations

You'll notice differences in the thickness, coarseness, and distribution patterns of your patients' hair. These factors vary according to race, sex, and age—whites, for example, typically have more body hair than Asians. Men and women also develop different distribution patterns. The pattern of hair growth in the male genital area is diamond-shaped, whereas the pattern in the female genital area is triangular. And in males, facial and chest hair gradually coarsen after puberty. A deviation from these normal male and female patterns could indicate an endocrine problem.

Aging causes further changes. Head hair loses pigment, volume, and thickness. The loss of scalp hair is, in both sexes, genetically determined. In men, the hairline starts to recede at the temples, and balding begins at the vertex—in some men as early as age 20. You may notice some hair loss in elderly female patients, but it's usually less severe. Older people also lose body hair on the trunk, pubic area, axillae, and the extremities. Women's facial hair sometimes coarsens by age 55.

Nails

Like the hair, fingernails and toenails are composed of keratin. Nails are made up of the nail root called the matrix, the nail plate, the nail bed, and the periungual tissue.

The nail root or matrix, where the nail plate is formed, isn't visible. The nail plate is the visible, hardened, horny layer attached to and covering the nail bed. The nail plate is roughly rectangular, 0.3 to 0.65 mm thick, and translucent. Its pinkish color results from the underlying blood vessels in the nail bed. (See *Reviewing nail structure*, page 72.)

With age, nail growth slows. You may notice flaking and brittleness in the elderly patient's nails, and the nails may split easily. Nails lose their luster, develop longitudinal ridges, and change in form and shape. Slower peripheral circulation can cause yellowing and thickening, especially in the toenails.

Health history

If you're taking a complete history, be sure to ask the patient if he has any problems or complaints associated with his skin, hair, and nails. Even if a skin, hair, or nail problem isn't the patient's chief complaint, important concerns may come up when you review his history. Keep in mind that skin abnormalities often stem from a separate medical problem and can be minimized or overlooked by the patient. When the patient does have a primary problem related to skin, hair, or nails, of

ANATOMY

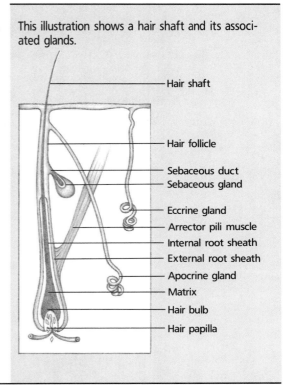

Reviewing hair structure

This illustration shows a hair shaft and its associated glands.

- Hair shaft
- Hair follicle
- Sebaceous duct
- Sebaceous gland
- Eccrine gland
- Arrector pili muscle
- Internal root sheath
- External root sheath
- Apocrine gland
- Matrix
- Hair bulb
- Hair papilla

course, you'll focus your history on his chief complaint.

Skin

If you're assessing a skin problem, you'll need to thoroughly explore the patient's chief complaint, medical history, family history, psychosocial history, and activities of daily living. As you question the patient, try to narrow down the possible causes of his skin problem.

Chief complaint
Ask the patient to describe his chief complaint in his own words. The most common skin problems include itching, rashes, lesions, abnormalities of pigmentation, and scaling. To investigate these or other chief complaints of the

ANATOMY

Reviewing nail structure

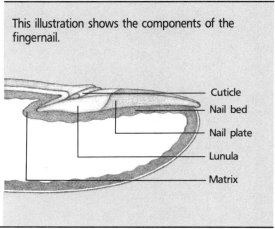

This illustration shows the components of the fingernail.

- Cuticle
- Nail bed
- Nail plate
- Lunula
- Matrix

skin, ask the patient relevant questions about such particulars as onset, duration, and severity. (See *Gauging pain.*) Also ask what precipitates the symptom, what makes it worse, and what makes it better. For more information on investigating chief complaints, see Chapter 3.

Medical history
Ask about the patient's medical history, including recent surgeries and dental work. Has he ever had a serious cut or burn? How well did it heal?

Try to identify risk factors for skin conditions. For instance, find out if the patient's skin reacts to certain substances. Has he ever had an allergic reaction to chemicals, paints, animals, or plants? Does a particular kind of clothing irritate his skin or cause a reaction? Explore possible environmental influences, such as exposure to extreme heat or cold, sun, or artificial tanning devices. Also ask if he's taking any medications. Skin reactions to drugs are common. (See *Possible causes of skin disorders,* page 74.)

Ask the patient how he has treated his symptoms at home. Has he used any creams, ointments, lotions, or special baths? Some home remedies can cause associated symptoms. Applying heat, for example, can enhance

healing, but the resulting vasodilation worsens edema and pruritus. In contrast, edema and pruritus can be decreased by applying cold, but healing will take longer.

Ask the patient to describe how his skin has changed over the years. Clarify the difference between normal and abnormal skin changes.

Family history
If anyone in the patient's family has a skin problem, ask him to describe it. Skin conditions such as acne, psoriasis, and allergic dermatitis may be hereditary. Other conditions, such as chicken pox and impetigo, are contagious. Always ask the patient if he's been in contact with a carrier of a contagious disease.

Psychosocial history
Because skin conditions are often noticeable, patients may be self-conscious about them. This self-consciousness can lead to depression and feelings of isolation if the condition is severe or the self-consciousness is ignored. Ask the patient if his skin condition has affected his self-esteem. Does he shun social contact because he or others think that his condition is ugly, unclean, unsafe, or contagious? Have his sexual relationships changed?

Activities of daily living
Ask which foods the patient eats. Does he know of any food allergies, especially to milk, wheat, or corn products?

Ask the patient to describe his daily skin care routine. Which types of soap, cream or lotion, and cosmetics does he use? If the patient shaves, does he use a blade or an electric razor? Do household cleaning agents irritate his skin and, if so, does he protect his hands with rubber gloves?

Hair

Loss of head hair and excessive hair on the body are the most common patient complaints. To investigate either, ask when the problem began.

If the patient has hair loss, is the loss complete, diffuse, or patchy? Overall hair loss may result from a systemic illness or a treatment, such as chemotherapy. Patchy hair loss can be caused by hair products, wigs, hairpieces, infections, and infestations, such as lice. Ask which shampoos, conditioners, and styling products the patient uses. Note if he uses chemical products, such as dyes, permanents, and straighteners.

Excessive hair growth, or hirsutism, can be hereditary or an effect of certain drugs. It can also signal an endocrine problem. Keep in mind that hirsutism can adversely affect self-image, especially in women.

For either complaint, ask the patient to describe his personal grooming habits. Try to determine his general level of health, fitness, and nutrition. And find out if he's taking any medications.

Nails

Common complaints include changes in nail color and growth. To investigate these complaints, ask the patient specific questions. For instance, ask if he bites his nails or cuticles. A nail can develop an infection from such biting.

Also have the patient describe his nail care and cosmetic use. Improper nail-cutting techniques can cause ingrown nails or infections. Nail polishes, especially those with hardening agents, can cause brittleness or discoloration. Polish removers that contain acetone cause dryness and brittleness. Nail wrappings and acrylic nails can result in infection and damage to the nail and surrounding tissue.

Systemic illnesses can also cause changes in the growth and color of nails. Aging and peripheral vascular disease can affect nail health as well.

Physical examination

Before beginning your examination, take a moment to check the surroundings. Make sure the lighting is adequate for inspection of the skin, hair, and nails. Because the patient will be par-

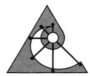

ASSESSMENT INSIGHT

Gauging pain

A subjective symptom like pain can be hard for the patient to describe. To help him rate the severity, offer him a numerical scale. Ask him to select a number on a scale of 1 to 5, with 1 representing the least severe pain he's ever felt and 5 representing the most severe.

tially undressed, also make sure the room temperature is comfortably warm. Then put on a pair of gloves to protect yourself during palpation.

Skin

To examine the patient's skin, you'll use both inspection and palpation—sometimes simultaneously. During your examination, you'll focus on such skin tissue characteristics as color, texture, turgor, moisture, and temperature. You'll also evaluate any skin lesions.

Color
Begin by systematically inspecting the skin's overall appearance. Remember, skin color reflects the patient's nutritional, hematologic, cardiovascular, and pulmonary status.

Observe general coloring and pigmentation, keeping in mind racial differences as well as normal variations from one part of the body to another. Examine all exposed areas of the skin, including the face, ears, back of the neck, the axillae, and the backs of the hands and arms.

Note the location of any bruising, discoloration, or erythema. Also look for pallor, a dusky appearance, jaundice, and cyanosis. Always ask the patient if he has noticed any changes in skin color anywhere on his body. (See *Evaluating skin color variations,* page 75.)

Dark skin and black skin
Some dark-skinned patients have a pigmented

Possible causes of skin disorders

Sometimes the cause of your patient's skin disorder won't be obvious. To help zero in on the cause, ask yourself these questions. Then review the list of possible causes beneath each one.

Does the patient have any of these disorders?
Acquired immunodeficiency syndrome
Allergies
Anemia
Arteriosclerosis
Bacterial infections
Cancer
Cardiopulmonary disorders
Cirrhosis
Dental caries or periodontal disease
Depression
Diabetes mellitus
Fungal infections
Hepatitis
Jaundice
Lupus erythematosus
Peripheral vascular disease
Renal failure
Scleroderma
Thyroid dysfunction
Venous stasis
Viral infections

Could an aspect of the patient's treatment be the cause?
Imposed immobility
Mechanical devices (orthopedic devices, restraints, dressings, tourniquets)
Medications
Radiation
Surgery
Therapeutic extremes in body temperature

Can you rule out these nutritional factors?
Dehydration
Edema
Emaciation
Malnutrition
Obesity

Has the patient been exposed to any of the following?
Animals or parasites
Chemicals or noxious substances
Poisonous plants
Radiation
Temperature or humidity extremes

Could any of the following personal factors be the cause?
Inadequate sleep
Poor personal hygiene
Stressful family life
Stressful job

line, called Futcher's line, extending diagonally from the shoulder to the elbow. This is normal. Also normal are deeply pigmented ridges in the palm.

To detect color variations in dark-skinned and black patients, examine the sclerae, conjunctivae, buccal mucosa, tongue, lips, nail beds, palms, and soles. A yellowish brown color in dark-skinned patients or an ashen grey color in black patients indicates pallor, which results from a lack of the underlying pink and red tones normally present in dark skin.

Among dark-skinned blacks, yellowish pigmentation isn't necessarily an indication of jaundice. To detect jaundice in these patients, examine the hard palate and the sclerae.

Look for petechiae by examining areas with lighter pigmentation, such as the abdomen, gluteal areas, and the volar aspect of the fore-

arm. To distinguish petechiae and ecchymoses from erythema in dark-skinned patients, apply pressure to the area. Erythematous areas will blanch, but petechiae or ecchymoses won't. Because erythema is commonly associated with an increased skin temperature, you can also palpate the skin for warmth.

When you assess edema in dark skin, remember that the affected area may have a decreased color because fluid expands the distance between the pigmented layers and the external epithelium. When you palpate the affected area, it may feel tight.

Cyanosis can be difficult to identify in both white and black patients. Because the lips and nail beds are often affected by factors such as cold, be sure you also assess the conjunctivae, palms, soles, buccal mucosa, and tongue.

To detect rashes in black- or dark-skinned

Evaluating skin color variations

COLOR	DISTRIBUTION	POSSIBLE CAUSE
Absent	Small, circumscribed areas	Vitiligo
	Generalized	Albinism
Blue	Around lips (circumoral pallor) or generalized	Cyanosis. *Note:* In blacks, bluish gingivae are normal.
Deep red	Generalized	Polycythemia vera (increased red blood cell count)
Pink	Local or generalized	Erythema (superficial capillary dilation and congestion)
Tan to brown	Facial patches	Chloasma of pregnancy; butterfly rash of lupus erythematosus
Tan to brown-bronze	Generalized (not related to sun exposure)	Addison's disease
Yellow	Sclera or generalized	Jaundice from liver dysfunction. *Note:* In blacks, yellowish brown pigmentation of the sclera is normal.
Yellow-orange	Palms, soles, and face; not sclera	Carotenemia (carotene in the blood)

patients, you'll need to palpate the area for skin texture changes.

Texture
Inspect and palpate the texture of the skin, noting thickness and mobility. Does the skin feel rough, smooth, thick, fragile, or thin? Changes can indicate local irritation or trauma, or they can be a result of problems in other body systems. For example, rough, dry skin is common in hypothyroidism; soft, smooth skin is common in hyperthyroidism. To determine if the skin over a joint is supple or taut, have the patient bend the joint as you palpate.

Turgor
Assessing the turgor, or elasticity, of the patient's skin helps you evaluate hydration. To assess turgor, gently squeeze the skin on the forearm. If it quickly returns to its original shape, the patient has normal turgor. If it resumes its original shape slowly or maintains a tented shape, the skin has poor turgor. Decreased turgor occurs with dehydration as well as with aging, whereas increased turgor is associated with progressive systemic sclerosis, a connective tissue disease.

To accurately assess skin turgor in an elderly patient, try squeezing the skin of the sternum or forehead instead of using the forearm. In an elderly patient, the skin of the forearms tends to be flaccid. So using this site to assess skin turgor wouldn't give you an accurate evaluation of the patient's hydration.

Moisture
Observe the skin for excessive dryness or moisture. If the patient's skin is too dry, you may see reddened or flaking areas. Elderly patients frequently have dry, itchy skin. Moisture that appears shiny may result from oiliness.

If a patient is overhydrated, the skin may be edematous and spongy. Localized edema can occur in response to trauma or skin abnormalities, such as ulcers. When you palpate local edema, be sure to document any associated discoloration or lesions.

(Text continues on page 78.)

Identifying primary and secondary lesions

Use these descriptions and drawings to help identify your patient's lesion. When examining a lesion, remember to keep your centimeter ruler with you so that measurements will be accurate.

PRIMARY LESIONS

Macule

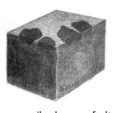

A flat, circumscribed area of altered skin color; generally less than 1 cm. Examples: freckle, flat nevus

Patch

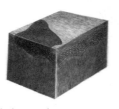

A macule larger than 1 cm. Example: herald patch (pityriasis rosea)

Papule

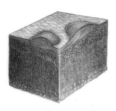

Raised, circumscribed, solid area; generally less than 1 cm. Examples: elevated nevus, wart

Pustule

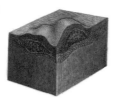

Raised lesion containing purulent fluid; varying in size. Examples: acne pustulosa, impetigo, furuncle

Nodule

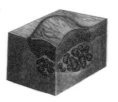

Raised or solid area; generally greater than 1 cm. Examples: acne pustulosa, epithelioma

Tumor

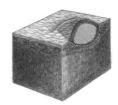

Solid lesion extending into dermal and subcutaneous layers; can be raised, level with skin, or beneath skin; larger than 1 cm. Example: tumor stage of mycosis fungoides

Plaque

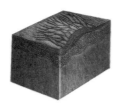

Circumscribed, superficial, solid elevation; larger than 1 cm. Examples: localized mycosis fungoides, neurodermatitis

Vesicle

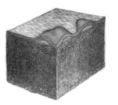

Circumscribed, elevated lesion; contains serous fluid; less than 1 cm. Examples: early chicken pox, contact dermatitis

Bulla

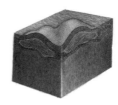

Vesicle larger than 2 cm. Examples: pemphigus, second-degree burn

SECONDARY LESIONS

Scale

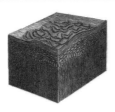

Thickened, desiccated epithelial cells that flake off. Examples: dandruff, psoriasis

Crust

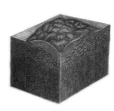

Dried serum, blood, or purulent exudate. Examples: impetigo, infectious dermatitis

Fissure

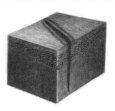

Deep linear break in the skin, extending into the dermis. Examples: congenital syphilis, athlete's foot

Erosion

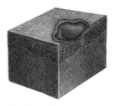

Circumscribed, moist, depressed lesion. Example: abrasion

Keloid

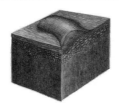

Thick, firm, reddened scar formed by hyperplasia of fibrous tissue; more common among blacks and Asians. Example: surgical incision

Ulcer

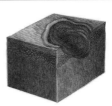

Localized tissue destruction that can extend into mucous membrane or through epidermis, dermis, and underlying tissue. Example: tertiary syphilis

Scar

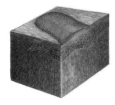

Area of replacement connective tissue, resulting from damage or disease. Example: healed surgical incision

Excoriation

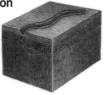

Abrasion or scratch mark. Example: eczema

Lichenification

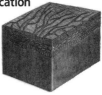

Thickened, rough skin with obvious lines. Example: chronic atopic dermatitis

ASSESSMENT INSIGHT

Macule or papule?

To determine whether a lesion is a macule or a papule, try this test. Reduce direct light, and shine a penlight or flashlight at a right angle to the lesion. If the light casts a shadow, the lesion is a papule. Macules are flat and won't produce a shadow.

Temperature

To assess skin temperature, touch the surface, using the backs of your fingers. Inflamed skin will feel warm because of increased blood flow. Cool skin results from vasoconstriction. With hypovolemic shock, for instance, the skin feels cool and clammy.

Make sure you distinguish between generalized and localized warmth or coolness. Generalized warmth, or hyperthermia, is associated with fever stemming from a systemic infection or hyperthyroidism. Localized warmth occurs with a burn or localized infection. Generalized coolness occurs with hypothyroidism; localized coolness, with arteriosclerosis.

Skin lesions

During your inspection, you may note vascular changes in the form of red, pigmented lesions. Among the most common are hemangiomas, telangiectases, petechiae, purpura, and ecchymoses. Keep in mind that these lesions may or may not indicate disease. You'll see telangiectases, for instance, in pregnant patients as well as in those with hepatic cirrhosis.

When you do detect a lesion, identify the type and provide an accurate description. Document the lesion's location, distribution pattern, and configuration as well as any associated symptoms.

Begin by classifying the skin lesion as primary or secondary. A primary lesion is the initial lesion that develops. When changes take place in the primary lesion, they constitute the secondary lesion. (See *Identifying primary and secondary lesions,* pages 76 and 77.)

Document a primary lesion as solid or fluid-filled. Macules, papules, nodules, wheals, and hives are examples of solid lesions. Vesicles, bullae, pustules, and cysts are fluid-filled lesions. (See *Macule or papule?*)

Once you've determined the type of lesion, note the following information, using the ABCD mnemonic device:
• A = Asymmetry. Is the lesion symmetrical or asymmetrical?
• B = Border. Note whether the border is well defined.
• C = Color. Describe the lesion's color.
• D = Diameter. Measure the diameter using a centimeter ruler. Don't estimate.

If you note drainage, document the type and amount. Note also if the lesion has an odor. Because most skin lesions don't have an odor, the presence of a noxious smell could indicate a superimposed infection, such as that found with open, oozing wounds. This commonly occurs with a gangrenous wound (necrotizing fasciitis) or with stasis ulceration of the legs.

If you note multiple lesions, identify the location of each one as well as the pattern of distribution. If the lesions affect a discrete area, the pattern is localized. The area may be small, such as the hand or the elbow. Or it may be large, such as the front or back of the trunk. If you detect lesions over the entire body, document the pattern as generalized.

Also note the configuration of the lesions. Are they separate from one another, or do they appear fused together? (See *Recognizing common lesion configurations.*)

A patient with lesions may complain of pruritus or a burning sensation. Itching, burning skin can interfere with your patient's sleep and daily activities as well as his overall emotional health. If the patient doesn't mention these symptoms, be sure to ask about them. Have him quantify the severity of the burning or itching, using a scale of 1 to 5.

Hair

Examine the hair over the patient's entire body, not just his head hair. Be sure you assess the distribution, quantity, texture, and color. The quantity and distribution of body hair vary among individuals and are, to some extent, determined by race.

Examine the pattern of the patient's hair growth and loss. If you note patchy hair loss, look for regrowth. Check the scalp for erythema, scaling, and encrustations. Excessive hair loss with scalp crusting could indicate ringworm infestation. But you can detect this only in a darkened room using a Wood's light, a specially filtered ultraviolet light. Also look for excessive hair growth.

Differences in grooming and hairstyling can also affect the scalp and quality of the hair. Repeated braiding, for example, pulls the hair and can cause hair loss. Feel the hair for dryness, brittleness, thickness, and oiliness. Dryness or brittleness can result from using harsh treatment products, or it might be caused by a systemic illness. Excessive oiliness usually is related to sebaceous gland production of sebum.

Nails

Examining the patient's nails is a vital part of your assessment because they can be a critical indicator of a systemic illness. Plus, their overall condition tells you much about the patient's grooming habits and level of self-care.

Color

First look at the color of the patient's nails. Whites generally have pinkish nails, and blacks and dark-skinned people have brown nails, typically with longitudinal lines.

Note if the nails are blue-black, purple, brown, or yellow-gray. Changes in nail color can result from contact with silver nitrate, gentian violet, and cosmetics, as well as from poisons, drugs, endocrine or cardiovascular disorders, lymphatic disease, infections, and trauma. White spots or streaks, for example, can be caused by trauma or by cardiovascular, hepatic, or renal disease. Yellow nails can result from thyrotoxicosis or from the nicotine in cigarettes. Blue nails can stem from vascular diseases, and green nails are usually a sign of *Pseudomonas* infection.

Recognizing common lesion configurations

Identify the configuration of your patient's skin lesions by matching it to one of these diagrams.

Discrete
Individual lesions are separate and distinct.

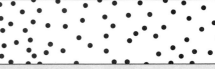

Grouped
Lesions are clustered together.

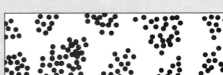

Confluent
Lesions merge so that individual lesions aren't visible or palpable.

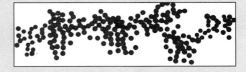

Linear
Lesions form a line.

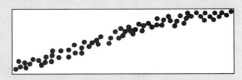

Annular
Lesions are arranged in a single ring or circle.

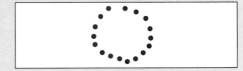

Polycyclic
Lesions are arranged in concentric circles.

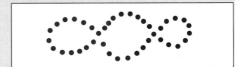

Arciform
Lesions form arcs or curves.

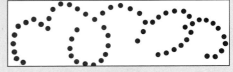

Reticular
Lesions form a mesh-like network.

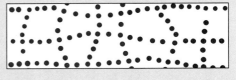

Shape and texture

Inspect the shape and texture of the patient's nails, noting any brittleness, cracking, or peeling. Are there striations, ridges, or depressions in the nails? What about any swollen, erythematous, or oozing tissue surrounding the nails?

To check for finger clubbing, you'll inspect and palpate. With clubbed fingers, you'll see obvious changes: The nail will be thickened, hard, shiny, and curved at the end. Press the nail base to determine firmness, and press the nail to determine the strength of its attachment to the nail bed.

To assess capillary refill, press the tip of the nail plate and check for blanching. The color should return in less than 1 second after you release the pressure. A delay could indicate cardiovascular disease.

Abnormal findings

Disorders of the skin, hair, and nails are classified according to cause, location, or type of lesion. Sometimes, two patients with identical diagnoses will have very different signs and symptoms. And you've probably noticed that the reverse can also be true: Two patients with the same signs and symptoms may not have the same disorder. Always document all signs and symptoms, and include as much information as possible about the cause of a patient's disorder.

Skin disorders

The signs and symptoms you detect during your assessment may be caused by widely varying skin disorders. This section describes allergic dermatoses, pruritic dermatoses, vascular dermatoses, papulosquamous dermatoses, acne, bacterial infections, viral infections, fungal infections, scabies, pemphigus vulgaris, pigmentation disorders, burns, and skin tumors. (See *Recognizing common disorders*, pages 87 to 90.)

Allergic dermatoses

These disorders result from allergic reactions. They include contact dermatitis, atopic eczema, nummular eczema, and dermatoses caused by drugs.

Contact dermatitis

A common disorder, contact dermatitis is an inflammation of the skin that results from contact with certain irritants or allergenic substances. It can develop in any area of the body as a result of contact with soaps, deodorants, creams, shampoos, clothing, jewelry, or plants.

The primary lesions include red macules, which appear as localized areas of redness; vesicles; and large, oozing bullae. Secondary lesions, such as crusting and excoriations, can result from bacterial infections. Lichenification may also occur as a secondary lesion.

Atopic eczema

Known as atopic dermatitis, this form of eczema occurs in both adults and infants. A patient with atopic eczema will have extreme pruritus. Some patients have a single mild episode, whereas others have chronic patterns.

Atopic eczema results from an inherited characteristic that increases the skin's sensitivity to irritants and allergens. The condition is aggravated by dry weather and emotional stress. A patient with atopic eczema may have a family history of asthma, eczema, or hay fever.

In infants, the characteristic lesions of atopic eczema cause blisters, oozing, and crusting on the face, scalp, or extremities. In adults, extreme dryness, thickening, and excoriation of the skin can be generalized but mainly affects the cubital and popliteal fossae.

Nummular eczema

You can identify nummular eczema by the presence of coin-shaped papulovesicular patches on the skin of the extremities. It mainly affects young adults and elderly patients. Although the exact cause is unknown, factors associated with this type of eczema include a history of asthma, hay fever, atopic eczema and, in elderly patients, a low-protein diet. As with atopic eczema, itching is severe.

Adverse skin reactions to drugs

The list below shows you common dermatoses and the drugs that typically cause them.

Allergic dermatoses (fixed eruption)
barbiturates
meprobamate (Equanil, Miltown)
ovulation stimulants
phenolphthalein (Alophen)
phenylbutazone (Azolid, Butazolidin)
salicylates
sulfonamides
tetracyclines

Vascular dermatoses (erythema multiforme)
barbiturates
chlorpropamide (Diabinese)
griseofulvin microsize (Fulvicin-U/F)
hydantoin derivatives
penicillins
phenothiazines
sulfonamides
thiazide diuretics

Papulosquamous dermatoses (lichenification)
chlordiazepoxide hydrochloride (Librium)
chloroquine hydrochloride (Aralen HCl)
gold salts
para-aminosalicylate sodium (PAS)
quinacrine hydrochloride (Atabrine)
quinidine (Cardioquin)
thiazide diuretics

Acne
corticosteroids
corticotropin (ACTH)
dactinomycin (Cosmegen)
hydantoin derivatives
iodides
lithium (Eskalith)
ovulation stimulants

Patients may develop secondary lichenification and infection.

Drug reactions
As you know, drugs can cause various skin reactions. The type and severity of the reaction depend on several factors, including the drug, the patient's overall health, and the timing and appropriateness of the intervention. (See *Adverse skin reactions to drugs.*)

Pruritic dermatoses
Generalized pruritus refers to extreme itching without a skin disorder. You'll often see it in older patients, especially during the dry winter months. Although the cause of pruritus isn't known, it's usually associated with dry skin and contact with exogenous irritants.

Pruritus also occurs with anaphylactic reactions and in chronic illnesses, such as uremia and biliary cirrhosis. In these cases, the skin will show excoriations and scaling plaques.

Neurodermatitis is a fairly common condition characterized by small, localized patches of thickened, scaly, dry skin. It occurs mainly on the neck, wrists, ankles, ears, and anal area. The disorder often results from a patient's con-tinuous cycle of itching and scratching, and its secondary lesions include excoriations and lichenification.

Vascular dermatoses
Vascular dermatoses occur in many forms, each of which produces some type of lesion. The vascular dermatoses you may encounter include urticaria, erythema multiforme, stasis dermatitis, purpuric dermatoses, and telangiectases.

Urticaria
Commonly known as hives, urticaria occurs as part of a vascular reaction pattern. It's typically acute, although you may also see instances of chronic urticaria. Frequently caused by allergies, both chronic and acute urticaria can also result from cancer, hyperthyroidism, and juvenile rheumatoid arthritis.

The lesions associated with urticaria range from small red papules to larger circular patterns with red borders. In severe cases of hives, you may see vesicles and bullae. The lesions usually subside, although treatment may be necessary.

Erythema multiforme

This form of vascular dermatosis is characterized by red macules, papules, or bullae on the extremities, face, or lips. It primarily affects children and young adults.

The accompanying skin lesions may be associated with other diseases or syndromes, such as Stevens-Johnson syndrome. Many drugs also cause erythema multiforme, including sulfonamides, penicillins, phenytoin (Dilantin), and phenylbutazone (Azolid).

Stasis dermatitis

Often associated with varicose veins, stasis dermatitis results from impaired venous circulation in the legs. It appears initially as a red, scaly, pruritic area and then develops vesicles and becomes crusted. Hyperpigmentation, stasis ulcers, and infectious eczematous dermatitis are forms of secondary lesions that often accompany stasis dermatitis.

Purpuric dermatoses

These dermatoses include purpura, petechiae, ecchymoses, and hematomas—all of which are caused by red blood cells in the skin or mucous membranes and appear as red macules and papules. When you apply pressure, these lesions won't blanch.

Purpura and petechiae may be palpable or nonpalpable. The palpable variety is caused by allergic vasculitis, polyarteritis nodosa, and various types of emboli. Embolic lesions (purpura) can be found in acute meningococcemia and Rocky Mountain spotted fever. Nonpalpable purpura result from trauma, Cushing's syndrome, disseminated intravascular clotting, and reactions to warfarin (Coumadin).

Telangiectases

Permanently dilated small blood vessels, telangiectases often form a weblike pattern. You may see them in healthy older patients, but they also result from scleroderma, lupus erythematosus, and cirrhosis.

Papulosquamous dermatoses

The papulosquamous dermatoses you may detect during your assessment include psoriasis, pityriasis rosea, and seborrheic dermatitis.

Psoriasis

When you notice whitish scaly patches on the patient's elbows, knees, and scalp, they may result from psoriasis. The lesions of this chronic disorder vary in shape and size. Psoriasis may result from an upper respiratory tract infection caused by beta-hemolytic streptococci. About half of the people with psoriasis also have nail pitting or thickening, and many of these people have joint disease.

Pityriasis rosea

Pityriasis rosea consists of oval, macular, erythematous lesions that occur on the trunk and arms. A herald patch, which looks like ringworm, usually appears first. Distribution of the lesions occurs mainly on the chest and trunk. Sometimes, the lesions form a "Christmas tree branches" pattern, in which oval lesions are distributed along skin lines, resembling the branches of a fir tree.

Seborrheic dermatitis

A common chronic disorder called dandruff, or cradle cap in infants, seborrheic dermatitis most often occurs on the scalp. But you'll sometimes notice the redness and scaling of dandruff on the patient's face, axillae, and groin. For most people, dandruff doesn't result from an underlying disorder; however, it often accompanies Parkinson's disease and acquired immunodeficiency syndrome (AIDS).

Acne

Characterized by comedones (or blackheads), pustules, and cysts, acne vulgaris leaves varying degrees of scarring. You'll see acne most often in adolescents and young adults. Usually self-limiting, acne occurs primarily on the face and neck, although you'll also see it on the back, chest, and arms. Acne vulgaris results from overactive sebaceous glands.

Bacterial infections

These infections include impetigo, a primary bacterial infection; secondary bacterial infections; and scarlet fever, chancroid, and syphilis, which are systemic bacterial infections.

Impetigo

A superficial bacterial infection, impetigo most often affects children. It results from group A beta-hemolytic streptococci or *Staphylococcus aureus*.

The primary lesions range from small vesicles to large bullae that, when ruptured, ooze a honey-colored serous fluid that can become purulent. Typically, crusts form as secondary lesions. You'll detect lesions most often on the face, especially near the nose and mouth, as well as in creases on the hands and elsewhere.

Secondary bacterial infections

These infections can develop in any type of skin lesion, but growing evidence suggests that they are more likely to occur in long-term conditions than in short-term ones. Streptococci and staphylococci are most often the causative organisms in secondary bacterial infection.

Scarlet fever

A result of infection with group A beta-hemolytic streptococci, scarlet fever (or scarlatina) forms a rash of red macules over the entire body, with the exception of the area around the mouth. The rash lasts about 7 days, usually accompanied by a sore throat and high fever. If left untreated, scarlet fever can progress to rheumatic fever and glomerulonephritis.

Chancroid

A systemic bacterial infection caused by *Haemophilus ducreyi*, the venereal disease chancroid causes deep or superficial erosion primarily in the genital area. The primary lesions form a small area of redness and edema.

Chancroid can spread by autoinoculation to other areas of the body. In chronic cases, deep ulcers with purulent discharge, bleeding, fistulas, and gangrene may develop.

Syphilis

The spirochete *Treponema pallidum* causes syphilis. During primary syphilis, you may see a single small erosion or several ulcerated lesions in the genital area. With a female patient, however, you may not see any skin changes.

The macular, papular, pustular, or eroded lesions of secondary syphilis may occur before the primary chancre heals or after several weeks of latency, and may be generalized or localized. The characteristic moist, warty lesions in the genital area are known as condyloma lata.

Patients with tertiary syphilis, a late stage of the disease, will show skin changes 5 to 20 years after being infected. You may see nodular and gummatous ulcerations that scar on healing. Systemic changes related to the syphilis develop in many of the body systems.

Viral infections

Many of the common skin disorders you'll observe result from a particular virus. Most of these are contagious, and you should make sure your patient is aware of this.

Viral infections include herpes simplex, herpes zoster, chicken pox, warts, and measles.

Herpes simplex

This recurrent virus is characterized by an acute, moderately painful eruption of a single group of vesicles (fever blister). It occurs in two strains: Type 1 and Type 2. If the patient has a fever blister near his mouth, he has Type 1. If the lesions appear in the genital area, he has the sexually transmitted Type 2 virus.

Herpes zoster

Probably caused by the same virus that causes chicken pox, herpes zoster (or shingles) appears as multiple vesicles along a cutaneous nerve—mostly on the face, neck, and thorax. A patient with shingles will probably complain of pain.

Though fairly common, herpes zoster can become serious when it affects the ocular area or the eye itself.

Chicken pox

In chicken pox (varicella), a common childhood disease, vesicles develop over the body and cause itching. As the disease progresses, the vesicles change to pustules and develop a crust that falls off.

Warts

Papilloma viruses cause the common growths known as warts (verrucae). The clinical diagnosis of warts varies, depending on the appearance and location of the growth.

Measles

Rubeola, or measles, a common childhood disease, causes skin changes characterized by a faint, red, patchy rash.

Fungal infections

Known as tinea, superficial fungal infections of the skin can affect various sites on a patient's body. Athlete's foot, or tinea pedis, is probably the fungal infection you'll see most often. It causes blistering lesions, fissures, and cracks on the soles and sides of the feet and between the toes.

A deep fungal infection known as candidiasis causes lesions in the mouth and vagina and on the hands and nails. Candidiasis of the mouth, commonly known as thrush, appears as whitish flakes on reddened mucous membranes. You may also note associated fissures in the corners of the mouth. Candidal vulvovaginitis, often affecting pregnant or diabetic women, causes skin lesions with definite borders and a milklike vaginal discharge.

Scabies

Caused by a mite that burrows under the skin, scabies often occurs in school-age children. Scabies causes extreme itching and is characterized by vesicles or excoriation over the burrows.

Pemphigus vulgaris

A blistering skin disease, pemphigus vulgaris can be fatal if left untreated. Typically, it affects elderly people. At onset, small vesicles or bullae appear on otherwise normal skin. When the bullae rupture, large eroded areas result. You may also detect an odor from a secondary bacterial infection.

Pigmentation disorders

Chloasma, also known as melasma, is a hyperpigmentation of the skin on the sides of the face and neck and on the forehead. This common condition can result from excessive sun exposure, the estrogen in oral contraceptives, and pregnancy.

Patients with vitiligo, a slowly progressive disease of hypopigmentation, develop irregular areas of pigmented skin, commonly on the face, hands, and feet. Vitiligo probably results from the destruction of normal melanocytes caused by the immune response to malignant melanocytes.

Burns

Burns are usually classified by their cause and by the extent of damage. All burns are categorized as first-, second-, or third-degree. In a patient with a first-degree burn, only the epidermis is injured, leaving a red, slightly painful area. Second-degree burns involve the epidermis and part of the dermis, and the patient develops blisters. Third-degree burns cause complete destruction of the epidermis and dermis and even some underlying tissue.

A type of thermal burn, sunburn can range from mild to severe. Sunburned skin initially appears red and then vesicles develop. Later, scaling or peeling and, occasionally, an infection may occur.

Radiodermatitis, a skin disorder caused by ionizing radiation therapy, causes skin changes similar to those of thermal burns. In the first stage of radiodermatitis, patients develop erythema, hyperpigmentation, and hair loss. In the second stage, vesicles and erosions form. Hair loss, secondary infection, and delayed healing also distinguish the second stage. In the severest stage, the skin develops ulcerations, infection, and even more delayed healing.

Skin tumors

As you know, many types of skin tumors exist, some dangerous and some harmless. To help distinguish among the most common types, review the following discussion of pedunculated fibromas, actinic keratosis, basal cell carcinoma, squamous cell carcinoma, hemangiomas, melanocytic nevi, malignant melanomas, and Kaposi's sarcoma.

Pedunculated fibromas

These soft tumors, often called skin tags, develop the same color as the patient's skin. Occurring most often on the neck and axillae of middle-aged or elderly patients, these benign skin tags grow slowly and can be removed for cosmetic reasons.

Actinic keratosis
Considered a precancerous tumor, actinic keratosis appears as a faint red scaly area that gradually enlarges. You'll notice it most often on the sun-exposed skin surfaces of elderly patients. Occasionally, these lesions develop into squamous cell carcinomas.

Basal cell carcinoma
The most common skin cancer, basal cell carcinoma grows slowly and doesn't metastasize. Caused by sun exposure, it occurs most often on the head and neck. The type you'll see most frequently is the noduloulcerative basal cell carcinoma — a small, waxy-looking nodule that ulcerates, forming a central depression. Whenever you suspect basal cell carcinoma, a histologic study should be performed.

Squamous cell carcinoma
This malignant skin cancer, caused by direct exposure to the sun, can metastasize. Squamous cell carcinomas vary from fast-growing lesions to slowly developing raised growths. The degree of metastasis and malignancy also varies. The tumors have a raised border and a central ulcer, and they may develop on any area of the skin, especially the face and neck.

Hemangiomas
These benign vascular abnormalities of the skin come in several varieties, which are distinguished by their appearance and location. Two of the most common types are port-wine hemangiomas and spider hemangiomas. Port-wine hemangiomas usually are present at birth and often appear on the face and upper body as a flat purple mark. Spider hemangiomas are small, red lesions arranged in a weblike configuration.

Melanocytic nevi
These skin tumors contain nevus cells. They can develop as pigmented or unpigmented, flat or elevated, and with a wide or small base.

Nonhairy nevi that are flat or slightly elevated and brown or black are usually junctional nevi. A malignant melanoma can originate in junctional nevi.

Malignant melanomas
Malignant melanomas usually appear as black or purple nodules, although some are pink or red. They can develop anywhere on the body. Some melanomas may result from repeated sun exposure. But more often they develop in patients who've had a single, severe, blistering sunburn as a child.

Because a large percentage of melanomas develop from preexisting nevi, always document any changes in the size, shape, and pigmentation of nevi as well as any associated erythema. Early diagnosis and prompt treatment of these lesions can protect a patient from fatal skin cancer.

When a malignant melanoma is diagnosed, it will be classified according to the depth of growth, using Clark's system. This scale ranges from level I (indicating that the melanoma affects only the epidermis) to level V (indicating that the melanoma has penetrated the subcutaneous fat).

Kaposi's sarcoma
This multiple hemorrhagic sarcoma usually begins on the feet and ankles. Initially, you'll notice multiple bluish red or brown nodules and plaques. Visceral lesions may also develop.

A significantly different pattern of Kaposi's sarcoma affects patients with human immunodeficiency virus. In this pattern, the lesions are small, oval, pink papules that occur on any area of the body.

Hair disorders

Often stemming from other problems, hair disorders can cause your patient emotional distress. Among the most common hair abnormalities are hirsutism, alopecia, folliculitis, carbuncles, and pediculosis.

Hirsutism

Excessive hairiness in women, hypertrichosis can develop on the face and legs. Facial hirsutism may affect self-image.

You may see localized hirsutism associated with pigmented nevi. Generalized hirsutism results from drug therapy or endocrine problems, such as Cushing's syndrome and acromegaly.

Alopecia

Alopecia, or hair loss, occurs in both men and women, although you'll see it more often and more extensively in men.

Diffuse hair loss, while often a normal part of aging, may result from pyrogenic infections, chemicals and drugs, endocrinopathy, or other disorders. Tinea capitis, trauma, and third-degree burns can also cause patchy hair loss.

Folliculitis

Usually caused by staphylococci, this infection of the hair follicles can extend to the hair bulb. Scarring and patchy areas of alopecia may develop from deep forms of folliculitis.

Carbuncles

Extensive infection of several adjoining hair follicles can produce carbuncles. The lesions drain from multiple openings on the skin.

Pediculosis

Pediculosis, or lice infestation, usually occurs on the scalp but can occur anywhere a patient has body hair. Although you may not see the bites themselves, you'll probably see the white mites in the patient's hair. This disorder can result from crowded living conditions or lack of cleanliness. It affects people of all ages.

Nail disorders

Many nail abnormalities you encounter will be harmless, but some will point to serious underlying problems. To help distinguish the harmless from the serious, review the discussion below on contact reactions, onycholysis, Beau's lines, finger clubbing, koilonychia, racket nail, Terry's nails, and anonychia.

Contact reactions

Contact reactions may result from using nail polishes. These reactions commonly produce thickening and color changes in the nails.

Onycholysis

To detect onycholysis, look for a separation of the nail from its nail bed. This abnormality can result from trauma or numerous chronic disorders, including psoriasis and heart disease.

Beau's lines

Transverse depressions in the nails are known as Beau's lines. This abnormality may indicate a severe acute illness, malnutrition, or anemia.

Finger clubbing

In early clubbing, the nail bases feel spongy. In late clubbing, you'll see swelling. Associated with a decrease in oxygen supply, clubbing is common in chronic obstructive pulmonary disease, cardiovascular diseases, and cirrhosis.

Koilonychia

Koilonychia refers to spoon-shaped, white, opaque nails. It's associated with hypochromic anemias, chronic infections, malnutrition, pellagra, and Raynaud's disease.

Racket nail

A flattened and enlarged nail, racket nail usually affects the thumb. This abnormality can indicate secondary syphilis.

Terry's nails

In Terry's nails, bands of white and pink alternate. Hypoalbuminemia may produce this sign.

Anonychia

Usually congenital, anonychia refers to the complete absence of a nail.

(Text continues on page 91.)

Recognizing common disorders

Contact dermatitis

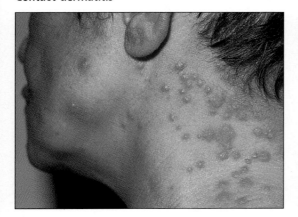

Purpura

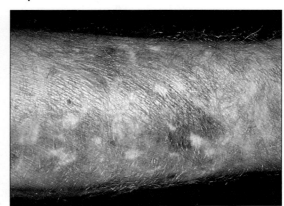

Eczema

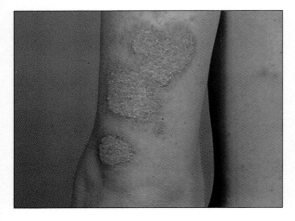

Telangiectasis

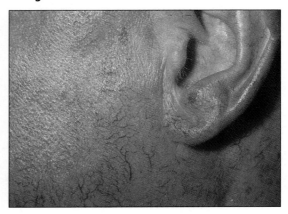

Urticaria

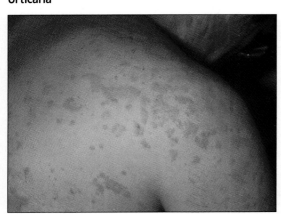

Psoriasis

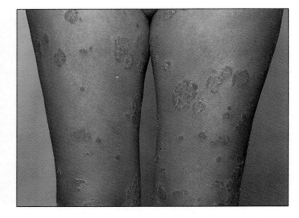

Recognizing common disorders *(continued)*

Acne

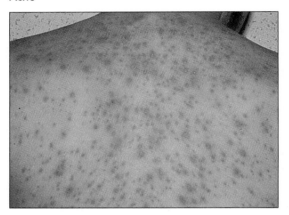

Verruca

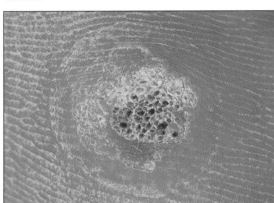

Cystic acne

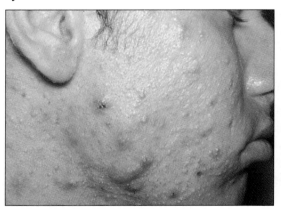

Candidiasis (monilial)

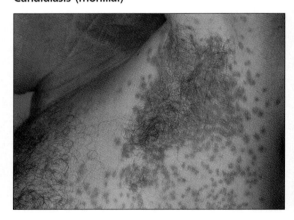

Impetigo

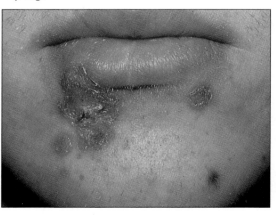

Herpes simplex

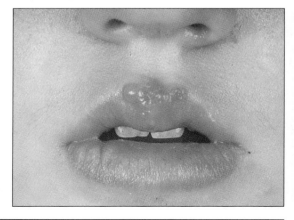

Recognizing common disorders *(continued)*

Herpes zoster

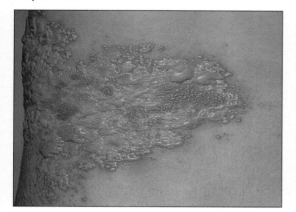

Vitiligo

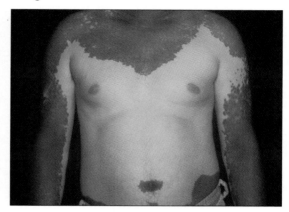

Scabies

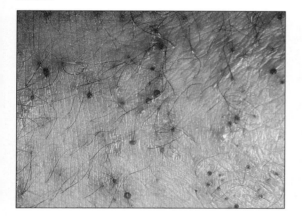

Lupus erythematosus (discoid or systemic)

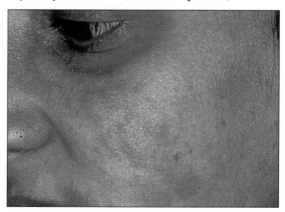

Tinea corporis

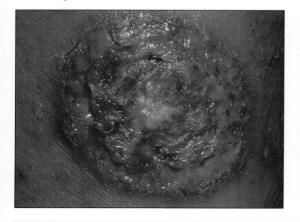

Seborrheic keratosis

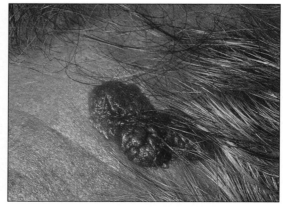

Recognizing common disorders *(continued)*

Cherry angioma

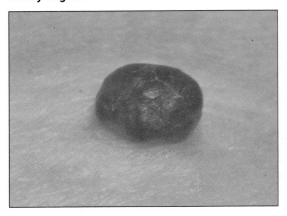

Squamous cell carcinoma

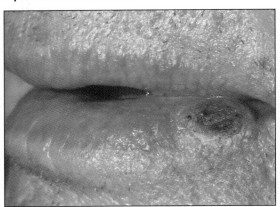

Spider nevus

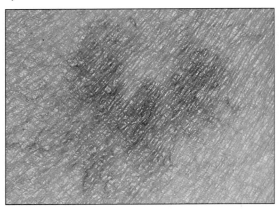

Malignant melanoma

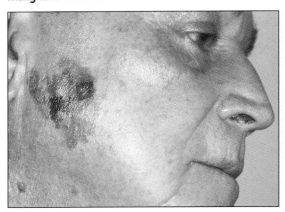

Basal cell carcinoma

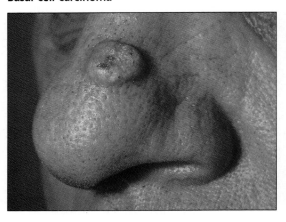

Kaposi's sarcoma

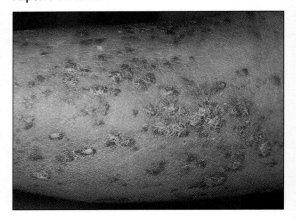

Pertinent diagnostic tests

Dermatologic testing primarily consists of identifying an allergen or a pathogen. The specimens may be obtained by drawing a blood sample, by scraping a lesion, or by swabbing a lesion. Also, a cerebrospinal fluid (CSF) specimen may be drawn or a biopsy specimen may be taken. Before collecting a specimen directly from an affected area, be sure to remove any medications, crusts, or exudates.

Among the most common dermatologic tests are the patch test, potassium hydroxide (KOH) preparation, culture, and histologic examinations, including dark-field microscopic examination and Gram stain.

Patch test

You may use a patch test to determine the cause of a patient's contact dermatitis. For this test, place the suspected allergen on the patient's skin—usually on his back—and cover it with an occlusive dressing. Leave the patch on for 48 hours, and then examine the skin for evidence of a delayed hypersensitivity reaction.

KOH preparation

When you suspect a fungal infection, you may use a KOH preparation. To collect a specimen for this test, scrape the edge of a scaling skin lesion and place the specimen on a glass slide. It will then be treated with KOH; if the fungus is present, it will be visible.

Culture

In some cases, a culture may be used to identify a pathogen. To obtain a specimen, scrape the edge of the lesion. Then place the specimen in a medium for laboratory examination.

Histologic examinations

When a lesion is associated with a drug reaction or vasculitis, either a punch biopsy or an excisional biopsy may be used to obtain a specimen. Histologic study and a culture can then be used to test the specimen for cell changes consistent with a specific disease.

A Gram stain is used to identify bacteria in the skin. To obtain the specimen, you may swab an oozing lesion, or a biopsy may be performed.

A dark-field microscope may be used to detect syphilis because the spirochete may not be visible under a regular microscope. To collect the specimen, you may swab the chancre, or draw a blood sample. Or a CSF or biopsy specimen may be obtained.

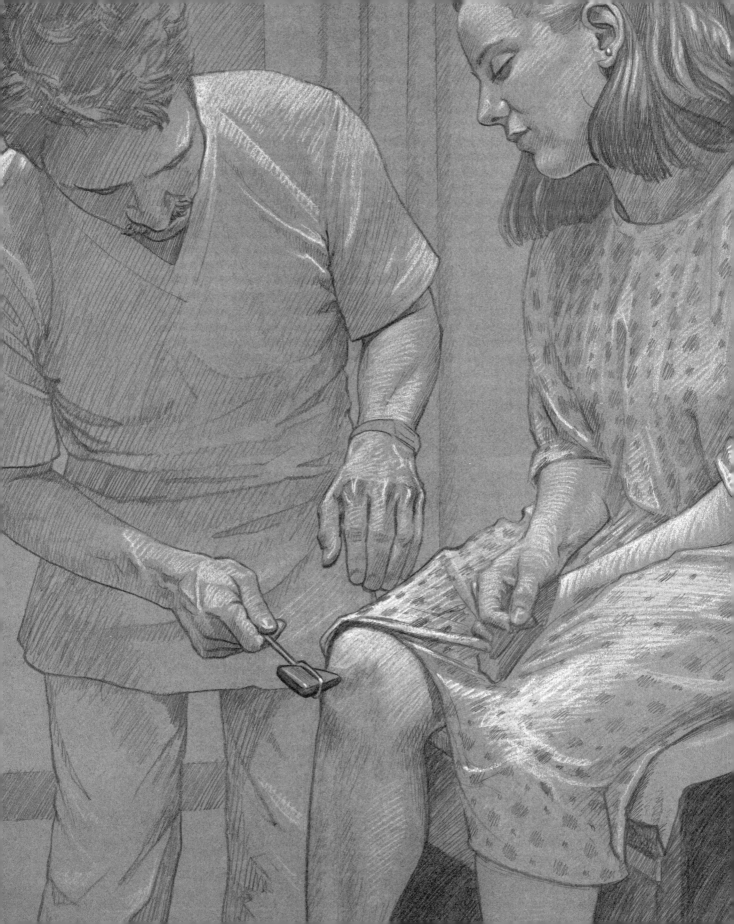

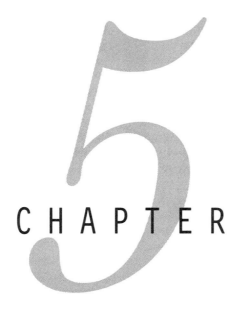

CHAPTER 5

Neurologic system

Signs and symptoms of a neurologic disorder can appear in patients of all ages. For instance, an elderly patient may show signs of neurologic dysfunction from a cerebrovascular accident (CVA), while a young adult may have neurologic problems from a traumatic brain injury. And patients of all ages can develop progressive deterioration of the nervous system.

You can identify such neurologic problems while performing a complete nursing assessment or a neurologic screening to investigate a complaint. With this screening, you can evaluate overall neurologic function and detect abnormalities, as you assess mental status, the cranial nerves, sensory system, motor system, and reflexes.

Before explaining how to perform this five-part examination, this chapter reviews neurologic anatomy and physiology and covers the health history questions you'll ask your patient. After the physical examination, you'll find a section that will help you analyze your abnor-

ANATOMY

Central nervous system

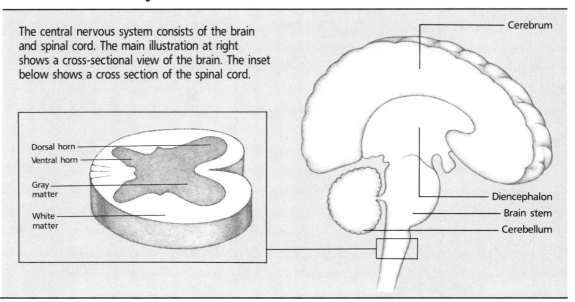

The central nervous system consists of the brain and spinal cord. The main illustration at right shows a cross-sectional view of the brain. The inset below shows a cross section of the spinal cord.

Dorsal horn
Ventral horn
Gray matter
White matter

Cerebrum
Diencephalon
Brain stem
Cerebellum

mal findings. Then, in the last section of the chapter, you'll find a brief overview of pertinent diagnostic tests.

Anatomy and physiology

The nervous system consists of the central nervous system, the peripheral nervous system, and the autonomic nervous system. Through complex and coordinated interactions, these three components integrate all physical, intellectual, and emotional activities.

Central nervous system

The central nervous system includes the brain and the spinal cord. These two structures are responsible for collecting and interpreting voluntary and involuntary sensory and motor signals. (See *Central nervous system.*)

Brain

As the highest functioning center of the nervous system, the brain collects, integrates, and interprets all stimuli. It also initiates and monitors voluntary and involuntary motor activity. The brain has three distinct regions: the cerebrum, brain stem, and cerebellum.

Encased by the skull and enclosed by three membrane layers called the meninges, the cerebrum is divided into right and left hemispheres. (See *Cranial meninges.*) Each hemisphere has four lobes: parietal, occipital, temporal, and frontal. The right cerebral hemisphere controls activities on the left side of the body, and the left hemisphere controls activities on the right side of the body.

The diencephalon, a division of the cerebrum, contains the thalamus, epithalamus, subthalamus, and hypothalamus. The thalamus and hypothalamus are particularly important: The thalamus serves as a relay station for sensory impulses, and the hypothalamus has many regulatory functions, including control of temperature and pituitary hormone production and regulation of water balance.

ANATOMY

Cranial meninges

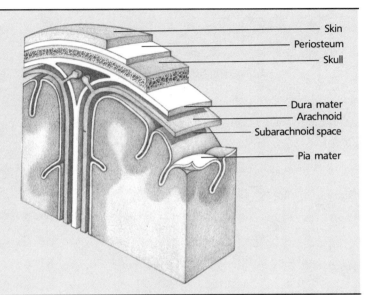

The three cranial meninges surround the brain and are continuous with the spinal meninges. The *dura mater,* the outermost layer, is adjacent to the skull. The epidural space lies above the dura and the subdural space lies below it. The *arachnoid* is the middle layer. The cerebrospinal fluid circulates below the arachnoid in the subarachnoid space. The *pia mater,* the innermost layer, lies adjacent to the brain tissue and extends into the multiple fissures (gyri) and grooves (sulci) of the brain.

Skin
Periosteum
Skull

Dura mater
Arachnoid
Subarachnoid space

Pia mater

Made up of the midbrain, pons, and medulla, the brain stem lies inferior to the diencephalon. The brain stem contains the nuclei of cranial nerves III through XII and is a major sensory and motor pathway for impulses running to and from the cerebrum. It also regulates basic body functions such as respiration, auditory and visual reflexes, swallowing, and coughing.

The cerebellum, the most posterior portion of the brain, contains the major motor and sensory pathways. It facilitates smooth, coordinated muscle movements and helps to maintain equilibrium.

Spinal cord

The spinal cord is the primary pathway for messages traveling between the peripheral areas of the body and the brain. It also mediates the reflex arc — the natural pathway used in reflex action. An elongated mass of neural tissue, the spinal cord extends from the upper border of the first cervical vertebra to the lower border of the first lumbar vertebra. It's enclosed by the three meninges and pro-

tected by the bony vertebrae of the spine.

A cross section of the spinal cord reveals a central H-shaped mass of gray matter, surrounded by a circle of white matter. The dorsal section of gray matter contains cell bodies of sensory (afferent) nerves, and the ventral section contains cell bodies of motor (efferent) neurons. The dorsal white matter contains the ascending sensory tracts that carry impulses up the spinal cord to the higher sensory centers. The ventral white matter contains the descending motor tracts that transmit motor impulses down from the higher motor centers to the spinal cord.

Peripheral nervous system

The peripheral nervous system includes the peripheral and cranial nerves. Peripheral sensory nerves transmit stimuli to the dorsal horn of the spinal cord from sensory receptors located in the skin, muscles, sensory organs, and viscera. The upper motor neurons of the brain and the lower motor neurons of the cell bodies in the ventral horn of the spinal cord carry impulses that affect movement.

The 12 pairs of cranial nerves are the primary motor and sensory pathways between the brain and the head and neck. (See *Cranial nerves.*)

Autonomic nervous system

Consisting entirely of motor neurons, the autonomic nervous system regulates the activities of the visceral organs by its effect on smooth muscle, cardiac muscle, and the glands. Its two divisions — sympathetic and parasympathetic — maintain internal homeostasis.

The sympathetic (or adrenergic) nervous system controls the body's fight-or-flight reaction to stress. The parasympathetic (or cholinergic) nervous system maintains baseline body functions.

Health history

Whether you're performing a complete nursing assessment or investigating a neurologic chief complaint, you'll need to begin with a thorough neurologic health history. Make sure the health history includes questions about your patient's chief complaint, medical history, family history, psychosocial history, and activities of daily living.

Chief complaint

The most common chief complaints of the neurologic system include headache, dizziness, faintness, confusion, impaired mental status, disturbances in balance or gait, and changes in consciousness. To investigate these or any other chief complaints, ask your patient relevant questions about such particulars as onset, duration, and severity. Also ask what precipitates the symptom, what makes it worse, and what makes it better. For more information on exploring chief complaints, see Chapter 3.

Medical history

Begin by asking about neurologic problems. For example, ask whether the patient has had transient ischemic attacks or CVAs, either of which can place him at risk for future CVAs. Ask, too, if he's ever had seizures. If so, ask about their characteristics. Has the patient ever had a head injury? If he has, did he lose consciousness? Has he ever had a malignant tumor? Such tumors tend to recur, can provoke seizures, and may cause neurologic deficits. Has the patient been diagnosed with Parkinson's disease, multiple sclerosis, or dementia?

Then, ask the patient about chronic conditions, such as hypertension, which is a major risk factor of cerebrovascular disease. Does he have a significant cardiac or pulmonary disease that would affect cerebral perfusion? What about chronic liver disease or renal failure? Either can produce apathy, fatigue, impaired mental status, stupor, and coma. Ask, too, about a history of diabetes mellitus, which can cause peripheral and autonomic neuropathies and impaired mentation, particularly in an elderly patient. Does the patient have hypothyroidism, a potential cause of ataxia, dementia, and psychiatric symptoms? Ask about anemia, which can produce apathy and confusion. Vitamin B_{12} deficiency (pernicious anemia) can also cause peripheral neuropathy, confusion, incoordination, and dementia.

Next, ask the patient about infectious diseases, such as meningitis and encephalitis — both causes of seizures and other neurologic sequelae. Also ask about acquired immunodeficiency syndrome (AIDS), which is accompanied by several neurologic disorders, including dementia and peripheral neuropathy. AIDS patients are also at great risk for contracting neurologic opportunistic infections from *Cryptococcus* and cytomegalovirus.

Family history

Ask the patient or a family member about hereditary conditions that can adversely affect neurologic function. These conditions include epilepsy, diabetes mellitus, migraine headaches,

Cranial nerves

This illustration shows the origin of each cranial nerve (CN) and describes its type (motor, sensory, or both) and function.

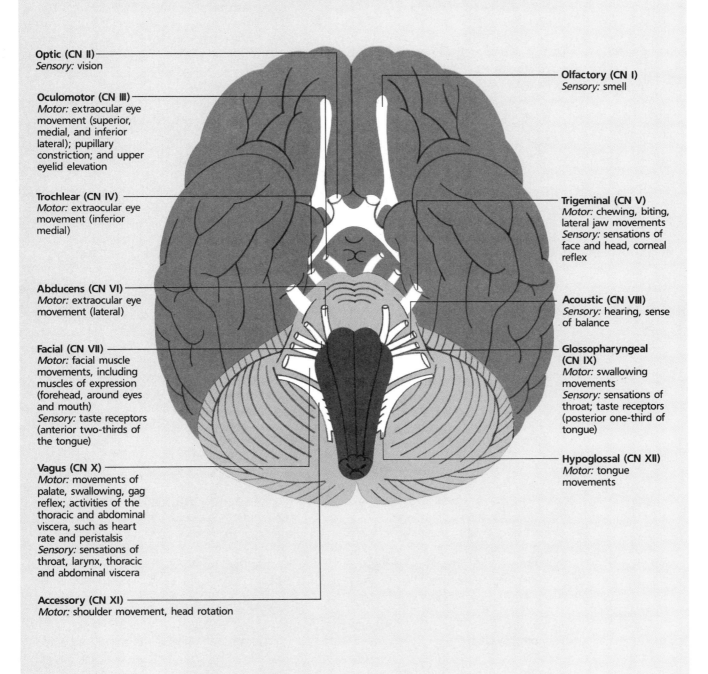

Optic (CN II)
Sensory: vision

Oculomotor (CN III)
Motor: extraocular eye movement (superior, medial, and inferior lateral); pupillary constriction; and upper eyelid elevation

Trochlear (CN IV)
Motor: extraocular eye movement (inferior medial)

Abducens (CN VI)
Motor: extraocular eye movement (lateral)

Facial (CN VII)
Motor: facial muscle movements, including muscles of expression (forehead, around eyes and mouth)
Sensory: taste receptors (anterior two-thirds of the tongue)

Vagus (CN X)
Motor: movements of palate, swallowing, gag reflex; activities of the thoracic and abdominal viscera, such as heart rate and peristalsis
Sensory: sensations of throat, larynx, thoracic and abdominal viscera

Accessory (CN XI)
Motor: shoulder movement, head rotation

Olfactory (CN I)
Sensory: smell

Trigeminal (CN V)
Motor: chewing, biting, lateral jaw movements
Sensory: sensations of face and head, corneal reflex

Acoustic (CN VIII)
Sensory: hearing, sense of balance

Glossopharyngeal (CN IX)
Motor: swallowing movements
Sensory: sensations of throat; taste receptors (posterior one-third of tongue)

Hypoglossal (CN XII)
Motor: tongue movements

dementia, psychiatric disorders (such as schizophrenia and mood disorders), hyperlipidemia, and hypertension.

Psychosocial history

Ask if the patient's current problem has affected his family relationships or required that family members take on responsibilities that he once handled. Does the patient receive adequate support from family members?

Activities of daily living

Ask the patient if his current neurologic problem has had an impact on his ability to perform his daily activities. Can he bathe, dress, and feed himself? Has he had to curtail any of his usual activities?

You also need to evaluate the patient's habits, including his use of illicit drugs, cigarettes, and alcohol. When inquiring about alcohol intake, determine the number of drinks he has daily, the type of drinks, and the number of ounces per drink. Also ask him about his lifetime drinking pattern. Chronic alcohol use can result in cerebellar degeneration, peripheral neuropathy, seizures, and dementia.

Physical examination

During the neurologic screening, you'll assess five areas: mental status, cranial nerves, sensory system, motor system, and reflexes. By using this sequence, you move from the most complex to the least complex functions. The mental status examination tests the cerebral cortex, the area of greatest neurologic complexity, whereas the examination of the patient's reflexes tests the simple reflex arc.

Mental status

Assess the patient's mental status as you listen to his answers during the health history. Con-

sider such factors as recent and remote memory, attention span, and coherence of thoughts. If confusion or deteriorating mental status is the patient's chief complaint, or if he has obvious neurologic deficits, you'll need a more detailed assessment of his mental status.

Depending on the circumstances, you may perform a complete mental status examination, evaluating level of consciousness (LOC), appearance and behavior, speech, cognitive function, emotional status, and constructional ability. Or you may perform a shortened version of the complete examination.

Level of consciousness
A patient's LOC is the earliest and most sensitive indicator of a change in his neurologic status. To describe the patient's LOC, you may use the following terms:
• *Alert.* The patient is awake and responds fully and appropriately to all stimuli.
• *Lethargic.* The patient is drowsy and indifferent, and his verbal responses to stimuli are delayed. He reacts to stimuli but falls asleep when stimulation stops.
• *Obtunded.* The patient is even more lethargic and sleeps unless aroused.
• *Stuporous.* The patient can be aroused from sleep only by vigorous stimulation.
• *Comatose.* The patient has lost consciousness and no longer interacts with the environment.

As an alternative to using these terms, you may use the Glasgow Coma Scale to assess and document your patient's LOC. (See *Glasgow Coma Scale*, opposite, and *Detecting increased ICP*, page 100.)

Appearance and behavior
Observe the patient's clothing, grooming, and personal hygiene. Are his clothes appropriate for the setting and the weather? A patient with organic mental syndrome may wear multiple layers of clothing. A manic patient may dress flamboyantly. Someone suffering from dementia or schizophrenia may have poor hygiene and grooming.

Observe the patient's posture and motor behavior. Look for a stiff posture and lack of movement—possible signs of Parkinson's disease or advanced dementia. Also, note any restlessness, pacing, or agitation.

Observe the patient's facial expression. Is it consistent with his mood and conversation?

Speech
Listen to the patient's speech, noting how well he expresses himself and how well he comprehends your speech. You can also incorporate writing and reading tests into your speech evaluation.

Note the pace, volume, clarity, and spontaneity of the patient's speech. To test for dysarthria or garbled speech, ask him to repeat the phrase "No if's, and's, or but's." Assess his comprehension by determining if he can follow instructions and cooperate with your examination.

Note whether the patient has aphasia, a speech impairment that usually results from an injury to the cerebral cortex. A CVA or brain tumor may cause such an injury. Types of aphasia include the following:
• *Expressive (Broca's) aphasia.* In a patient with this disorder, you'll note impaired fluency and word-finding ability. The patient may use single words without articles or prepositions. His ability to repeat words and to write may also be impaired. This type of aphasia results from damage to the anterior cerebral cortex.
• *Receptive (Wernicke's) aphasia.* A patient with this disorder can't understand written words or speech. He may use made-up words (neologisms). Receptive aphasia results from damage to the posterior cortex.
• *Global aphasia.* Damage to both the anterior and the posterior cortex results in the loss of expressive and receptive speech.

Writing and reading
Test writing ability by asking the patient to write a sentence. The sentence should have a subject and a verb and convey a complete thought. Keep in mind that a patient with a visual or musculoskeletal disability or without a formal education may not be able to complete this task.

Glasgow Coma Scale

The Glasgow Coma Scale provides an objective way to evaluate a patient's level of consciousness and to detect changes from the baseline. To use this scale, evaluate and score your patient's best eye-opening response, verbal response, and motor response. A total score of 15 indicates that he is alert; oriented to person, place, and time; and can follow simple commands. A comatose patient will score 7 points or less. A score of 3 indicates deep coma and a poor prognosis.

TEST	REACTION	SCORE
Eye-opening response	Open spontaneously	4
	Open to verbal command	3
	Open to pain	2
	No response	1
Verbal response	Oriented and converses	5
	Disoriented and converses	4
	Uses inappropriate words	3
	Makes incomprehensible sounds	2
	No response	1
Motor response	Obeys verbal command	6
	Localizes painful stimulus	5
	Flexion—withdrawal	4
	Flexion—abnormal (decorticate rigidity)	3
	Extension (decerebrate rigidity)	2
	No response	1

Test reading ability and comprehension by writing "Close your eyes." Then ask the patient to read the sentence and do what it says. Make sure that you print in large, clear letters, especially if you're testing a patient who's visually impaired.

Cognitive function
To test the patient's cognitive function, assess orientation, memory, attention span and calculation, thought content, abstract thought, judgment, and insight.

Detecting increased ICP

The earlier you recognize the signs of increased intracranial pressure (ICP), the quicker you can intervene, and the better the patient's chances of recovery. By the time late signs appear, intervention may be useless.

This chart shows you both early and late signs of increased ICP.

	EARLY SIGNS	LATE SIGNS
Level of consciousness	• Requires increased stimulation • Subtle orientation loss • Restlessness • Sudden quietness	• Unarousable
Pupils	• Pupil changes on side of lesion • One pupil constricts but then dilates (unilateral hippus) • Sluggish reaction of both pupils • Unequal pupils	• Pupils fixed and dilated ("blown" pupils)
Motor response	• Sudden weakness • Motor changes on side opposite the lesion • Positive pronator drift (with palms up, one hand pronates)	• Profound weakness
Vital signs	• Intermittent increases in blood pressure	• Increased systolic pressure, profound bradycardia, abnormal respirations (Cushing's response)

Orientation

Test orientation to time by asking the patient the time of day, day of the week, date (month and year), and season. Orientation to time is usually the first type of orientation to be lost when mental status becomes impaired.

When evaluating orientation to time, be sure to consider the patient's environment and physical condition. A patient who's been in the intensive care unit for a few days probably won't be oriented to time.

Test orientation to place by asking the patient to tell you where he is. Also ask for his home address, including the house number, street, city, and state.

To test orientation to person, ask the patient his name. Typically, this is the last type of orientation a patient loses.

Memory

Assess the patient's short-term and remote memory. To test short-term memory, ask him to tell you why he has been hospitalized. Make sure that you can verify his answers. Next, have the patient repeat a series of five nonconsecutive numbers. Say each number slowly and then ask him to repeat the sequence. The patient with an intact short-term memory and a good attention span can repeat a series of five to seven numbers.

You can also evaluate short-term memory by naming three unrelated objects—for example, table, candle, and apple—and asking the patient to repeat the series. Then tell him you'll ask him to repeat the series in 10 minutes. After covering other aspects of the examination for about 10 minutes, ask him to repeat the series.

Test the patient's remote memory by asking his date and place of birth or the names of his parents. Again, be sure to verify the accuracy of the information.

Attention span and calculation

As you assess the patient, note whether he is attentive and obeys your commands. To formally test attention span and calculation, ask the patient to count backward from 100 by 7's until he reaches 0. He should be able to complete this task in 1½ minutes with fewer than four errors. Keep in mind that anxiety and mathematical ability may affect the patient's performance.

As an alternative, you can ask him to count backward from 100 by 3's. If he can't do this, ask him to subtract one number at a time from 100 or to count forward from 1 to 100.

If the patient has difficulty with numerical computation, ask him to spell the word "world" backward. Note his performance on any of these tests, and evaluate his ability to maintain his attention throughout.

Thought content

Assessing thought content includes evaluating the clarity and cohesiveness of ideas. Note whether the patient's conversation has smooth, logical transitions between ideas. Does he have hallucinations (sensory perceptions that lack appropriate external stimuli) or delusions (beliefs not supported by reality)? Disordered thought patterns may indicate delirium or psychosis.

Abstract thought
Test the patient's ability to think abstractly by asking him to interpret a common proverb, such as "A stitch in time saves nine" or "A rolling stone gathers no moss." A patient with dementia, schizophrenia, or mental retardation may interpret the proverb literally, failing to comprehend its figurative meaning. Keep in mind that if English isn't the patient's first language, he may have difficulty interpreting a proverb.

Judgment
Test the patient's judgment by describing a hypothetical situation and asking him to tell you how he would respond. For example, ask what he'd do if he were in a public building and he heard the fire alarm go off. Evaluate the appropriateness of his answer.

Insight
Evaluate insight by assessing the patient's ability to understand the implications of his situation and to recognize any abnormalities in his perceptions, judgments, and thought content. When you ask why he has sought health care, a patient who lacks insight may tell you that nothing is wrong with him. A cognitively impaired elderly patient may lack insight into the risks of living alone and make decisions that put him at further risk.

Emotional status
You can evaluate the patient's emotional state throughout the interview by noting his mood, emotional lability or stability, and the appropriateness of his emotional responses. Also assess mood by asking him how he feels about himself and how he looks at the future.

If the patient is depressed, ask when his depression began. What caused it? Has he experienced insomnia, anorexia, or fatigue? Also, ask about suicidal ideation. Keep in mind that an elderly person may have atypical symptoms of depression, such as decreased function or increased agitation, rather than the usual sad affect.

Constructional ability
Observe the patient's motor skills as he performs a simple task and determine his ability to understand the purpose of various objects. Apraxia—an inability to perform purposeful movements, especially to make proper use of objects—often results from parietal lobe damage. You may note the following types:
• *Ideomotor apraxia.* The patient has lost his understanding of the effect of a motor activity. He may be able to perform automatic, simple motor activities, such as waving or crossing his arms, but is unaware that he is doing so. He's also unable to imitate these actions on command.
• *Ideational apraxia.* The patient is aware of movements that need to be accomplished, but he can't perform them. For example, he may be unable to fold a piece of paper according to your directions.
• *Constructional apraxia.* The patient is unable to copy a design, such as the face of a clock. He's also not able to arrange two- or three-dimensional shapes to match a common pattern.
• *Dressing apraxia.* The patient is unable to understand the purpose of various articles of clothing or the sequence of actions required to get dressed.

Agnosia, an inability to identify common objects, may indicate a lesion in the sensory cortex. You may note the following types of agnosia:
• *Visual agnosia.* The patient is unable to recognize common objects by sight. For example, he won't be able to identify a key just by looking at it. However, he will be able to name it after he touches it.
• *Auditory agnosia.* The patient is unable to identify common sounds, such as the telephone ringing or the sound made by paper crumpling.
• *Body-image agnosia.* The patient is unable to identify his body parts by sight or touch. He may deny the existence of half of his body, or he may be unable to localize a stimulus. When you apply stimuli simultaneously to contralat-

eral body parts, the patient may not feel the stimulus on the side opposite the cerebral lesion.

Cranial nerves

The 12 pairs of cranial nerves transmit motor and sensory messages between the brain and the head and neck. The cranial nerves are designated by both a name and a Roman numeral. The names of the nerves indicate their function. The Roman numerals indicate the order in which the nerves are found in the brain, from anterior to posterior.

Olfactory nerve
Before testing the olfactory nerve, or cranial nerve (CN) I, check the patency of the patient's nostrils. Ask him to occlude one nostril as he inhales through the other and vice versa. Olfactory nerve testing will be impaired if the nostrils are blocked by edema of the mucosa or turbinates, or by nasal polyps or discharge.

Use at least two common substances with recognizable odors, such as coffee, cloves, or cinnamon. Vaporous substances, such as oil of peppermint or ammonia, stimulate the nerve endings of the trigeminal nerve (CN V), producing irritation that may be mistaken for odor perception.

Place the container of the first aromatic substance under the patient's nostril and ask him to identify the odor. Using a different substance, test the other nostril.

Optic nerve
Test the optic nerve, CN II, by assessing visual acuity and visual fields, as described in Chapter 6. Then, using the ophthalmoscope, examine the optic fundi for indications of arteriosclerotic small vessel disease and diabetic or hypertensive retinopathy. Swelling of the optic disk, or papilledema, marked by fuzziness of the disk margins, may indicate an obstruction to venous outflow caused by increased intracranial pressure (ICP). Papilledema also is indicated by the curving of the disk vessels over the edges of the disk and absence of the physiologic cup.

Oculomotor, trochlear, and abducens nerves
Usually, you'll test these three nerves—CN III, CN IV, and CN VI—together. Begin by evaluating extraocular eye movement, as described in Chapter 6. All three of these nerves control these movements.

The oculomotor nerve also controls the muscles that elevate the eyelids and produce pupillary constriction. So observe the patient for ptosis. Then inspect his pupils. Are they the same size?

Next, assess the patient's pupillary reaction to light, as described in Chapter 6. This reaction depends on the optic nerve's ability to transmit the light stimulus to the visual center and the oculomotor nerve's ability to produce pupillary constriction.

Trigeminal nerve
Test the sensory component of the trigeminal nerve, CN V, by assessing the patient's response to pain and light touch. If the patient's pain sensation is intact, you won't assess temperature sensation because they are carried by the same sensory pathways.

Before testing for pain, demonstrate the examination technique to the patient. After he closes his eyes, lightly apply the tip of a safety pin to the back of his hand and ask him if he feels a sharp sensation (from the tip of the pin) or a dull one (from the blunt end of the pin). After your demonstration, have the patient close his eyes again, and test for pain sensation bilaterally over the two facial dermatomes, using the tip of the safety pin. While you test for pain, also touch the two facial dermatomes bilaterally with the blunt end of the pin to ensure that the patient can distinguish pain from light-touch sensation. Keep in mind that a patient with neuropathy may maintain light-touch sensation after he's lost pain sensation. (See *Dermatome distribution*.)

To test light touch, instruct the patient to say "now" when he feels a cotton wisp on his face. Then touch the same two facial dermatomes with a wisp of cotton.

Next, test the patient's corneal reflex. If he wears contact lenses, have him remove them.

Dermatome distribution

The body is divided into dermatomes, each of which represents an area of the skin supplied with afferent (sensory) nerve fibers from an individual spinal root—cervical (C), thoracic (T), lumbar (L), or sacral (S). These illustrations show the dermatomes of the body.

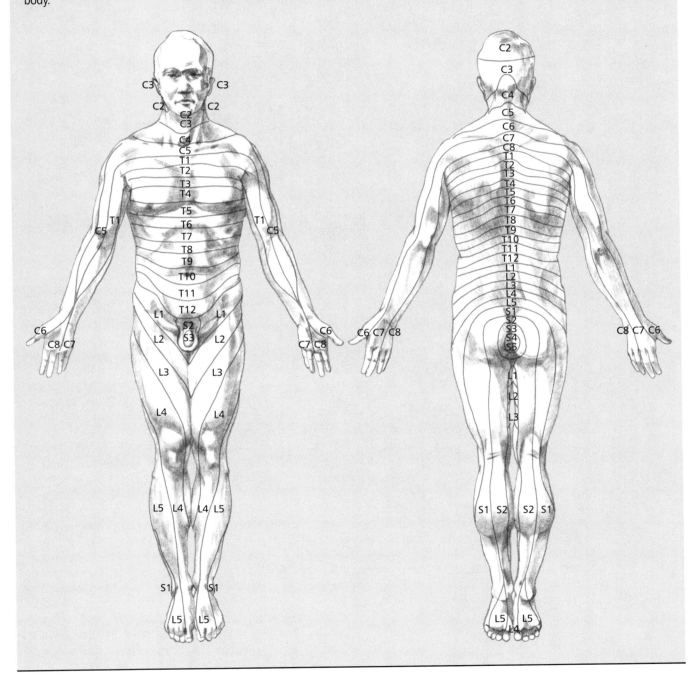

Assessing the trigeminal nerve

To assess the motor component of the trigeminal nerve, palpate the temporal and the masseter muscles. The first photograph shows the area you'll palpate to assess the temporal muscles. The second photograph shows a nurse palpating the masseter muscles.

Temporal muscles

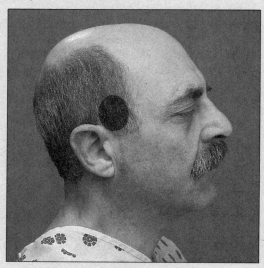

Masseter muscles

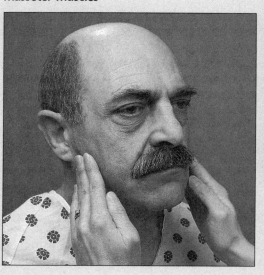

Then tell him to look up and to one side, and lightly touch the cornea with the cotton wisp. Blinking and tearing is the normal corneal reflex response.

Test the motor component of the trigeminal nerve by assessing the strength and symmetry of the patient's jaw muscles. Ask him to open and close his mouth and to move his jaw from side to side. Have him repeat these movements against your resistance. His jaw movements should be strong and symmetrical.

Next, palpate the temporal and masseter muscles. Do so with the muscles at rest and as the patient moves his jaw from side to side and opens and closes his mouth. Again, these movements should be strong and symmetrical. (See *Assessing the trigeminal nerve.*)

Facial nerve

To test the motor component of the facial nerve, CN VII, observe the patient's face for symmetry. Compare the lower eyelids and check for drooping. Are the nasolabial folds symmetrical? Can the patient shed tears and salivate? Ask the patient to raise his eyebrows, smile, frown, puff out his cheeks, and wrinkle his forehead. As he does, observe for symmetry.

To test muscle strength, ask the patient to close his eyes tightly and to try to keep them closed while you attempt to force them open. Then place your hand against the patient's puffed cheeks and compare the muscle mass and strength of the cheeks.

Depending on the circumstances, you may need to test taste sensation. This portion of the test is usually omitted from a neurologic screening examination because the procedure is tedious and the results are often inconclusive. To test the patient's sense of taste, have him close his eyes. Then test each side of the tongue separately, using cotton-tipped applicators dipped in water, salt, sugar, vinegar, and quinine. Ask the patient to rinse his mouth between each taste. Ideally, the patient should identify the taste by pointing to index cards labeled "salty," "sweet," "sour," and "bitter."

Acoustic nerve

During a neurologic screening, you'll usually test only the cochlear branch of the acoustic nerve, CN VIII. To do so, evaluate the patient's hearing, using the techniques described in Chapter 6. To distinguish sensorineural from conductive hearing loss, perform the Weber and Rinne tests, also explained in Chapter 6.

If a patient complains of vertigo, dizziness, imbalance, or a gait disturbance, you'll also evaluate the vestibular branch of the acoustic nerve. Instruct the patient to sit upright on the examination table with his legs and feet resting on the table. Ask him to look to the left and hold his head in that position. Observe for nystagmus. Then ask him to lie down and turn his head to the left. Have him lower his head to a 45-degree angle below the plane of the table. Keep him in that position for 30 seconds. Again, look for nystagmus, and ask him if he's experiencing vertigo. Help him to sit up with his head still turned to the left, and assess him again for nystagmus and vertigo. Repeat the procedure with the patient's head turned to the right, but only after any sensations from the first test have subsided. (See *Assessing the acoustic nerve.*)

Glossopharyngeal and vagus nerves

The glossopharyngeal and vagus nerves, CN IX and X, are usually tested together because their functions overlap. Begin by listening to the patient's voice for dysphonia. Next, check the gag reflex by touching the tip of the tongue blade against the posterior pharynx. Then ask the patient to say "ah" and note whether the soft palate and uvula rise symmetrically and if the uvula is at the midline.

Accessory nerve

The accessory nerve, or CN XI, innervates the sternocleidomastoid and upper portion of the

Assessing the acoustic nerve

To evaluate the vestibular branch of the acoustic nerve, perform positional testing. The illustration below shows a key step of positional testing. Note that the patient's head is turned to the left and her neck is at a 45-degree angle.

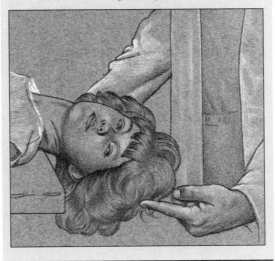

trapezius muscles, which govern shoulder movement and neck rotation.

Test sternocleidomastoid muscle strength by placing your palm against the patient's cheek and asking him to turn his head against the resistance of your hand. Repeat the test on the other side, comparing muscle strength. Test the trapezius muscles by placing your hands on the patient's shoulders and asking him to raise or shrug his shoulders against your resistance.

Hypoglossal nerve

The hypoglossal nerve, CN XII, controls tongue movements involved in swallowing and speech. Test this nerve by asking the patient to stick out his tongue and noting whether it's at the midline. After the patient has retracted his tongue, look for tremors or fasciculations. Next, test tongue strength by asking the patient to lift his tongue against the resistance you apply with a tongue blade. To check the strength of

Assessing vibratory sense

To evaluate vibratory sense, apply the base of a vibrating fork to the interphalangeal joint of the patient's great toe, as shown.

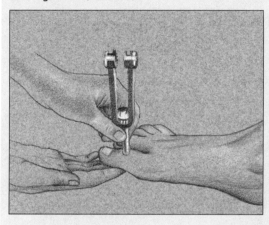

each side of the tongue, ask the patient to press it against his cheek as you apply resistance.

Test lingual speech by asking the patient to repeat the sentence "Round the rugged rock the ragged rascal ran."

Sensory system

Your examination of the patient's sensory system includes testing his ability to feel pain and light touch. You'll also evaluate the patient's vibratory sense, position sense, and discriminative sensations.

Pain

To test for pain, use the same technique you used to evaluate the sensory component of the trigeminal nerve. Ask the patient to close his eyes, and then touch the major dermatomes of the trunk and limbs with the tip of a pin. Again, ask him to indicate whether he feels a sharp or a dull sensation. If he has diminished pain sensation (hypesthesia) or no pain sensation (anesthesia), determine the borders of the

area of sensory deficit by applying pinpricks at short intervals, starting in the area of anesthesia and working outward until he can perceive the stimulus.

You can test most of the major dermatomes by applying the pin to the patient's shoulders, the inside and outside of the upper and lower arms, the thumbs, the fifth fingers, the anterior chest, the anterior and posterior thighs, the inside and outside of the thighs and lower legs, and the great toes. A more detailed examination can be performed on patients who have deficits on the screening examination. Be sure to test for pain sensation on the tips of both fingers and toes. The patient with peripheral neuropathy develops hypesthesia first in the most distal aspects of the extremities, the so-called glove-and-stocking distribution.

Light touch

To test for light-touch perception, touch the major dermatomes with a wisp of cotton. Don't swab or sweep with the cotton because you might miss an area of sensory loss. If you do detect a sensory deficit, determine the borders of the area.

Some patients with peripheral neuropathy retain their light-touch sensation after they've lost their pain sensation. However, pain, temperature, crude light touch, tickle, and itch sensations are all transmitted up the spinal cord by the same sensory pathways. Therefore, when one sensation is affected, the others may be as well.

Vibratory sense

To test vibratory sense, you'll apply a tuning fork over certain bony prominences. First, ask the patient to close his eyes. Then, strike the tines of the tuning fork against your hand and apply the base of the vibrating fork to the interphalangeal joint of the patient's great toe. Make sure you hold the fork on the stem; holding the tines will dampen the vibration. Ask the patient what he feels. Typically, he should report a vibration or buzzing. (See *Assessing vibratory sense* and *Vibratory sense: Ensuring accurate findings.*)

If the patient doesn't feel the vibration over the interphalangeal joint, move to the medial malleolus of the ankle. If he still doesn't feel it, apply the vibrating fork to the anterior tibia. Move the fork proximally until he can feel the vibration. Then note where he felt it. Repeat the test on the other leg.

Assess for vibratory sense on the arms. Start at the distal interphalangeal joint of the index finger and move proximally, as necessary.

Position sense

A patient needs intact position sense, known as proprioception, together with intact vestibular and cerebellar function to maintain balance. When testing the patient's position sense, you'll evaluate both his arms and his legs.

To test each arm, ask the patient to close his eyes, and then grasp the sides of his index finger. Move the finger up or down and ask the patient to tell you the direction in which you moved the finger.

If the patient doesn't answer correctly, repeat the test at his wrist. If he still doesn't answer correctly, test his elbow and, if necessary, his shoulder. Note where he's able to perceive position change.

To evaluate the legs, grasp the sides of the great toe, move it up and down, and ask the patient to tell you the direction of the movement. If necessary, proceed to the ankles, the knees, and the hips until the patient gives you a correct response. Always grasp the sides of the body part, not the top and bottom. If you grasp the top and bottom of the toe, for instance, the pressure you apply may signal the position to the patient even though he has diminished position sense.

The same sensory pathway transmits position and vibratory sensations. Thus, peripheral neuropathy may diminish both, even though the patient's ability to feel pain, temperature, and light touch remain intact. In some disorders, vibratory sense may diminish sooner than position sense.

Discriminative sensations

If peripheral sensations are intact, test the more finely tuned integrative functions of the cerebral cortex. Begin by evaluating stereog-

nosis, the ability to discriminate shape, size, weight, texture, and form of an object by touching and manipulating it. Ask the patient to close his eyes and open his hand. Then place a small, common object, such as a coin or key, in his palm and ask him to identify it.

If he can't identify the object or perform the fine motor movements necessary to identify a small object, test graphesthesia. Have him hold out his hand. Then trace a large number on his palm using the eraser of a pencil. Ask him to identify the number.

Stereognosis and graphesthesia test the ability of the sensory cortex to integrate sensory input. An inability to recognize the object by touch, called tactile agnosia, may indicate a parietal lobe lesion.

Next, test point localization by asking the patient to close his eyes; then touch one of his limbs and ask him to point to the spot you touched. His inability to do so may indicate a lesion in the sensory cortex.

Finally, test extinction by touching the patient simultaneously in contralateral areas. He should be able to feel both touches. If he only feels one, he may have a cortical lesion on the other side.

Motor system

Assessing the motor system includes inspecting the muscles, testing muscle tone, and testing

Testing muscle strength

To evaluate the motor system, you'll test the strength of the major muscle groups of the patient's arms and legs. These illustrations show you four of the techniques you'll use.

Biceps strength

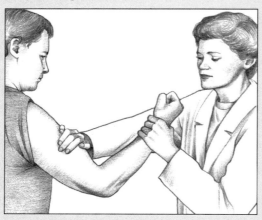

Triceps strength

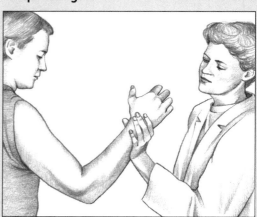

muscle strength. You'll also evaluate cerebellar function because the cerebellum plays a role in smooth-muscle movements, balance, and gait.

Inspection

Observe the symmetry of large contralateral muscle masses, noting any atrophy. In some cases, you may need to measure muscle mass to compare contralateral sides. To do so, wrap a tape measure around the widest circumference of the muscle on each side. Muscle atrophy may result from decreased neural input, as occurs in paraplegia.

Look too for any abnormal muscle movements, such as tics, tremors, or fasciculations.

Testing muscle tone

Muscle tone represents muscular resistance to passive stretching. To test arm muscle tone, move the patient's shoulder through passive range-of-motion (ROM) exercises. You should feel slight resistance to your movements. Next, let the arm drop to the patient's side. Typically, it should fall easily. If the arm is rigid, the pa-

tient has heightened muscle tone, which may result from an upper motor neuron lesion. If the arm is flaccid, the patient has diminished tone, which may result from a lower motor neuron lesion.

To test leg muscle tone, guide the hip through passive ROM exercises; then let the leg fall to the bed or examination table. If the leg falls into an externally rotated position, note it as an abnormal finding.

Testing muscle strength

You can evaluate general muscle strength as you observe the patient's gait and his motor activities. To test specific muscle groups, have the patient use the muscles against your resistance, as described below. Always compare the strength of contralateral muscle groups.

For a neurologic screening, you need to test the strength of only the major muscle groups. Grade muscle strength on a scale of 0 to 5, with 0 indicating no strength and 5 indicating maximum strength. You can document your findings as a fraction, with the patient's

Ankle strength: Plantar flexion

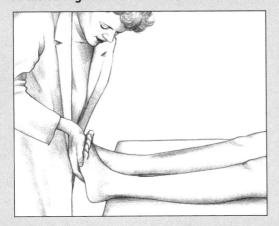

Ankle strength: Dorsiflexion

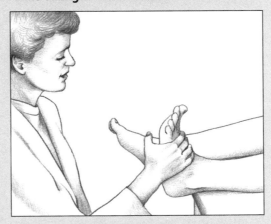

score as the numerator and the maximum strength as the denominator, for example, $2/5$ or $5/5$.

Arms

To test shoulder girdle strength, instruct the patient to extend his arms with his palms up and to maintain this position for 30 seconds. If he has shoulder girdle weakness in one arm, he may be unable to lift it. Or he may be unable to lift it as high as he can lift the other arm. If he does lift both arms equally, look for pronation of the hand and downward drift of the arm on the weaker side. If he is able to maintain his arms outstretched, further test his strength by placing your hands on his forearms and pressing down as he resists.

To test biceps and triceps strength, ask the patient to hold his arm up in front of him with his elbow flexed and to maintain this position while you try to move his arm. Test biceps strength by pulling down on the flexor surface of his forearm as he resists. Test triceps strength by pushing against the extensor sur-

faces of his forearms as he tries to straighten his arms. (See *Testing muscle strength.*)

To test wrist flexion, ask the patient to flex his wrist against your resistance. Test wrist extension by asking him to extend his wrist as you push down. Test handgrip, finger abduction, and thumb opposition in the same way.

Legs

Begin by asking the patient to lift both legs off the bed simultaneously. If he's hemiplegic, he may not be able to lift the affected leg, to lift it as high, or to hold it up. To check quadriceps strength, ask him to lift his legs as you press down on his anterior thighs.

Next, ask him to flex his legs at the knees and put his feet flat on the bed. To check lower leg strength, try to pull his lower leg forward as he resists. Then try to push his lower leg backward as he tries to extend his knee.

Finally, evaluate ankle strength by asking the patient to push his foot down (plantar flexion) as you resist. Then ask him to push his foot up (dorsiflexion) as you press down on the dorsum of his foot.

Cerebellar testing

Before you test cerebellar function, observe the patient's general balance and coordination. Can he sit upright without support? Can he sit on the edge of the bed? Stand at the bedside? Remember that the ability to sit on the edge of the bed and to stand may be diminished by weakness unrelated to cerebellar dysfunction.

To assess the patient's cerebellar function, you'll evaluate his whole-body coordination and extremity coordination.

Whole-body coordination

Assessing whole-body coordination includes evaluating the patient as he walks and performs certain maneuvers. Observe the patient as he walks across the room, turns, and walks back. Note any imbalance or abnormalities in his gait. He should be able to maintain his posture, his arms swinging in tandem with his leg movements. His movements should be smooth and rhythmic, without hesitation or jerkiness. A patient with cerebellar dysfunction will exhibit a wide-based, unsteady gait. Deviation to one side may indicate a cerebellar lesion on that side.

Ask the patient to walk heel to toe and observe his balance. Although he may be slightly unsteady, he should be able to walk forward and maintain his balance. (See *Assessing cerebellar function*.)

Next, perform the Romberg test. Ask the patient to stand with his feet together, his eyes open, and arms at his side. Hold your outstretched arms on either side of him so you can support him if he sways to one side or the other. Observe his balance, and then ask him to close his eyes. Note whether he loses his balance or sways. If he falls to one side, the Romberg test is positive. Patients with cerebellar dysfunction have difficulty maintaining balance with their eyes closed because they cannot use the visual cues that orient them to the upright position.

You can also test whole-body coordination by asking the patient to do deep knee bends

or to hop first on one foot and then the other. Keep in mind that patients with arthritis or other musculoskeletal disorders may have difficulty with these tests.

Extremity coordination

To evaluate the patient's extremity coordination, you'll test point-to-point movements, and rapid skilled and rapid alternating movements.

Point-to-point movements. Have the patient sit about 2' (0.6 m) away from you. Hold your index finger up, and ask him to touch the tip of his index finger to the tip of yours and then to touch his nose. Now, move your finger and ask him to repeat the maneuver. Gradually, have him increase his speed as you repeat the test. Then test his other hand. Expect the patient to be more accurate with his dominant hand. A patient with cerebellar dysfunction will overshoot his target, and his movements will be jerky.

Next, ask the patient to touch the heel of his right foot to his left shin and to run his heel down his shin. Then have him repeat the maneuver with his left foot. If he has cerebellar dysfunction, he'll have difficulty placing his heel on his shin and maintaining the position. Plus, his movements will be jerky.

Rapid skilled and rapid alternating movements. To further test cerebellar function, observe rapid skilled movements and rapid alternating movements of the arms and legs.

Test rapid skilled movements by asking the patient to touch the thumb of his right hand to his right index finger and then to each of his remaining fingers. Then instruct him to increase his speed. Observe his movements for smoothness and accuracy. Repeat the test on his left hand.

To test rapid alternating movements, have the patient sit and place his palms down on his thighs. Now, tell him to turn his palms first up and then down. Instruct him to gradually increase his speed.

Have the patient lie supine. Then stand at the foot of the bed and hold your palms near his soles. Instruct him to alternately tap the sole of his right foot and then his left foot

Assessing cerebellar function

To evaluate cerebellar function, you'll test the patient's balance and coordination. The illustrations below show you four of the tests you'll use.

Heel-to-toe walking

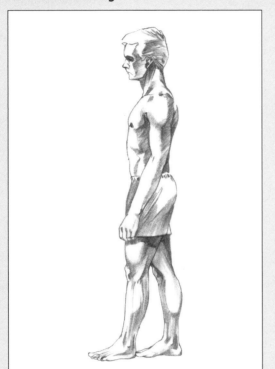

Romberg test

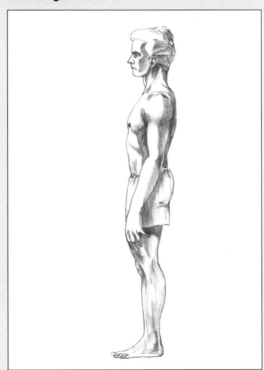

Point-to-point movements

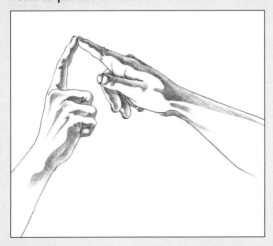

Rapid skilled movements

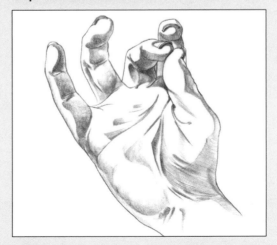

Grading deep tendon reflexes

This figure indicates normal deep tendon reflex activity. When testing the patient's deep tendon reflexes, use the following grading scale.

0 absent
1+ present but diminished
2+ normal
3+ increased but not necessarily pathologic
4+ hyperactive; clonic

Record the patient's reflex scores by drawing a stick figure and entering the scores at the proper location.

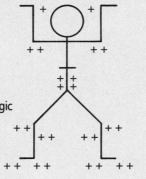

sponse on a scale of 0 (no response) to 4+ (hyperactive). (See *Grading deep tendon reflexes.*)

Biceps reflex

Position the patient's arm so his elbow is flexed at a 45-degree angle and his arm is relaxed. Place your thumb or index finger over the biceps tendon and your remaining fingers loosely over the triceps muscle. Strike your thumb or index finger with the pointed tip of the reflex hammer, and watch and feel for contraction of the biceps muscle and flexion of the forearm. (See *Assessing reflexes.*)

Triceps reflex

Have the patient abduct his arm and place his forearm across his chest. Strike the triceps tendon about 2" (5 cm) above the olecranon process on the extensor surface of the upper arm. Watch for contraction of the triceps muscle and extension of the forearm.

If you don't elicit the triceps reflex, try this alternative technique: Ask the patient to abduct his arm at the shoulder. If you're right-handed, support his upper arm with your left arm. Ask him to let his arm hang loosely over yours. With the hammer in your right hand, strike the triceps tendon briskly, using either the blunt or the pointed end. Again, watch for contraction of the triceps and extension of the forearm at the elbow.

Brachioradialis reflex

Instruct the patient to rest the ulnar surface of his hand on his knee and to partially flex his elbow. With the tip of the hammer, strike the radius about 2" proximal to the radial styloid. Watch for supination of the hand and flexion of the forearm at the elbow.

Patellar reflex

Have the patient sit on the side of the bed with his legs dangling freely. If he can't sit up, flex his knee at a 45-degree angle and place your nondominant hand behind it for support. Strike the patellar tendon just below the patella, and look for contraction of the quadriceps muscle in the anterior thigh and for extension of the leg.

against your palms. Tell him to increase his speed as you observe his coordination. A patient with cerebellar dysfunction exhibits dysdiadochokinesia (an inability to perform coordinated alternating movements).

Reflexes

Evaluating your patient's reflexes includes testing deep tendon and superficial reflexes as well as observing for primitive reflexes.

Deep tendon reflexes

Before you test a deep tendon reflex, be sure the limb is relaxed and the joint is in the midposition; for instance, the knee or elbow should be flexed at a 45-degree angle. Then distract the patient by asking him to focus on an object across the room. If he focuses on his performance, the cerebral cortex may dampen his response. You can also distract the patient by using Jendrassik's maneuver. Simply instruct him to clench his teeth or to squeeze his thigh. Be sure to document which technique you used to distract the patient.

Always test deep tendon reflexes, moving from head to toe, and, of course, compare contralateral reflexes. To elicit the reflex, tap the tendon lightly but firmly with the reflex hammer. Then grade the briskness of the re-

Assessing reflexes

During your neurologic examination, you'll evaluate your patient's reflexes. These photographs show 6 reflexes you'll test.

Biceps reflex

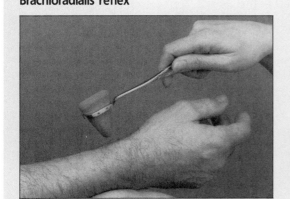

Triceps reflex

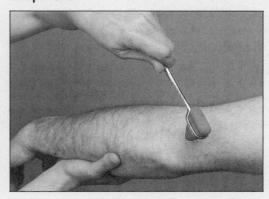

Brachioradialis reflex

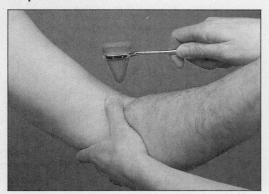

Patellar reflex

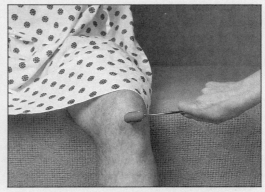

Achilles reflex

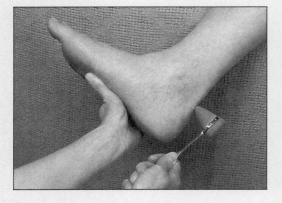

Grasp reflex

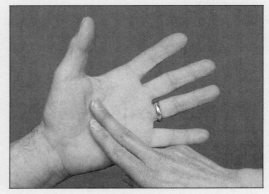

Achilles reflex

Slightly flex the foot and support the plantar surface. Using the pointed end of the reflex hammer, strike the Achilles tendon. Watch for plantar flexion of the foot at the ankle.

If the patient is bedridden, position him with his hip externally rotated and his foot resting on his other knee. Slightly flex the foot at the ankle and strike the tendon briskly.

Superficial reflexes

These reflexes include the plantar, cremasteric, and abdominal reflexes. To elicit these reflexes, you'll stimulate the patient's skin or mucous membranes. To document your findings, use a plus sign (+) to indicate that a reflex is present and a minus sign (−) to indicate that it's absent.

Plantar reflex

Using an applicator stick, a tongue blade, or a key, slowly stroke the lateral side of the patient's sole from the heel to the great toe. The normal response is plantar flexion of the toes. In an elderly patient, this normal response may be diminished because of arthritic deformities of the toe or foot.

In patients with disorders of the pyramidal tract (such as CVA), the Babinski's reflex, an abnormal response, is elicited. The patient responds to the stimulus by dorsiflexion of his great toe. You may also see a more pronounced response in which the other toes extend and abduct. In some cases, you may even see dorsiflexion of the ankle, knee, and hip.

Cremasteric reflex

With a male patient, use an applicator stick to lightly stimulate the inner thigh. Watch for contraction of the cremaster muscle in the scrotum and prompt elevation of the testicle on the side of the stimulus. This reflex may be absent in upper or lower motor neuron disease.

Abdominal reflex

Place the patient in the supine position with his arms at his sides and his knees slightly flexed. Using the tip of the reflex hammer, a key, or an applicator stick, briskly stroke both sides of the abdomen above and below the umbilicus, moving from the periphery toward the midline. After each stroke, watch for abdominal muscle contraction and movement of the umbilicus toward the stimulus. If you're evaluating an obese patient, retract the umbilicus to the side opposite the stimulus and note whether it pulls toward the stimulus. Aging and diseases of the upper and lower motor neurons cause an absent abdominal reflex.

Primitive reflexes

Although normal in infants, primitive reflexes are pathologic in adults. They include the grasp, snout, sucking, and glabellar reflexes.

Grasp reflex

Apply gentle pressure to the patient's palm with your fingers. If he grasps your fingers between his thumb and index finger, suspect cortical (pre-motor cortex) damage.

Snout reflex

Tap lightly on the patient's upper lip. Lip pursing, known as the snout reflex, indicates frontal lobe damage.

Sucking reflex

Observe the patient while you are feeding him or suctioning his mouth. If he begins sucking, you've elicited the sucking reflex—an indication of cortical damage typically seen in the patient with advanced dementia.

Glabellar reflex

Repeatedly tap the bridge of the patient's nose. A persistent blinking response indicates diffuse cortical dysfunction.

Abnormal findings

During your assessment, you may detect abnormal findings caused by neurologic dysfunction. The most common ones include decreased LOC, cranial nerve impairment, abnormal muscle movements, abnormal gaits, and abnormal reflexes.

Decreased level of consciousness

LOC can be impaired by various disorders that diffusely affect the cerebral hemispheres, such as toxic encephalopathy, hemorrhage, and extensive, generalized cortical atrophy. Compression of brain stem structures by either a tumor or hemorrhage can also depress consciousness by affecting the reticular activating system, which is responsible for maintaining wakefulness. What's more, various drugs, such as sedatives and narcotics, can diminish LOC.

Cranial nerve impairment

Damage to the cranial nerves may cause numerous abnormalities including olfactory, visual, auditory, and muscular problems. Vertigo and dysphagia also indicate cranial nerve damage.

Olfactory impairment
If the patient can't detect odors with both nostrils, he may have a disorder of the olfactory nerve (CN I). The symptom can result from a lesion in the olfactory tract caused by an intracranial mass, a hemorrhage, or a fracture of a facial bone.

Visual impairment
Visual fields are affected by a variety of lesions, such as tumors or infarcts of the optic nerve (CN II) head, optic chiasm, or optic tracts.

Pupillary changes
If the patient's pupillary response to light is impaired, he may have damage to both the optic and the oculomotor nerve (CN III). Increased ICP can cause bilateral dilation of the pupils. (See *Understanding pupillary changes,* page 116.)

Eye muscle impairment
Weakness or paralysis of eye muscles or eyelids can result from cranial nerve damage. Increased ICP and intracranial lesions can affect the motor nuclei of the oculomotor, trochlear, and abducens nerves (CN III, IV, and VI).

Nystagmus
In nystagmus, the patient's eyes drift slowly in one direction and then jerk back in the other direction. Nystagmus is associated with nerve damage in a number of sites, but the most common are the peripheral labyrinth (inner ear), the brain stem (CN III, IV, and VI), and the cerebellum.

Ptosis
A drooping eyelid on one side, or ptosis, results from a defect of the oculomotor nerve. You may detect it more readily when the patient is sitting up, rather than reclining. The pupil may also be dilated on the affected side.

Facial sensory impairment
If the patient responds inadequately to sensory stimuli of the skin or eye, the trigeminal nerve (CN V) may be damaged. Lesions of the sensory division of the nerve may cause decreased skin perception of pain, temperature, and light touch.

Facial pain
Trigeminal neuralgia, or tic douloureux, causes severe, lancinating pain over one or more of the facial dermatomes.

Hearing loss
Sensorineural hearing loss can result from lesions of the cochlear branch of the acoustic nerve (CN VIII) or from lesions in any part of the nerve's pathway to the brain stem. A patient with this type of hearing loss may have trouble hearing high-pitched sounds, or he may lose all hearing in the affected ear. Sensorineural hearing loss can occur in one or both ears.

Vertigo
The illusion of movement, or vertigo, can result from a disturbance of the vestibular centers. If the patient has a peripheral lesion (labyrinthine system), vertigo and nystagmus will occur 10 to 20 seconds after he changes position, and the symptoms will diminish with repetition of the position change. If the vertigo is of central origin (brain), there is no latent period and the symptoms will not diminish with repetition.

Understanding pupillary changes

Use this chart as a guide to the significance of pupillary changes.

PUPILLARY CHANGE	POSSIBLE CAUSES
Unilateral, dilated (4 mm), fixed, and nonreactive 	• Uncal herniation with oculomotor nerve damage • Brain stem compression from an expanding lesion or an aneurysm • Increased intracranial pressure • Tentorial herniation • Head trauma with subsequent subdural or epidural hematoma • May be normal in some people
Bilateral, dilated (4 mm), fixed, and non-reactive 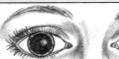	• Severe midbrain damage • Cardiopulmonary arrest (hypoxia) • Anticholinergic poisoning
Bilateral, midsize (2 mm), fixed, and non-reactive 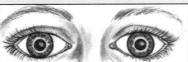	• Midbrain involvement caused by edema, hemorrhage, infarctions, lacerations, contusions
Bilateral, pinpoint (< 1 mm), and usually nonreactive 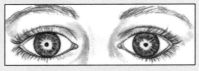	• Lesion of pons, usually after hemorrhage, leading to blocked sympathetic impulses • Opiates, such as morphine (pupils may be reactive)
Unilateral, small (1.5 mm), and non-reactive 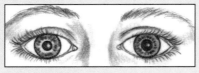	• Disruption of sympathetic nerve supply to the head caused by spinal cord lesion above the first thoracic vertebra

Dysphagia

Damage to the glossopharyngeal and vagus nerves (CN IX and X) may cause dysphagia. A diminished gag reflex may be normal and may not cause swallowing problems. In multi-infarct dementia and bilateral cortical or subcortical disease, the gag reflex may increase.

Abnormal muscle movements

Neurologic disorders may cause a wide range of abnormal muscle movements, from facial tics to motor restlessness. These abnormalities may or may not indicate a serious neurologic disease.

Tics

These sudden, uncontrolled movements of the face, shoulders, or extremities are caused by abnormal neural stimuli. Tics actually are normal movements that appear repetitively and inappropriately. They include blinking, shoulder shrugging, and facial twitching.

Tremors

Like tics, tremors are involuntary, repetitive movements usually seen in the fingers or wrists as well as in the eyelids, tongue, and legs. They can occur when the affected body part is at rest (resting tremors) or when it is voluntarily moved (intention tremors). The patient with Parkinson's disease has a characteristic "pill-rolling" resting tremor.

The patient with cerebellar disease has tremors when he voluntarily reaches for an object. A sustained posture, such as holding the arms outstretched, indicates postural tremor. This tremor may occur in some elderly patients and in patients with anxiety or hypermetabolic states, such as hyperthyroidism.

Fasciculations

These fine twitchings in single small muscle groups are most commonly associated with lower motor neuron dysfunction. You may detect fasciculations in the patient with tongue dysfunction, which results from a disorder of the hypoglossal nerve.

Akathisia

In motor restlessness, or akathisia, the patient feels agitated and has the compelling need to walk around. You may see this disorder in patients with Parkinson's disease or those who are taking neuroleptic drugs.

Oral-facial dyskinesias

Tardive dyskinesia—repetitive chewing motions accompanied by intermittent darting movements of the tongue—represents a late, irreversible complication of neuroleptic drugs.

Abnormal gaits

During your assessment, you may identify one of these four gait abnormalities: hemiparetic, parkinsonian, ataxic, or steppage gait. These gaits may result from disorders of the cerebellum or posterior columns, disorders of the corticospinal tract, basal ganglia defects of Parkinson's disease, and lower motor neuron lesions. The abnormality can reflect both the site and degree of neurologic damage.

Hemiparetic gait

Characteristics of the hemiparetic gait vary according to the amount of damage to the upper motor neurons. The severely affected patient walks with the affected arm abducted and the elbow, wrist, and fingers flexed. His upper body is somewhat stooped, and he tilts slightly toward the opposite side. As he walks, he extends his leg and inverts his foot at the ankle. The leg swings in a semicircular motion, first away from and then toward the trunk, and the foot drags along the floor.

Parkinsonian gait

The patient with Parkinson's disease bends over when walking. The neck and thoracic spine are flexed forward, and the elbows, hips, and knees are also flexed. The patient doesn't swing his arms as he walks. His steps are short and shuffling, and he has difficulty both initiating and stopping movement.

Ataxic gait

The patient with cerebellar ataxia has difficulty maintaining balance both while standing still and while walking. Ambulation is characterized by a wide-based, reeling, "drunken" gait.

In sensory ataxia, the patient must watch his feet because he can't feel where he is placing them. His legs are partially flexed at the hips, and he lifts his legs up and slaps his feet on the floor with each step.

Steppage gait

A patient with a steppage gait purposefully lifts his legs up, and then slaps them down on the floor. This gait is associated with lower motor neuron disease and is often accompanied by muscle weakness and atrophy, and fasciculations.

Abnormal reflexes

Impaired reflexes may result from upper and lower motor neuron lesions as well as from damage to the dorsal and ventral roots of the spinal nerves. Abnormal reflexes include deep tendon reflex impairments, superficial reflex impairments, and the presence of primitive reflexes.

Deep tendon reflex impairment
Deep tendon reflexes should be symmetrical. A markedly brisk hyperreflexic response indicates an upper motor neuron lesion. Such lesions can also cause clonus at the ankle—a repetitive, alternating movement between dorsiflexion and plantar flexion. Diminished or absent deep tendon reflexes indicate damage to the lower motor neurons.

Superficial reflex impairment
In Babinski's reflex, the patient dorsiflexes his great toe when you attempt to elicit the plantar reflex. This abnormal finding occurs with disorders of the pyramidal tract.

Primitive reflexes
The appearance of primitive reflexes—grasp, snout, sucking, and glabellar—is abnormal in adults, resulting from one of several neurologic disorders. Frontal lobe damage, widespread cortical atrophy, bilateral thalamic degeneration, and occipital lobe dysfunction can cause the reappearance of the primitive reflexes.

Pertinent diagnostic tests

Because of the complexity of neurologic dysfunction and the far-reaching implications of many neurologic symptoms, you may need to recommend the patient for further testing. Diagnostic tests used in the evaluation of neurologic disorders range from basic X-rays to complex computer imaging studies and electrical recordings of brain functions.

Radiography
Although tests that use more sophisticated technology are often preferred to X-rays, skull and spine radiography are still used to evaluate some specific neurologic disorders.

Skull X-rays diagnose skull fractures and the bony changes associated with Paget's disease, hyperostosis, and osteolytic disease. Calcifications seen in the brain on skull films may indicate an intracranial mass, although their pathologic significance can't be identified by X-ray alone. Alteration in bony contours, sutures, and bony cavities may result from increased ICP or displacement of cranial contents by a mass.

Spinal X-rays show the structure of a patient's vertebrae, the intervertebral disk spaces, the vertebral foramina, and the width of the spinal canal. They can aid the diagnosis of fractured vertebrae as well as herniated disks, bone spurs, spinal cord masses, and structural abnormalities, such as scoliosis and kyphosis.

CT scan
Computed tomography (CT) scan produces a computer image of the brain, showing the precise location and extent of intracranial pathology. Cranial contents, such as bone, blood vessels, and brain tissue, have different densities and absorb varying amounts of radiation during the scan. Contents of greatest density (bone) appear white and those of lesser density (air) appear darker. The quality of the scan can be enhanced by injecting iodine-based contrast material.

Lumbar puncture
In lumbar puncture, a small amount of cerebrospinal fluid is withdrawn and tested for glucose, protein, and electrolyte levels; the presence of red and white blood cells; and bacteria. The lumbar puncture is used to detect subarachnoid hemorrhage; infectious encephalopathy; demyelinating processes, such as

multiple sclerosis; Guillain-Barrè syndrome; or a tumor of the spinal cord or cerebrum.

Magnetic resonance imaging

Within the magnetic resonance imaging (MRI) scanner, a magnetic field is created around the patient. Radio frequency pulses are applied to the brain, causing groups of atomic nuclei within it to resonate. Energy signals resulting from this process are analyzed by a computer and copied onto film.

MRI offers several advantages over CT scanning. It doesn't expose the patient to radiation, and it offers better contrast images of soft tissues. MRI can also differentiate between the brain's gray and white matter and is therefore better than the CT scan in diagnosing demyelinating processes, tumors, vascular infarctions, arteriovenous malformations, and aneurysms.

Positron emission tomography

In positron emission tomography (PET) scanning, molecules in the brain are labelled with a radioactive isotope and followed by radiation-sensitive detectors in the scanner. The scanner follows the activity of the isotope within the patient's brain cells, and provides information about protein synthesis and energy production within the brain. By identifying chemical tissue changes, such as the use of glucose by tumor cells, PET can help evaluate the effectiveness of antineoplastic drug therapy. It can also confirm the presence or absence of Alzheimer's disease as well as localize epileptogenic foci.

Single-photon emission computed tomography

The single-photon emission computed tomography (SPECT) scan uses a more readily available radioisotope than the PET scan. The SPECT scan can detect perfusion defects in CVA patients before there is CT evidence of infarction and during transient ischemic attacks. Like PET, SPECT has proved effective in localizing seizure foci.

Cerebral arteriography

The more precise and less invasive CT and MRI scans are now preferred to cerebral arteriogra-

phy. But the test is still useful in diagnosing atherosclerosis of the extracranial vessels and in evaluating a patient scheduled for vascular surgery, such as endarterectomy.

Disadvantages of arteriography include anaphylactic reaction to the contrast dye, embolization of clots, and dislodgment of arterial plaques. Bleeding and localized spasm at the injection site (usually the femoral artery) can cause occlusion of arterial flow in the affected extremity.

Doppler ultrasound

A noninvasive test, Doppler imaging can accurately detect atheromatous plaques within the carotid arteries. The Doppler ultrasonic probe is placed over the common carotid artery and moved to the bifurcation of the internal and external carotid arteries to determine lumen patency.

Digital subtraction angiography

This procedure uses computer imaging to enhance arteriographic images of extracranial blood vessels. Pictures of the vessels are taken before and after injection of contrast material into the antecubital vein. The images taken without contrast are then "subtracted" from the images taken with contrast and the vessels are more clearly visualized.

Electroencephalography

With this test, electrodes attached to the patient's scalp detect electrical impulses generated by the brain cells. Lead wires then transmit these impulses to an electroencephalographic machine, which translates them into waveforms. Altered waveforms occur with seizures, hypoxia, hypothermia, hypoglycemia, hypotension, and toxic or metabolic encephalopathy.

Evoked potential studies

Evoked potential studies record the brain's responses to external visual, auditory, or somatic stimuli. The tests are used to evaluate the effects of multiple sclerosis, to detect brain stem lesions, and to evaluate the extent of damage produced by demyelinating spinal cord lesions.

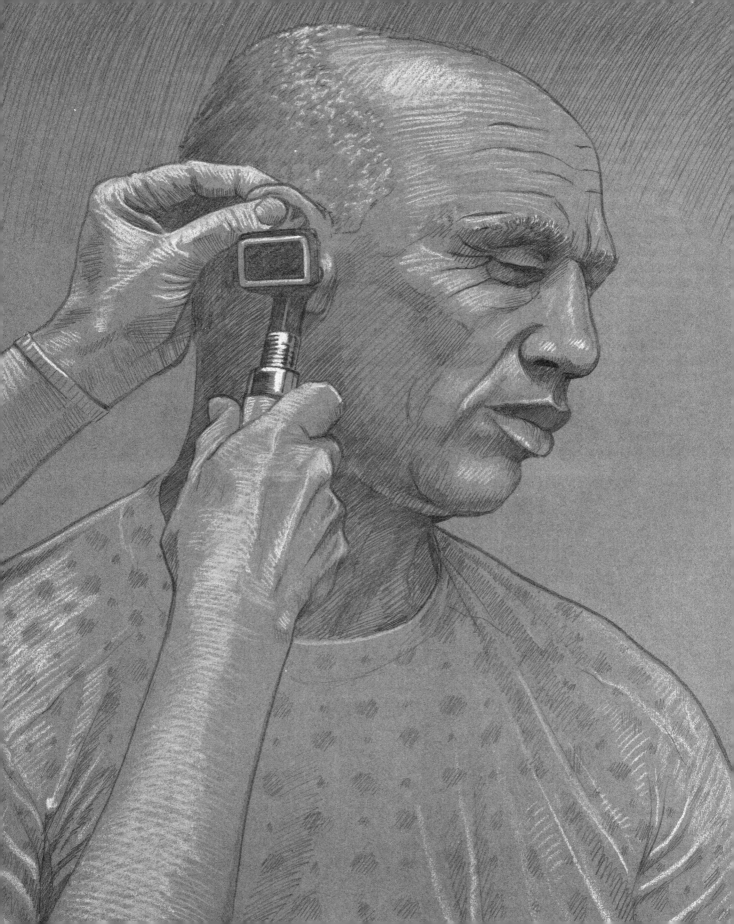

CHAPTER

Eyes, ears, nose, and throat

Because roughly 70% of all sensory information reaches the brain through the eyes, visual disorders can interfere with a patient's ability to function independently, perceive meaning in the world, and enjoy aesthetic pleasure. Disorders of the ears, nose, and throat can cause a patient considerable pain and severely impair his ability to communicate. Thus, when a patient complains of a specific problem or when you're performing a complete assessment, you need to carefully evaluate one or all of these important structures.

In this chapter, you'll find pertinent reviews of the anatomy and physiology of the eyes, ears, nose, and throat. Then come sections describing how to conduct the health history and perform the physical examination. To help you interpret your assessment findings, the chapter also covers common abnormal findings for the eyes, ears, nose, and throat. Finally, it identifies pertinent diagnostic tests that may be performed after you've analyzed your assessment findings.

ANATOMY

Structures of the eye

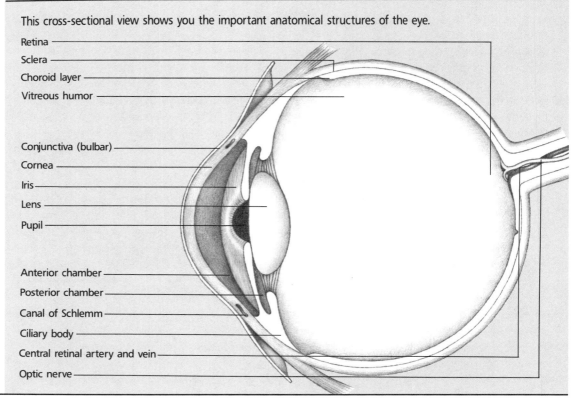

This cross-sectional view shows you the important anatomical structures of the eye.

Retina
Sclera
Choroid layer
Vitreous humor

Conjunctiva (bulbar)
Cornea
Iris
Lens
Pupil

Anterior chamber
Posterior chamber
Canal of Schlemm
Ciliary body
Central retinal artery and vein
Optic nerve

Eyes

Although fewer people lose their sight from infections or injuries today than in the past, the overall incidence of blindness is rising as the population ages. The primary causes of vision loss include diabetic retinopathy, glaucoma, cataracts, and macular degeneration—conditions that occur more frequently in elderly patients. Other conditions that don't cause blindness (such as strabismus, amblyopia, and refractory errors) may limit a person's ability to function.

By thoroughly assessing your patient's eyes and vision and then analyzing your findings, you may identify one of these conditions. In many cases, your early detection can lead to successful, sight-saving treatment.

Anatomy and physiology

The eyes are delicate sensory organs equipped with a number of protective structures. The bony orbits, eyelids (palpebrae), lashes (cilia), and lacrimal apparatus all protect the eyes against injury, dust, and foreign agents.

Bony orbits

The bony orbits hold the eyes in place and protect them from injury. These orbits have four walls (medial, lateral, roof, and floor) that partially surround the maxillary sinuses, the frontal lobe, and the lateral wall of the nose. (See *Structures of the eye*.)

Eyelids and lacrimal apparatus

Normally, the open eyelid covers a small part

of the iris and doesn't cover the pupil. Eyelashes are attached to the lid margins. The area between the top and bottom eyelids is known as the palpebral fissure.

The palpebral conjunctiva — a thin, transparent membrane — lines the undersurface of the eyelid. The bulbar conjunctiva lines the anterior surface of the eyeball up to the edge of the cornea.

The series of ducts and glands that secrete and drain tears is known as the lacrimal apparatus. Located in the superior, lateral portion of each orbit, the lacrimal gland is about the size of an almond. A series of lacrimal ducts allow tears (or lacrimal fluid) to flow onto the conjunctiva, keeping it moist. The lacrimal sac is a canal that drains tears away from the eyes, into the nasolacrimal duct, and then into the nose.

Tears help to protect the eye by washing away foreign matter and acting as a lubricant. Tears are bacteriostatic, protecting the eye from infection.

Layers of the eyeball

An adult's eyeball is about 1″ (2.5 cm) in diameter, with only one-sixth visible. The eyeball consists of three layers: the fibrous tunic, the vascular tunic, and the retina.

Fibrous tunic

Covering the outer eyeball, the fibrous tunic is divided into two regions: the sclera and the cornea. The sclera covers the white of the eye, giving the eyeball shape and protecting its inner structures. The cornea, which is rich in nerve endings and sensitive to touch and trauma, protects the iris.

Vascular tunic

The middle layer of the eyeball, the vascular tunic consists of three structures: the choroid, the ciliary body, and the iris. The choroid lines most of the inner sclera. This structure has many pigment cells that absorb light as it enters the eye, preventing it from being lost by reflection. The choroid's rich blood supply helps nourish the retina.

The anterior portion of the choroid forms the ciliary body. Muscles within this structure

alter the shape of the lens, enabling the lens to accommodate for near and far vision.

Located between the lens and the cornea, the iris consists of smooth-muscle fiber. Its color is determined by the amount and distribution of melanin. The iris's smooth-muscle cells regulate the amount of light that enters the eye by controlling pupil size.

Behind the pupil and iris lies the lens. Consisting of layers of protein fibers, the lens normally is transparent. The lens and cornea work together to allow light to bend so that it can be focused on the retina and produce clear vision. The lens's ability to change shape also helps to accomplish this.

Retina

The eye's innermost layer, the retina receives visual stimuli, partially analyzes the images, and sends the information to the brain for interpretation. (See *How an image is formed,* page 124.) Ten inner retinal layers contain photoreceptor neurons known as rods and cones. Rods, located in the periphery, enable vision in dim light and discrimination between shades of dark and light as well as identification of shapes and movement. Cones provide detailed color vision and visual acuity and are densely concentrated in the central fovea, a small depression in the macula lutea.

The macula lutea, most often simply called the macula, is a yellow spot in the center of the retina. The central fovea and its concentration of cones make the macula the site of sharpest vision. The axons of the photoreceptor neurons exit the eye posteriorly at the optic disk, which is known as the blind spot because this part of the retina has no neuroreceptors for light.

Chambers

The interior of the eye contains three chambers: anterior, posterior, and vitreous. The anterior and posterior chambers are filled with aqueous humor and known collectively as the aqueous chamber. This chamber is located in front of the lens. The aqueous humor is secreted into the posterior chamber and circulates through the anterior chamber. It drains through the canal of Schlemm, which leads to

How an image is formed

A visual image is created when light is reflected off an object and focused on the retina after passing through the cornea, aqueous humor, lens, and vitreous humor. Nerve impulses travel from the retina through the optic nerve and optic tract to the visual cortex of the occipital lobe, which then interprets the image.

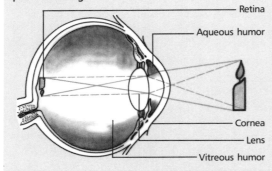

the vascular system. The amount of aqueous humor in circulation is controlled so that intraocular pressure is maintained. This pressure keeps the retina smooth, providing clear visual images.

The vitreous chamber, which occupies four-fifths of the eyeball, is located behind the lens. The vitreous humor, a gelatinous substance that fills the chamber, helps give the eyeball its shape and enables it to resist extraocular pressure.

Extraocular muscles

Six extraocular muscles, which are innervated by cranial nerves (CNs), control the movements of each eye. The coordinated action of these muscles allows the eyes to move in tandem, ensuring clear vision. The following list identifies the function of the six muscles:
• superior rectus—moves the eye upward and inward
• inferior rectus—moves the eye downward and outward
• lateral rectus—moves the eye outward
• medial rectus—moves the eye inward
• superior oblique—moves the eye downward and inward
• inferior oblique—moves the eye upward and outward.

Health history

Regardless of the patient's diagnosis and chief complaint, you should ask him about his eyes and vision. Remember, poor vision may contribute to a patient's signs and symptoms and interfere with his ability to comply with treatment. Of course, if the patient's chief complaint is related to his eyes or vision, you'll focus on his immediate problem.

Chief complaint

The most common chief complaints of the eye include diplopia, visual floaters, vision loss, and eye pain. To investigate these or any chief complaints, ask the patient relevant questions about such particulars as onset, duration, and severity. Also ask what precipitates the symptom, what makes it worse, and what makes it better. For more information on exploring the chief complaint, see Chapter 3.

Medical history

Does the patient wear corrective lenses? If so, when was his last eye examination? An elderly patient or one with limited income or mobility may not undergo regular eye examinations.

Ask the patient if he's ever had a central nervous system disorder, such as a cerebrovascular accident (CVA). A CVA may cause visual disturbances, such as double vision or blind spots. Paralysis of the oculomotor, trigeminal, or abducens nerve (CN III, V, or VI) may impair extraocular muscle movement.

Does the patient have high blood pressure? If so, how long has it been high? How well is it controlled? Persistent, poorly controlled hypertension can lead to severe hypertensive retinopathy, arteriosclerosis of the retinal vessels, or visual disturbances.

Determine whether the patient has diabetes mellitus. If so, how long has he had it and how well is it controlled? Ask about his usual blood glucose level. Does he see an ophthalmologist regularly? Diabetic retinopathy is the most common cause of blindness in adults.

Certain medications can affect vision, so find out which ones the patient is taking. Digoxin (Lanoxin), for instance, may cause the patient to see yellow halos around bright lights. Be sure you ask about over-the-counter eyedrops and eyewashes, too.

Family history
Find out if the patient's family has a history of early vision loss, retinitis pigmentosa, glaucoma, or cataracts. Such a history may predispose the patient to these conditions.

Activities of daily living
Ask the patient what kind of work he does and what he does for recreation. Are his eyes exposed to chemicals, fumes, flying debris, or infectious agents? If so, does he wear eye protection?

Ask the patient if he drinks alcohol. If so, how much and how often? Some alcoholics may, when regular alcohol supplies aren't available, drink wood alcohol or another type of poisonous alcohol, which can cause blindness.

Does the patient smoke tobacco? If so, how much? How long has he been smoking? Tobacco smoking can accelerate vascular disease and increase the risk of vision damage.

Ask a visually impaired patient how he manages his daily needs. With whom does he live? Does his vision loss interfere with the activities of daily living? Consider whether the patient and his family need help learning to use adaptive devices or need a referral to an agency that helps visually impaired people.

Physical examination

For most of the examination, the patient should be comfortably seated so that when you stand, your eyes are at his eye level. Asking him to sit at the end of an examination table usually accomplishes this. This arrangement will help you to avoid neck and back strain during the examination.

You'll begin your examination by testing the patient's visual acuity, fields of vision, and extraocular muscle function. Then you'll inspect and palpate the external eye. Finally, if appropriate, you'll examine the patient's internal eye, using an ophthalmoscope.

Visual acuity
If the patient can stand, use the standard Snellen chart at a distance of 20' (6 m). If he can't stand, hold a Snellen card 14" (35.6 cm) from his eyes. Ask the patient to read the smallest line possible, first using both eyes and then using each eye individually with the other eye covered. If the patient uses corrective lenses, test him both with and without them.

When measuring visual acuity, the first number you report will always be 20, meaning that vision was tested at 20'. The second number reflects how well the patient sees at 20' compared with a person who has normal vision. For example, a person who has 20/40 vision sees at 20' what a person with normal vision sees at 40' (12 m).

Fields of vision
The test of visual acuity that you just performed evaluates the patient's central retinal function. By testing his fields of vision, you evaluate the function of his outer retina. This examination also tests the function of the optic nerve (CN II).

The normal peripheral range is a circle of about 4' (1.2 m) at a distance of 20" (51 cm) from the eye. Each eye has its own peripheral visual field. With both eyes open, the two fields overlap.

Have the patient cover one eye and look straight ahead with the other. Then hold a finger at the upper edge of his expected visual field and ask him to tell you how many fingers you're holding up. If the patient can't see your finger, slowly move it into the expected visual field, noting the point where he can see it. Now move to the lower edge of the expected visual field, hold up a different number of fingers, and ask the same question. Do the same thing at the left and right borders of his expected visual field. Repeat the test on the

Corneal light reflex test

Ask the patient to look straight ahead while you shine a penlight on the bridge of her nose from a distance of 12″ to 15″ (30.5 to 38 cm). The corneas should reflect the light in exactly the same place in both eyes.

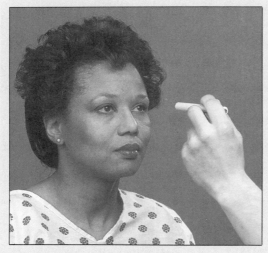

other eye and on both eyes together.

Alternatively, you can test visual fields by using confrontation. With this technique, you bring your finger from outside the patient's expected visual field into the field and ask him to tell you when he can see your finger. Although this technique determines the range of the visual field, it doesn't test the patient's acuity because you don't ask him how many fingers you're using.

Extraocular muscle function

A thorough assessment of the eyes should include an evaluation of the extraocular muscles. To evaluate these muscles, you'll examine the corneal light reflex and assess the cardinal positions of gaze. Depending on your findings, you may also perform the cover-uncover test.

Corneal light reflex

While the patient looks straight ahead, shine a penlight on the bridge of his nose from about

12″ to 15″ (30.5 to 38 cm). The light should fall at the same spot on each cornea. If it doesn't, the eyes aren't being held in the same plane by the extraocular muscles. This finding is most common in patients with strabismus. (See *Corneal light reflex test*.)

Cardinal positions of gaze

This test of coordinated eye movements evaluates the oculomotor, trigeminal, and abducens nerves as well as the extraocular muscles. To perform the test, sit directly in front of the patient and ask him to remain still. Hold a small object, such as a pencil, directly in front of his nose at a distance of about 18″ (46 cm). Ask him to follow the object with his eyes, without moving his head. Then move the object to each of the six cardinal positions, returning it to midpoint after each movement. The patient's eyes should remain parallel as they move. Note any abnormal findings, such as nystagmus or the failure of one eye to follow the object. (See *Testing the cardinal positions of gaze*.)

Cover-uncover test

Typically, you'll use this test only if you detect an abnormality during one of the two previous tests. Have the patient stare at a distant object, perhaps something on the wall on the other side of the room. Then cover one eye and watch for movement in the uncovered eye. Remove the eye cover, again watching for movement.

Repeat the test on the other eye. Any eye movement while covering or uncovering is considered abnormal. Such movement may result from weak or paralyzed extraocular muscles, which in turn may be caused by cranial nerve impairment.

Inspecting the external eye

Observe the patient's face. His eyes should be about one-third of the way down from the scalp line. They also should be about one eye's width apart from each other.

The upper eyelid should cover the top quarter of the iris bilaterally so that the eyes appear alike. Do you note an excessive amount of sclera (lower lid lag)? Or excessive drooping

Testing the cardinal positions of gaze

For this test, you'll move a small object to each of the six cardinal positions of gaze: the left lateral, the left inferior, the right inferior, the right lateral, the right superior, and the left superior. These illustrations show a nurse testing the three left cardinal positions of gaze.

Left lateral

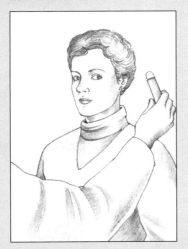

Left inferior

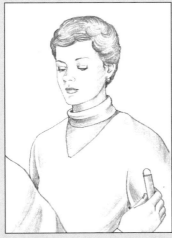

Left superior

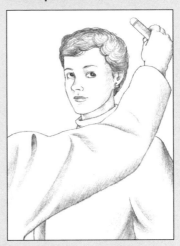

of the upper lid (ptosis)? Do the lids close completely? Note any redness, edema, inflammation, or lesions. Also inspect the eyes for excessive tearing and dryness.

Are the lashes and brows distributed equally? Note areas where hairs are missing and any redness at the follicles.

While wearing gloves, pull the lower eyelid down and inspect the bulbar conjunctiva. It should be clear and shiny. If a foreign body is suspected or the patient complains of pain, raise the upper lid to inspect the palpebral conjunctiva. It should be uniformly pink in White patients, red-orange in Black patients, and yellow-orange in Asian patients. Look for color changes, foreign bodies, and edema. (See *Inspecting the conjunctivae*, page 128.)

Observe the sclera's color, which should be white to buff. In Blacks, you may see flecks of tan. A bluish discoloration may indicate scleral thinning.

Now examine the cornea, shining a pen-

light first from both sides and then from straight ahead. Note whether the cornea is clear and observe for lesions.

Also examine the anterior chamber of the eye, which is bordered anteriorly by the cornea and posteriorly by the iris. The iris should appear flat; the cornea normally is convex. Excess pressure within the eye — such as that caused by acute angle-closure glaucoma — may cause the iris to be pushed forward, making the anterior chamber appear very small.

The irises should be the same size, color, and shape. The pupils should be about one-quarter the size of the irises in normal room light and round. The two pupils should be the same size as well. About one in four persons has asymmetrical pupils without having any kind of disease.

Pupillary response
Now test the pupils for direct and consensual response. In a slightly darkened room, hold a

Inspecting the conjunctivae

Bulbar conjunctiva
Gently evert the lower eyelid with the thumb or index finger of a gloved hand, as shown. Ask the patient to look up, down, left, and right as you examine the bulbar conjunctiva.

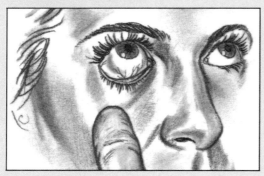

Palpebral conjunctiva
Check the palpebral conjunctiva only if you suspect a foreign body or if the patient complains of eyelid pain. To perform this examination, ask the patient to look down while you gently pull the medial eyelashes forward and upward with your thumb and index finger.

While holding the eyelashes, press on the tarsal border with a cotton-tipped applicator to evert the eyelid, as shown. Hold the lashes against the brow and examine the conjunctiva, which should be pink and unswollen.

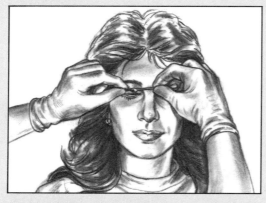

To return the eyelid to its normal position, release the eyelashes and ask the patient to look upward. If this doesn't invert the eyelid, grasp the eyelashes and gently pull them forward.

penlight about 20″ (51 cm) from the patient's eyes and bring the beam of light in from the side. Note the reaction of both the pupil you're testing (direct response) and the untested pupil (consensual response). They should react in the same way. Note any sluggishness or inequality in the response. Repeat the test, bringing the beam in from the other side.

To test the pupils for accommodation, ask the patient to look first at a fixed object in the distance and then to look at an object nearby. The pupils should dilate when he looks at the distant object and constrict when he looks at the near object. The eyes also should converge when focusing on the near object.

Palpation
After telling the patient what you'll be doing, gently palpate his eyelids and note any tenderness or swelling. Then, while he looks down with his eyelids closed, palpate the eyeballs. They should feel firm.

Next, palpate the lacrimal sac by pressing your index finger against the patient's lower orbital rim on the side close to his nose. As you're pressing, examine the punctum for abnormal regurgitation of purulent material or excessive tears, which could indicate blockage of the nasolacrimal duct.

Ophthalmoscopic examination
The ophthalmoscope allows you to directly observe the internal structures of the patient's eye. To see these structures properly, you must adjust the lens disk for near and far objects. Use the positive (black) numbers on the lens disk to focus on near objects, such as the patient's lens, and the negative (red) numbers to focus on distant objects, such as his retina.

Before the examination, have the patient remove his contact lenses or eyeglasses. (Some practitioners don't ask patients to remove contact lenses, but most patients find them uncomfortable during the examination.) Darken the room. This will dilate the patient's pupils, making your examination easier. (See *Promoting patient cooperation*.)

Near structures

Begin by asking the patient to focus on a point beyond you. Warn him that you'll be moving into his visual field and blocking his view. Explain that you'll be shining a bright light into his eye, which may be uncomfortable but isn't dangerous.

With the lens disk set at zero, hold the ophthalmoscope about 12" (30.5 cm) from the patient's eye and slightly lateral to it. Locate the red reflex, a reflection of light off the retina. Its presence indicates a clear cornea and lens. Now move the ophthalmoscope closer to the eye and, using the positive numbers on the lens disk, focus on the lens and anterior chamber. Look for clouding, foreign matter, or opacities. If the lens is opaque—indicating a cataract—completion of the ophthalmoscopic examination may not be possible. (See *Positioning for the ophthalmoscopic examination,* page 130.)

Retina

To examine the retina, turn the dial back to zero. As you rotate the dial, observe the vitreous body for transparency. The first retinal structures you'll see will be the blood vessels. Rotate the dial as needed into the negative numbers to focus on the blood vessels. The arteries will look thinner and brighter than the veins. Follow a vessel along its path toward the nose until you reach the optic disk, where all vessels in the eye originate. Note all arteriovenous (AV) crossings, watching for tapering of veins that might indicate AV nicking.

The optic disk is a creamy pink to yellow-orange structure, slightly concave, with clear borders and a round-to-oval shape. With practice, you'll be able to identify the physiologic cup, a small depression that occupies about one-third of the disk's diameter. Note that the nasal border of the disk may be somewhat blurred. (See *Viewing the optic disk,* page 131.)

Then follow four blood vessels from the optic disk to different peripheral areas so that you completely scan the retina. It should have a uniform color and be free of scars and pigmentation. As you scan, note any AV crossings.

Promoting patient cooperation

When you approach the patient with a bright light, his natural reflex will be to turn away. So warn him beforehand. Also, when you're ready to perform the examination, place one hand on his shoulder. That will remind him to remain still even though you'll be getting extremely close.

Macula

For the last part of this examination, move the light laterally from the optic disk to locate the macula, the most light-sensitive portion of the eye. It will appear as a bright spot of light, free from blood vessels. Your view of it may be fleeting because most patients can't cooperate with the examination once a beam of light falls on the macula. If you can't locate the macula, ask the patient to shift his gaze into the light.

Abnormal findings

During your assessment of the eyes, you may detect several abnormalities, including periorbital edema, ptosis, acute hordeolum, conjunctivitis, cataracts, macular degeneration, diabetic retinopathy, glaucoma, irregular pupil, strabismus, arteriolar narrowing, and AV nicking. (See *Common eye abnormalities,* page 132.)

Periorbital edema

Swelling around the eyes may result from allergies, local inflammation, or fluid-retaining disorders. Crying may also cause such edema.

Ptosis

A drooping upper eyelid may be caused by an interruption in sympathetic innervation to the eyelid, muscle weakness, or damage to the oculomotor nerve.

Acute hordeolum

Also called a stye, this bacterial infection of a sebaceous gland on the eyelid can be painful. The affected area becomes reddened and ten-

Positioning for the ophthalmoscopic examination

Have the patient sit across from you so that his eyes are at your eye level. To start the examination, set the lens disk at zero and hold the ophthalmoscope about 12" to 15" (30.5 to 38 cm) from the patient's eye and slightly lateral to it.

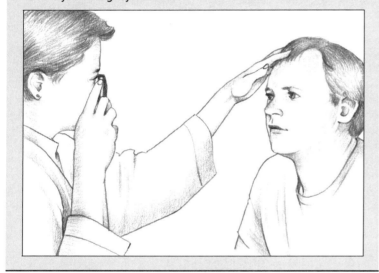

der, and you may observe greenish or yellowish discharge.

Conjunctivitis

With this disorder, the blood vessels of the conjunctiva become inflamed and clearly visible to the unaided eye. The patient may complain of irritation, and you may note discharge that's either clear and watery (usually indicating an allergic or viral cause) or purulent (typically associated with a bacterial infection).

Cataracts

During your examination, you may observe these opacities of the lens. Commonly seen in elderly patients, cataracts are associated with the aging process.

Macular degeneration

The formation of drusen, small raised areas within the macula, is characteristic in the

atrophic form. In the exudative form, subretinal hemorrhage and fluid accumulation are present, leading to retinal scarring.

Diabetic retinopathy

In nonproliferative, or background, retinopathy, microaneurysms and small retinal hemorrhages can be seen in the macular area. In proliferative retinopathy, new blood vessels and fibrous tissue grow along the retinal surface.

Glaucoma

Symptoms of chronic open-angle glaucoma include mild aching in the eyes, loss of peripheral vision, and halos around lights. In acute angle-closure glaucoma, eye pain is unilateral and pupils are moderately dilated and nonreactive to light. This acute form causes blindness in 3 to 5 days if untreated.

Irregular pupil

If an iridectomy has been performed to treat glaucoma, the pupil of the affected eye will be irregular.

Strabismus

In this disorder, the eyes deviate from their normal gazing positions. Strabismus may result from extraocular muscle weakness or paralysis or from an imbalance in ocular muscle tone. Early detection of this abnormality in a child can lead to successful treatment without surgery.

Arteriolar narrowing

Typically, arterioles are between two-thirds and three-fourths the width of veins, and they have a brighter appearance. When these minute arteries narrow, they appear to be about half as wide as the veins. This finding is common in patients who have hypertension.

AV nicking

In AV nicking, a vein appears to taper where the arteriole crosses it. This abnormality is common in patients who have poorly controlled hypertension.

Pertinent diagnostic tests

During your thorough physical examination, you may have detected abnormalities that require further testing. Among the tests that may be ordered are exophthalmometry, tonometry, fluorescein angiography, orbital radiography, orbital computed tomography (CT), and ocular ultrasonography.

Exophthalmometry

This test determines the degree of exophthalmos, the relative forward protrusion of the eye from its orbit. Exophthalmometry helps detect and evaluate thyroid disease, tumors of the eye, and any condition that displaces the eye in the orbit.

The exophthalmometer, a horizontal calibrated bar with movable carriers on both sides, measures the distance from the apex of the cornea to the lateral orbital margin. These carriers hold mirrors inclined at 45-degree angles that reflect both the scale readings and the corneal apex in profile.

Tonometry

An effective screen for the early detection of glaucoma, tonometry also provides an indirect measurement of intraocular pressure. A rise in intraocular pressure may cause the eyeball to harden and become more resistant to extraocular pressure. Indentation tonometry tests this resistance by measuring how deeply a known weight depresses the cornea. Applanation tonometry provides the same information by measuring the amount of force required to flatten a known area of the cornea.

Fluorescein angiography

In this test, rapid-sequence photographs of the fundus are taken with a special camera after an I.V. injection of sodium fluorescein, a contrast medium. Fluorescein angiography documents retinal circulation to help evaluate intraocular abnormalities, such as retinopathy, tumors, and circulatory or inflammatory disorders.

Orbital radiography

Because portions of the eye's orbit are made of

ANATOMY

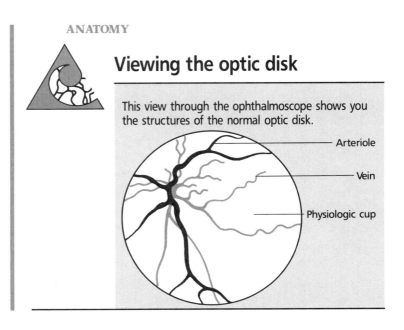

Viewing the optic disk

This view through the ophthalmoscope shows you the structures of the normal optic disk.

- Arteriole
- Vein
- Physiologic cup

thin, easily fractured bone, radiographs of these structures are commonly taken after facial trauma. Radiographs are also useful in diagnosing ocular and orbital pathology. Special radiographic techniques can visualize foreign bodies in the orbit or eye that can't be seen with an ophthalmoscope.

Orbital CT

Detection of abnormalities not readily seen on standard radiographs is possible with orbital CT. The orbital CT scan, a series of tomograms reconstructed by a computer and displayed as anatomic slices on an oscilloscope screen, identifies space-occupying lesions earlier and more accurately than other radiographic techniques. CT also provides three-dimensional images of orbital structures, especially the ocular muscles and optic nerve. With contrast enhancement, it can define ocular tissues and evaluate a patient with a circulatory disorder, hemangioma, or subdural hematoma.

Ocular ultrasonography

In ocular ultrasonography, high-frequency sound waves are transmitted through the eye and measurements are made of their reflections. The procedure is especially helpful in identifying cataracts undetectable by ophthal-

Common eye abnormalities

During an eye examination, you may observe the following disorders.

Periorbital edema

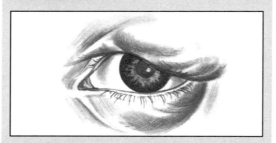

Ptosis

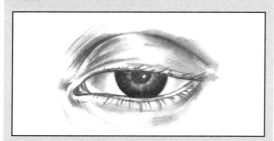

Acute hordeolum

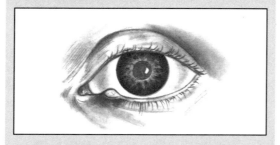

Cataract

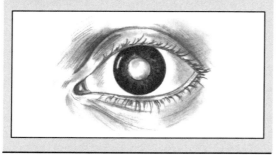

moscopy. Ultrasonography can also diagnose vitreous disorders, a detached retina, and intraocular and orbital lesions. Plus, it can detect the presence of intraocular foreign bodies.

Ears

Most commonly associated with hearing, the ears also maintain the body's sense of equilibrium. Thus, disorders of the ear can affect a patient's ability to communicate as well as his ability to function. When a patient complains of a problem with his ears, his hearing, or his equilibrium, you need to investigate by asking pertinent history questions and performing a thorough physical examination of the ear.

With your accurate nursing assessment, you may identify an infectious disorder early enough to prevent permanent damage. Or you may detect a hearing loss that can be treated medically or surgically, restoring the patient's ability to hear.

Anatomy and physiology

The ear has three parts: external, middle, and inner. The external ear structures transmit sound waves to the tympanic membrane. The vibrations caused by sound waves on the tympanic membrane are then transmitted through the middle ear to the inner ear, where the sensory structures control hearing and balance. (See *Structures of the ear.*)

External ear
Elastic cartilage forms most of the outer ear, making it a flexible appendage. The external structures consist of the ear flap, also known as the auricle or pinna, and the auditory canal. The outer third of this canal has a bony framework.

The tympanic membrane separates the external ear from the middle ear. This pearl gray structure is composed of three layers: fibrous tissue, skin, and a mucous membrane. Its upper portion, the pars flaccida, has little support, whereas the lower portion, the pars tensa, is

ANATOMY

Structures of the ear

Use this illustration to review the structures of the ear.

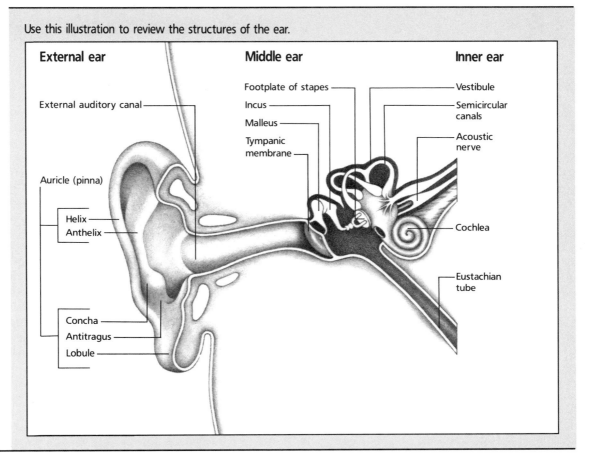

External ear

External auditory canal

Auricle (pinna)

Helix
Anthelix

Concha
Antitragus
Lobule

Middle ear

Footplate of stapes
Incus
Malleus
Tympanic membrane

Inner ear

Vestibule
Semicircular canals
Acoustic nerve
Cochlea
Eustachian tube

---

held taut. The center, or umbo, is attached to the tip of the long process of the malleus on the other side of the tympanic membrane.

Middle ear

A small, air-filled structure, the middle ear performs three vital functions. It transmits sound vibrations across the bony ossicle chain to the inner ear. It protects the auditory apparatus from intense vibrations. And it equalizes the air pressure on both sides of the tympanic membrane to prevent it from rupturing.

The middle ear contains the three small bones of the auditory ossicles: the malleus (hammer), the incus (anvil), and the stapes

(stirrup). These bones are linked like a chain and can move in place in a vibrating motion. As mentioned, the long process of the malleus is attached to the inner surface of the tympanic membrane. The head of the malleus fits into the incus, forming a true joint, so that the two structures move as a single unit.

The incus is attached to the posterior wall of the middle ear and connects with the stapes at the incudostapedial joint—the smallest joint in the body. The proximal end of the stapes fits into the oval window, an opening that joins the middle and inner ear.

The eustachian tube connects the middle ear with the nose and nasopharynx, equalizing air pressure on either side of the tympanic membrane. This prevents sudden atmospheric changes from rupturing the tympanic membrane. Swallowing and yawning open and close the tube, helping to equalize pressures within the ear. The eustachian tube also connects the ear's sterile area to the nasopharynx. A normally functioning eustachian tube keeps the middle ear free of contaminants from the nasopharynx. But upper respiratory tract infections can affect the tube, causing otitis media.

Inner ear
The inner ear consists of closed, fluid-filled spaces within the temporal bone. It contains the bony labyrinth, which includes three connected structures: the vestibule, the semicircular canals, and the cochlea. These structures are lined with the membranous labyrinth, with perilymph fluid circulating between the layers. The vestibule and semicircular canals help maintain equilibrium; the cochlea, a spiral chamber that resembles a snail shell, is the organ of hearing. The organ of Corti, also part of this membranous labyrinth, contains hair cells that act as receptors of auditory sensations.

Hearing process
Sound waves that reach the external ear are directed into the auditory canal, where they cause a chain reaction among the structures of the middle and inner ear. First, the tympanic membrane begins to vibrate. These vibrations are continued in the malleus, picked up by the incus, and transmitted to the stapes. The stapes then moves the oval window in and out, increasing the pressure in the fluid that circulates through the cochlea and stimulating the hair cells of the organ of Corti. Finally, the cochlear branch of the acoustic nerve transmits the vibrations to the temporal lobe of the cerebral cortex where the brain interprets the sound.

Equilibrium
Within the semicircular canals, endolymph fluid bathes the cristae, which alert the brain to rotational movements. When a person moves, hair cells within the cristae also bend, releasing impulses that stimulate the vestibular nerves,

allowing the brain to orient him to motion. When he's stationary, the pressure of gravity on the inner ear hair cells helps him maintain balance. The vestibular portion of the acoustic nerve (CN VIII) also sends this impulse to the brain, which then orients the person to the stationary position and the forces of gravity.

Health history

Begin your health history by asking the patient how well he can hear you. A hearing loss may prevent him from understanding the questions you ask or the information you give him.

If the patient can hear you, have him describe his chief complaint. Then ask about his medical history, family history, and activities of daily living.

Chief complaint
The most common chief complaints associated with the ear are hearing loss, tinnitus, pain, discharge, and dizziness. Whereas hearing loss and tinnitus typically indicate long-term problems, pain, discharge, and dizziness usually point to short-term conditions. To investigate the patient's chief complaint, ask relevant questions about such particulars as onset, duration, and severity. Also ask what precipitates the symptom, what makes it worse, and what makes it better. For more information on exploring the chief complaint, see Chapter 3.

Medical history
Ask the patient if he's ever had problems with his ears before. Has he been ill recently? Does he have a chronic disorder? Diabetes can cause ear infections. Hypothyroidism can cause reversible hearing loss. Hypertension occasionally causes high-pitched tinnitus. If the patient has one of these disorders, ask about his medical regimen, including treatments and medications.

Note any allergies the patient has. Serous otitis media is common in people who have environmental allergies, seasonal allergies, or both. Allergic reactions to hair dyes, cosmetics, and other personal care products can cause external otitis.

Family history

Ask the patient about the health of his immediate family. Make sure you ask if anyone in the family has a hearing disorder.

Activities of daily living

Ask the patient to describe his work environment and his recreational activities. Does he attend rock concerts? Often, such factors contribute to hearing disorders. Ask about his diet, exercise routine, and oral hygiene. Find out if he smokes.

Physical examination

You'll begin your examination by observing the patient's ears, noting characteristics such as position and symmetry. Next, you'll examine his external auditory canal and tympanic membrane, using the otoscope. Then, you'll conduct several tests of the patient's hearing.

Throughout the examination, you can also evaluate the patient's equilibrium. Unless he's bedridden, you can observe his balance as he moves to the examination table or in and out of bed.

Inspecting the ears

Observe the position of the ears. The top of the ear should line up with the outer corner of the eye. Low-set ears commonly accompany congenital disorders, including congenital kidney problems. The ears should look symmetrical, and the angle of attachment should be no more than 10 degrees.

Check the auricle for lesions and redness. Inspect and palpate the mastoid area, noting any tenderness, redness, or warmth. Manipulate the auricle, noting any discomfort—a common finding in external otitis. Finally, inspect the opening of the ear canal, noting any discharge, redness, or odor.

Otoscopic examination

Perform an otoscopic examination to assess the external auditory canal, tympanic membrane, and malleus. Before inserting the speculum into the patient's ear, check the canal opening for foreign particles or discharge. Palpate the tra-

Using the otoscope

Before inserting the speculum into the ear, straighten the canal by grasping the auricle and pulling it up and back, as shown.

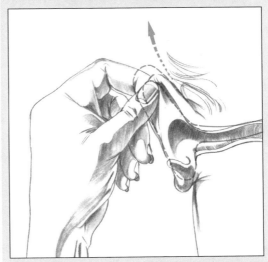

To examine the ear's external canal, hold the otoscope as shown below, with the handle parallel to the patient's head. Hold the otoscope firmly against his head to prevent hitting the canal with the speculum.

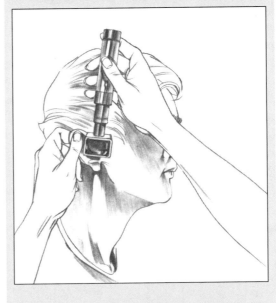

Weber's test: Positioning the tuning fork

With the tuning fork vibrating lightly, position it on the patient's forehead at the midline, as shown. As an alternative, you can place the tuning fork on the top of the patient's head.

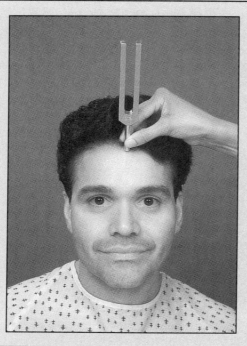

gus and pull up the auricle. If this area is tender, don't insert the speculum. The patient may have external otitis, and inserting the speculum could be painful. Inspect the external auditory canal and the tympanic membrane before proceeding.

After you've determined that inserting the otoscope is safe, tilt the patient's head toward the ear you'll be assessing. Straighten the canal by grasping the superior posterior auricle with your thumb and index finger and pulling it up and back. Each ear canal is shaped differently; you'll have to vary the angle of the speculum until you can see the tympanic membrane. (See *Using the otoscope,* page 135.)

External auditory canal
Hold the otoscope with the handle parallel to the patient's head and the speculum at his ear. Hold the otoscope firmly against his head to prevent any jerking against the external canal. Insert the speculum to about one-third its

length when inspecting the canal. Because the inner two-thirds of the ear canal is sensitive to pressure, you must insert the speculum gently. Usually, the canal will contain varying amounts of hair and cerumen. Note the color of the cerumen—old cerumen is usually dry and grayish brown. In the distal third of the canal, you'll see hair follicles and sebaceous and ceruminous glands. The external canal should be free from inflammation and scaling.

Excessive cerumen can conceal the tympanic membrane and contribute to conductive hearing loss. If a large, firm plug of cerumen obstructs your view of the tympanic membrane, don't try to remove it with an instrument—you could cause the patient great pain, and you might not be able to get the cerumen out. Rather, remove a cerumen impaction by using ceruminolytic drops and a warm water irrigation. You may remove a small amount of soft cerumen with an ear curette.

Tympanic membrane and malleus
For a complete view of the tympanic membrane, carefully rotate the speculum. The tympanic membrane should be pearl gray and glistening, with the annulus white and denser than the rest of the membrane. Look for bulging, retraction, or perforations at the periphery.

Then check the light reflex. If the tympanic membrane is correctly positioned, a bright cone of light will be clearly visible between the 4 and 6 o'clock positions in the right ear and between the 6 and 8 o'clock positions in the left ear. If the cone of light is displaced or absent, the patient's tympanic membrane may be bulging, retracted, or inflamed.

Next, look for the bony landmarks. The malleus will appear as a dense, white streak at the 12 o'clock position. At the top of the light reflex, you will find the umbo, the inferior point of the malleus.

Hearing tests
Evaluate the patient's hearing using qualitative tests. Start with two simple tests: the watch-tick test and the whisper-check test. These are gross measures of your patient's ability to hear. If he has a hearing loss, you may already have noticed it in conversation. If you haven't, these

Rinne test: Positioning the tuning fork

After striking it against your hand, hold the tuning fork behind the patient's ear, as shown.

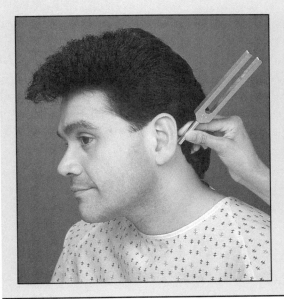

When your patient tells you the tone has stopped, move the still-vibrating tuning fork to the opening of his ear, as shown.

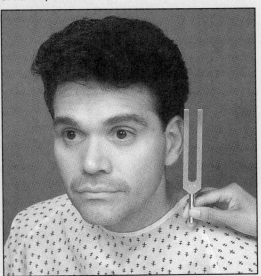

tests may detect a problem, and you can recommend further testing. You may use Weber's test and the Rinne test to assist in determining which type of hearing loss the patient has.

Watch-tick test
Hold a ticking watch at the patient's ear and slowly move it away. Note the distance at which he can no longer hear the ticking.

Whisper-check test
Ask the patient to cover the ear you're not testing. Then stand 1' to 2' (0.3 to 0.6 m) away where he can't see you and whisper a common two-syllable word, such as "baseball" or "airplane." If the patient can't hear you, move closer and repeat the word. Note the distance at which the patient can hear you. If he can't hear a softly whispered word at any distance, use a louder whisper. If necessary, use a normal or loud voice.

Weber's test
If you've detected a hearing deficit, you can evaluate bone conduction using Weber's test. To do so, obtain a tuning fork that's within the frequency of normal human speech (512 cycles/second). Lightly strike it against your hand and place it on the patient's forehead at the midline or on the top of his head. (See *Weber's test: Positioning the tuning fork*.)

If the patient hears the tone equally well in both ears, record this normal finding as a negative Weber's test. If he hears the tone better in one ear, record the result as right or left lateralization. With this abnormality, the tone actually sounds louder in the ear with more hearing loss because the bone conducts the tone to this ear. Because the unaffected ear picks up other sounds, it doesn't hear the tone as clearly.

Characteristics of hearing loss

Use this chart to review the causes, types, characteristics, and associated signs and symptoms of hearing loss.

CAUSE	TYPE	ONSET (SUDDEN OR GRADUAL)	LOCATION (UNILATERAL OR BILATERAL)	ASSOCIATED SIGNS AND SYMPTOMS
EXTERNAL EAR				
Cerumen impaction	Conductive	Either	Either	Itching
Foreign body	Conductive	Sudden	Unilateral	Discharge
External otitis	Conductive	Sudden	Unilateral	Pain, discharge
MIDDLE EAR				
Serous otitis media	Conductive	Either	Either	Fullness, itching
Acute otitis media	Conductive	Sudden	Either	Pain, fever, upper respiratory tract infection symptoms
Perforated tympanic membrane	Conductive	Sudden	Either	Trauma, discharge
INNER EAR				
Presbycusis	Sensorineural	Gradual	Bilateral	None
Drug-induced loss	Sensorineural	Either	Bilateral	Tinnitus, other adverse drug effects
Ménière's syndrome	Sensorineural	Sudden	Unilateral	Dizziness
Acoustic neuroma	Sensorineural	Gradual	Unilateral	Vertigo

Rinne test
The Rinne test compares air conduction of sound with bone conduction of sound. To perform the test, strike the tuning fork against your hand and then place it over the mastoid process. Ask the patient to tell you when the tone stops. Note the time in seconds.

Immediately, move the vibrating tuning fork to the opening of the ear without touching the ear. (See *Rinne test: Positioning the tuning fork,* page 137.) Ask the patient if he can hear the tone. If he can, have him tell you when it stops. Normally, the patient will hear the air-conducted tone twice as long as the bone-conducted tone. If the patient has a conductive hearing loss, he'll hear the bone-conducted tone as long as or longer than the air-conducted tone. Document this as a negative Rinne test.

Abnormal findings

During the otoscopic examination, you may detect abnormalities of the patient's internal ear. You'll detect hearing loss informally through conversation with the patient as well as from the more formal tests you administer.

Internal ear abnormalities
Your otoscopic examination may reveal signs of these common conditions: a perforated tympanic membrane, acute otitis media, and infectious myringitis.

Perforated tympanic membrane
With this condition, you'll usually see a hole in the tympanic membrane surrounded by reddened tissue. You may also see discharge draining through the perforated area. Typically, this abnormality results from a middle ear infection.

Acute otitis media

More common in children than in adults, acute otitis media causes the tympanic membrane to bulge and become inflamed. The patient may also have an earache, a fever, and hearing loss.

Infectious myringitis

A patient may develop this disorder after having acute otitis media or an upper respiratory tract infection. Infectious myringitis causes inflammation and hemorrhage. You may also see fluid leaking into the distal end of the external ear canal and the tympanic membrane.

Hearing loss

Hearing loss can be classified as conductive or sensorineural. Conductive hearing loss results from abnormal function of the external or middle ear, resulting in impaired transmission of sound to the inner ear. In sensorineural hearing loss, there is a problem with auditory nerve conduction or inner ear function. (See *Characteristics of hearing loss*.)

Conductive hearing loss

Several factors can interfere with the ear's ability to conduct sound waves. The ear canal may be obstructed by a cerumen impaction, foreign body, or polyp. Otitis media can cause a thickening of the fluid in the middle ear, which interferes with the vibrations that transmit sound. Otosclerosis, or the sclerosing of the bones within the middle ear, also interferes with the transmission of sound vibrations. A disruption of the middle ear's bony chain may also result from trauma.

Sensorineural hearing loss

Sensorineural hearing loss usually results from the loss of hair cells in the organ of Corti. In elderly people, presbycusis is a common cause of this type of loss. Hearing loss can also result from trauma to the hair cells caused by loud noise or ototoxicity. Drug toxicity can cause a rapid loss of hearing. The medication must be discontinued as soon as the hearing loss is detected. Drugs that may affect hearing include aspirin, aminoglycosides, loop diuretics, and several chemotherapeutic agents, including cisplatin.

Pertinent diagnostic tests

When the hearing tests you conducted during the physical examination reveal a hearing loss, you may need to refer the patient for further tests. These may include pure tone audiometry, electronystagmography, and site-of-lesion tests.

Pure tone audiometry

This test should be used for anyone who needs quantitative hearing assessment. Using an audiometer, the examiner will obtain a record of the lowest intensity levels at which a patient can hear a set of tones.

Electronystagmography

This battery of tests can identify the causes of dizziness, vertigo, or tinnitus, or help diagnose unilateral hearing losses of unknown origin. The process can also determine the presence and cause of a lesion.

Using a variety of techniques, electronystagmography measures nystagmus, or the involuntary back-and-forth movements of the eye. The tests used in electronystagmography include calibration, gaze, pendulum, tracking, optokinetics, positional methods, and caloric tests.

Site-of-lesion tests

These tests should be given when the patient's history or a pure tone audiogram suggests that he has a lesion. If the patient has trouble understanding you, and the difficulty is disproportionate to the amount of his pure tone loss, site-of-lesion tests may be necessary. A patient with dizziness, tinnitus, or sudden or fluctuating hearing loss may also require these tests.

For the tests, the examiner uses an audiometer, and the patient wears earphones. Although the site-of-lesion test battery can't diagnose a disorder by itself, it can suggest the location and extent of damage to the auditory system.

Nose and throat

The sensory organ of smell, the nose also plays an important role in the respiratory system, as

ANATOMY

Structures of the nose, sinuses, and throat

These three illustrations show you the key structures of the nose, sinuses, and throat.

Nose

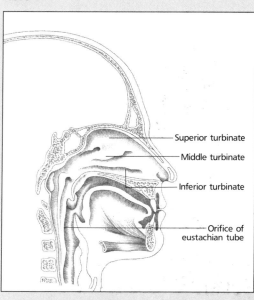

- Superior turbinate
- Middle turbinate
- Inferior turbinate
- Orifice of eustachian tube

Sinuses

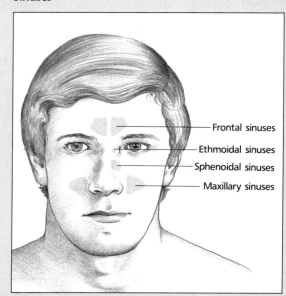

- Frontal sinuses
- Ethmoidal sinuses
- Sphenoidal sinuses
- Maxillary sinuses

it filters, warms, and humidifies inhaled air. The throat, of course, acts as part of both the respiratory and the GI systems, allowing air to pass into the larynx and food to pass into the esophagus.

Whether you're investigating a specific complaint or performing a complete nursing assessment, you need to evaluate these structures thoroughly. Frequently, when you assess the nose and throat, you'll also assess the paranasal sinuses and the thyroid gland.

Anatomy and physiology

The nose and sinuses are lined with a mucous membrane that continues into the throat and throughout the respiratory system. Located in

the neck, the thyroid gland is part of the endocrine system.

Nose
The lower two-thirds of the external nose consists of flexible cartilage; the upper third is rigid bone. Posteriorly, the internal nose merges with the pharynx; anteriorly, it merges with the external nose. The internal and external nose are divided vertically by the nasal septum.

Air entering the nose passes through the vestibule, which is lined with coarse hairs that help filter out large dust particles. The olfactory receptors lie above the vestibule in the roof of the nasal cavity and the upper third of the septum. Known as the olfactory region, this area is rich in capillaries and mucus-producing goblet cells that help heat, moisten,

Mouth and throat

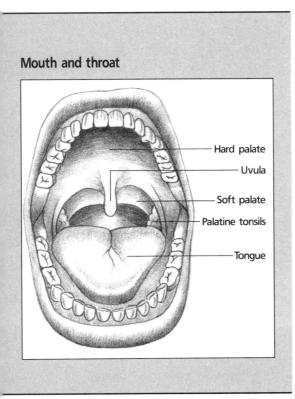

- Hard palate
- Uvula
- Soft palate
- Palatine tonsils
- Tongue

and further clean inhaled air. (See *Structures of the nose, sinuses, and throat*.)

Sinuses
Four pairs of paranasal sinuses open into the internal nose. The largest pair, the maxillary sinuses lie within the maxilla. The smaller ethmoidal sinuses are located between the orbits and the upper nasal cavity. The frontal sinuses lie within the frontal bone, whereas the sphenoidal sinuses lie within the sphenoid bone. The small openings between the sinuses and the nasal cavity can easily become obstructed because they're lined with mucous membrane that can become inflamed and swollen.

Throat
The throat, or pharynx, is divided into the nasopharynx, the oropharynx, and the laryngopharynx. Located within the throat are the hard and soft palate, the uvula, and the tonsils. The mucous membrane lining the throat normally is bright pink to light red.

Thyroid gland
The thyroid lies in the anterior neck, just below the larynx. Its two cone-shaped lobes are located on either side of the trachea and have a connecting isthmus inferior to the cricoid cartilage, which gives the gland its butterfly shape. The outer borders of the two thyroid lobes are covered by the sternocleidomastoid muscle.

The largest endocrine gland, the thyroid produces the hormones triiodothyronine (T_3) and thyroxine (T_4), which affect the metabolic reactions of every cell in the body. (See *Thyroid gland,* page 142.)

Health history

When investigating a problem related to the nose or throat, you'll conduct a fairly brief health history. After exploring the chief complaint itself, ask pertinent questions about the patient's medical history, psychosocial history, and activities of daily living.

Chief complaint
The most common chief complaints of the nose and throat include nasal stuffiness and discharge, epistaxis, and throat pain. To investigate these or any chief complaint, ask the patient relevant questions about such particulars as onset, duration, and severity. Also ask what precipitates the symptom, what makes it worse, and what makes it better. For more information on exploring the chief complaint, see Chapter 3.

Medical history
Ask the patient if he has any allergies. Environmental allergies can cause nasal stuffiness and discharge, limiting the passage of air. Stagnant nasal discharge acts as a culture medium, leading to sinusitis and other infections.

Depending on the patient's complaint and age, ask if he was ever treated with radiation to shrink enlarged tonsils. During the 1940s

ANATOMY

Thyroid gland

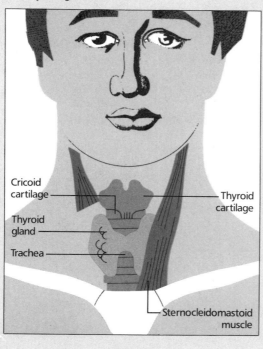

This illustration shows the structure and location of the thyroid gland.

Cricoid cartilage

Thyroid cartilage

Thyroid gland

Trachea

Sternocleidomastoid muscle

and 1950s, this was a common treatment. Patients who were treated in this manner are now at high risk for thyroid cancer and need regular evaluation for signs of this problem.

As appropriate, ask about changes in the way the patient tolerates hot and cold weather. Hyperthyroidism is associated with heat intolerance. Hypothyroidism, on the other hand, is associated with poor cold tolerance; the patient may become hypothermic if he's in a cold environment for a prolonged period.

Ask if the patient has noticed any skipped heartbeats or breathing difficulty. Hyperthyroidism may cause premature ventricular contractions or atrial fibrillation. In extreme cases of hypothyroidism, bradycardia with accompanying dyspnea may result from low cardiac output.

Ask women about changes in their menstrual pattern. Hyperthyroidism may produce short periods with scant flow. Hypothyroidism can cause prolonged periods (7 to 8 days) with heavy flow, often without ovulation.

Investigate any unexplained change in weight or appetite. Hyperthyroidism may be responsible for a 5- to 10-lb (2.2- to 4.5-kg) weight loss despite an increase in appetite. Hypothyroidism usually causes a 5- to 10-lb weight gain.

Psychosocial history

Has the patient experienced mood changes recently? Those with hyperthyroidism often are nervous, irritable, and emotionally labile. People with hypothyroidism may feel depressed.

Activities of daily living

Find out whether the patient smokes. Smokers have more frequent and longer-lasting upper respiratory tract infections. Such infections commonly lead to sinus infections.

Ask about any change in the patient's energy level. A patient with hyperthyroidism may experience a high level of nervous energy and have difficulty concentrating on a task. Hypothyroidism leaves a patient with low energy and makes performance of daily tasks difficult.

Has the patient noticed any changes in his sleep patterns? Does he feel rested after sleeping? Hyperthyroidism is associated with sleeping difficulties. Patients with hypothyroidism feel that they need more sleep, yet they feel poorly rested after sleeping.

Physical examination

To examine the nose, you'll use inspection, olfactory function tests, and direct inspection. When you assess the nose, you'll usually examine the sinuses too, using inspection and palpation. Depending on the purpose of your assessment, you may also inspect the patient's throat and palpate his thyroid gland.

Performing direct inspection

This illustration shows the proper placement of the nasal speculum during direct inspection. The inset shows the structures you should be able to see during this examination.

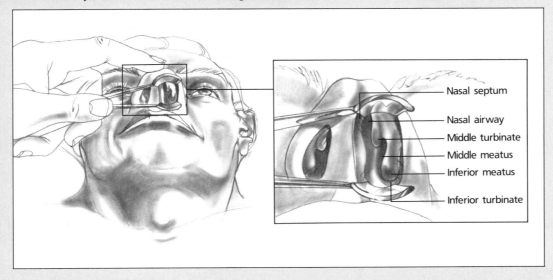

Nasal septum
Nasal airway
Middle turbinate
Middle meatus
Inferior meatus
Inferior turbinate

Nose

Begin by inspecting the nose for deviations in shape and size and for color. If you observe nasal discharge, note the color, quantity, and consistency. Also observe for nasal flaring, a sign of respiratory distress.

To test both nasal patency and olfactory nerve (CN I) function, have the patient block one nostril and inhale a familiar aromatic substance through the open nostril. Appropriate substances include soap, coffee, tobacco, and nutmeg. Some examiners use isopropyl rubbing alcohol (70%), but it can irritate the nasal mucosa, and many patients don't recognize its scent.

Ask the patient to identify the aroma. Then have him block the other nostril and repeat the test, using a different aroma.

When you're ready to inspect the nasal cavities, ask the patient to tilt his head back slightly. Using the light from an otoscope, illuminate the cavities while pushing the tip of the nose up slightly. Note the position of the nasal

septum and any deviation or perforation. Examine the vestibule and turbinates for excessive redness, softness, and discharge. In children and developmentally disabled adults, look for foreign bodies—a common cause of unilateral, purulent nasal discharge.

Direct inspection

To examine the nostrils closely, you may use direct inspection. For this technique, you'll need a nasal speculum and a small flashlight or penlight. (See *Performing direct inspection*.)

Have the patient sit in front of you. Then insert the tip of the closed speculum into one of his nostrils until you reach the point where the blade widens. Slowly open the speculum as wide as you can without causing discomfort. To improve visibility, ask the patient to tilt his head back. Now shine the flashlight in the nostril to illuminate the area.

Note the color and patency of the nostril and the presence of any exudate. The mucosa should be moist, pink to red, and free of le-

Palpating the maxillary sinuses

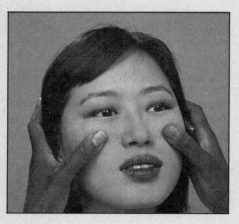

To palpate the maxillary sinuses, place your thumbs, as shown. Then apply gentle pressure.

sions and polyps. Normally, you won't see any drainage, edema, or inflammation of the nasal mucosa, although some tissue enlargement is normal in a pregnant patient.

You should see the choana (posterior air passage), cilia, and the middle and inferior turbinates. Below each turbinate will be a groove, or meatus, where the paranasal sinuses drain.

When you've completed your inspection of one nostril, close the speculum and remove it. Then inspect the other nostril.

Sinuses

You'll be able to examine the frontal and maxillary sinuses, but not the ethmoidal and sphenoidal sinuses. However, if the frontal and maxillary sinuses are infected, you can assume that the ethmoidal and sphenoidal are as well.

Begin by inspecting for swelling around the eyes, especially over the sinus area. Then palpate the frontal and maxillary sinuses for tenderness and warmth.

To palpate the frontal sinuses, place your thumbs above the patient's eyes, just under the bony ridges of the upper orbits. Place your fingertips on his forehead and apply gentle pressure. Then palpate the maxillary sinuses by gently pressing your thumbs (or index and middle fingers) on each side of the nose just be-

low the zygomatic bone (cheekbone). (See *Palpating the maxillary sinuses.*)

Throat

To examine the throat, have the patient open his mouth, stick out his tongue as far as possible, and say "Ah." This should open the pharynx enough to allow you to see the soft palate, uvula, tonsils, and posterior pharynx. Look for redness and exudate—indicators of infection. Also note any unusual breath odors.

Thyroid gland

To locate the thyroid gland, observe the lower third of the patient's anterior neck. Have him extend his neck slightly so you can look for masses or asymmetry in the gland. Then, ask him to take a sip of water, with his neck still slightly extended, while you watch the thyroid rise and fall with the trachea. You should see slight, symmetrical movement. A fixed thyroid lobe may indicate the presence of a mass.

Next, palpate the thyroid gland while standing in front of the patient. Many examiners stand behind the patient to palpate the thyroid, but standing behind someone and pressing on his throat can seem threatening.

Locate the cricoid cartilage first, and then move one hand to each side to palpate the thyroid lobes. The lobes can be difficult to feel because of their location and overlying tissues.

To evaluate the size and texture of the thyroid gland, ask the patient to tilt his head to the right. Then gently displace the thyroid toward the right. Have the patient swallow as you palpate the thyroid's lateral lobes. Displace the thyroid toward the left to examine the left side. (See *Palpating the thyroid gland.*)

Abnormal findings

During your assessment of a patient's nose and throat, you may detect certain abnormalities. Some of the most common include nasal flaring, nasal drainage, paranasal sinus tenderness, pharyngitis, and peritonsillar abscess.

Nasal flaring

In adults, some nasal flaring is normal during

quiet breathing. Nasal flaring is also normal in children. But marked, regular flaring in an adult may be a sign of respiratory distress.

Nasal drainage

The appearance of nasal drainage may help you determine its cause. Bloody drainage may result from frequent nose blowing or from spontaneous, traumatic epistaxis. Thick white or yellow drainage usually occurs with infection. Clear, thin drainage may simply indicate rhinitis. Or it may suggest cerebrospinal fluid leakage from a basilar skull fracture.

Paranasal sinus tenderness

Local sinus tenderness accompanied by fever and nasal drainage suggests acute sinusitis. This form of sinusitis usually involves the frontal or maxillary sinuses.

Pharyngitis

A patient with viral pharyngitis will typically have slight swelling and inflammation of the pharynx. Streptococcal pharyngitis produces severer swelling and inflammation of the pharynx as well as exudate from the tonsils.

With infectious mononucleosis, the patient may have enlargement or tenderness of the auricular, inguinal, and axillary lymph nodes as well as exudative pharyngitis.

Peritonsillar abscess

Also called quinsy, a peritonsillar abscess usually results from acute tonsillitis and causes painful swallowing and potential airway obstruction. In this condition, the streptococcal infection spreads from the tonsils to the surrounding soft tissue.

Pertinent diagnostic tests

When the patient has nasal secretions, sinus tenderness, or throat pain, you may recommend further testing. Tests that may be used include nasopharyngeal culture, paranasal sinus radiography, and throat culture.

Nasopharyngeal culture

This test evaluates nasopharyngeal secretions

Palpating the thyroid gland

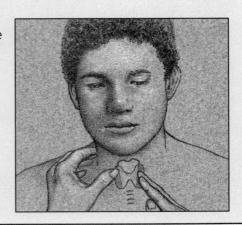

Ask the patient to swallow as you palpate his thyroid, as shown.

for the presence of pathogenic organisms. A Gram-stained smear of the specimen is examined under a microscope, providing a preliminary identification of the organisms present.

Nasopharyngeal culture can also be used to isolate viruses, especially in carriers of influenza virus A or B. Because the laboratory procedure required for virus testing is complex, time-consuming, and costly, these cultures are taken infrequently.

Paranasal sinus radiography

In paranasal sinus radiography, X-rays or gamma rays penetrate the paranasal sinuses and react on specially sensitized film, forming an image of the sinus structure. On this film, the air that normally fills the paranasal sinuses appears black. But fluid in a sinus appears as a cloudy or opaque density, revealing the level of air or fluid. A bone fracture appears as a linear, radiolucent defect. Cysts, polyps, and tumors are visible as soft-tissue masses.

Throat culture

A throat culture is used primarily to isolate and identify group A beta-hemolytic streptococci (most commonly *Streptococcus pyogenes*) to aid in the early treatment of pharyngitis. Throat cultures can also screen for carriers of *Neisseria meningitidis*.

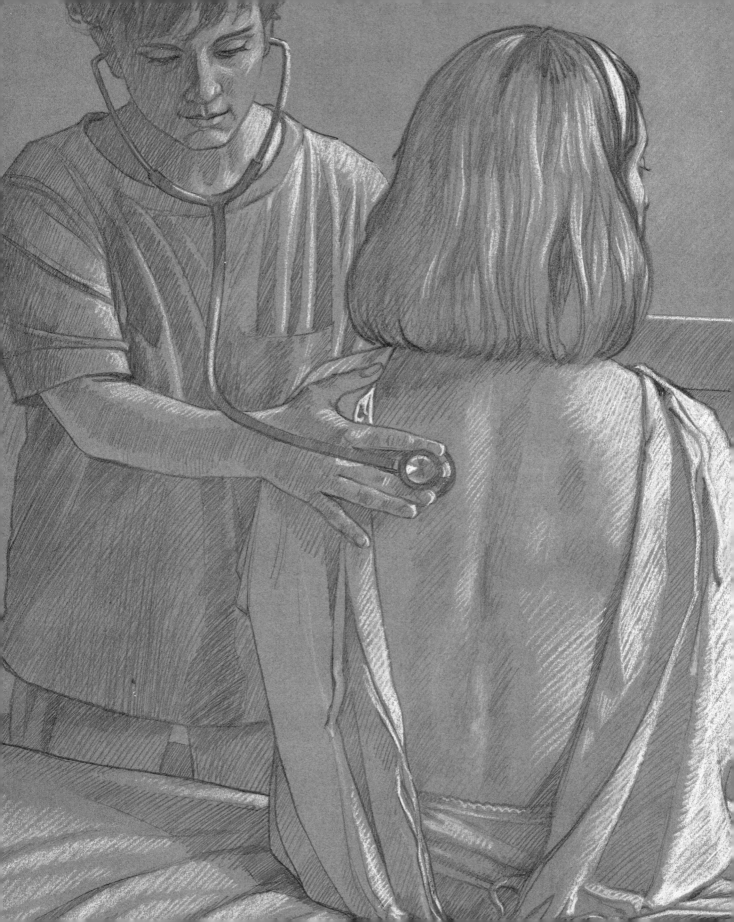

CHAPTER 7

Respiratory system

Any patient, regardless of his primary health problem, can develop respiratory complications. That's because a patient's respiratory status can be compromised by changes in any body system that influence:
• ventilation—movement of air into and out of the lungs
• diffusion—movement of oxygen (O_2) and carbon dioxide (CO_2) between the lungs and the bloodstream
• perfusion—circulation to the lungs, and transport of O_2 and CO_2 in the blood
• the control of normal ventilation.
    To detect either subtle or obvious respiratory changes, you need to perform a systematic assessment. This may be a complete assessment of the respiratory system or an investigation of a patient's chief complaint. The depth of your assessment will depend on several factors, including the patient's primary health problem and his risk of developing respiratory complications.

This chapter, which begins with a review of relevant respiratory anatomy and physiology, will guide you through a respiratory assessment, including the health history and the physical examination. After this information on assessment, you'll find a section designed to help you interpret common abnormal respiratory findings. The chapter then closes with an overview of pertinent diagnostic tests.

Anatomy and physiology

Consisting of the upper and lower airways and the lungs and pleura, the respiratory system performs the vital function of exchanging O_2 and CO_2. This system also helps regulate acid-base balance.

Normal breathing mechanics maintain adequate lung ventilation, while central and peripheral chemoreceptors control the rate and depth of respirations. In response to motor impulses from the respiratory center in the brain stem, the respiratory muscles accomplish the work of breathing.

Changes in a patient's lung function can result in acid-base disturbances, tissue hypoxia, and even sudden death. By using the correct assessment techniques, you can detect changes in a patient's respiratory system early and intervene quickly, perhaps preventing serious complications.

Upper airways

The nose, mouth, nasopharynx, oropharynx, laryngopharynx, and larynx make up the upper airways. These airways protect the lower airways, primarily by warming, humidifying, and filtering inhaled air.

The nose warms and humidifies air entering the nasal cavity, while the mucous membranes and hairs of the nose trap dust and dirt. Air flows from the nasal cavity into the nasopharynx, which contains the pharyngeal tonsils and the eustachian tube openings. The oropharynx (the posterior wall of the mouth) connects the nasopharynx with the laryngopharynx, the

lowest part of the pharynx, which extends down to the esophagus. The larynx contains the vocal cords. The epiglottis bends during swallowing to cover the larynx and protect the trachea from swallowed substances. (See *Upper and lower airways*.)

Lower airways

The lower airways begin at the top of the trachea and end at the alveoli. These airways are divided anatomically into the conducting airways, or the tracheobronchial tree (trachea, primary bronchi, and secondary bronchi) and the acinus (respiratory bronchioles, alveolar sacs, and alveoli). Gas exchange, the primary work of the respiratory system, takes place in the acinus. Mucous membranes line the lower airways, and the constant movement of mucus by ciliary action cleans the airways and carries foreign matter upward for swallowing or expectoration.

Lungs and pleura

The lungs and pleura are enclosed in the thoracic cavity. The right lung has three lobes and is larger than the left lung, which has two lobes. The diaphragm separates the inferior surfaces of the lungs from the abdominal viscera.

The visceral pleura envelops each lung and separates it from the mediastinal structures — the heart and its great vessels, the trachea, the esophagus, and the bronchi. The parietal pleura, which lines the thoracic cavity, covers all the areas that contact the lungs. The area between the visceral and the parietal pleura, known as the pleural space, is only a potential space. It contains a small amount of fluid that acts as a lubricant, allowing the two layers to slide smoothly over each other as the lungs expand and contract with respiration.

Mechanics of breathing

Voluntary and intercostal muscles, working with the diaphragm, produce normal inspira-

ANATOMY

Upper and lower airways

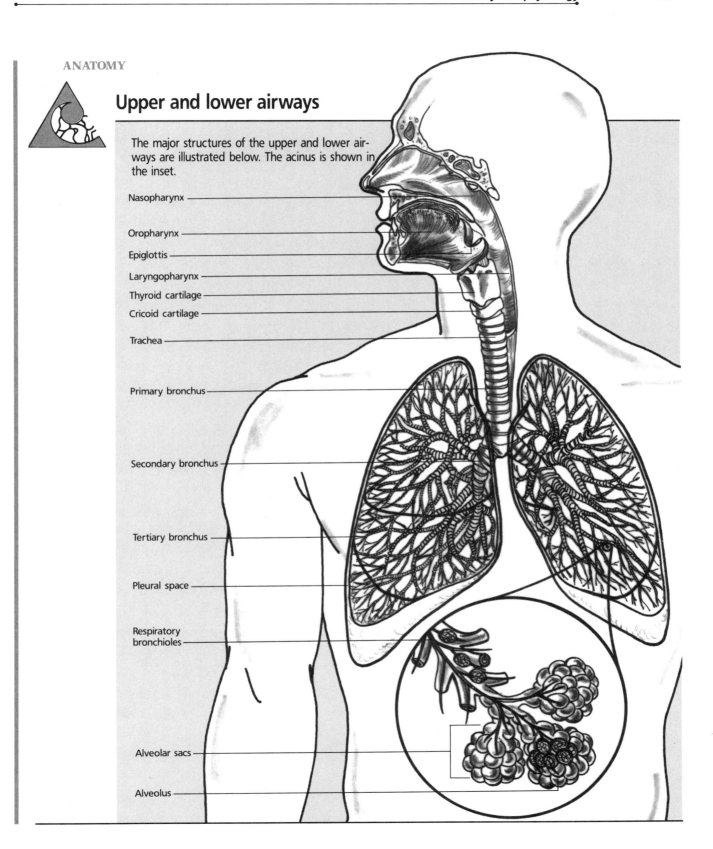

The major structures of the upper and lower airways are illustrated below. The acinus is shown in the inset.

Nasopharynx

Oropharynx

Epiglottis

Laryngopharynx

Thyroid cartilage

Cricoid cartilage

Trachea

Primary bronchus

Secondary bronchus

Tertiary bronchus

Pleural space

Respiratory bronchioles

Alveolar sacs

Alveolus

Understanding the mechanics of breathing

These illustrations show how mechanical forces, such as the movement of intercostal muscles and the diaphragm, produce inspiration and expiration. A plus sign (+) indicates positive pressure; a minus sign (−) indicates negative pressure.

At rest
• Inspiratory muscles relax.
• Atmospheric pressure is maintained in the tracheobronchial tree.
• No air movement occurs.

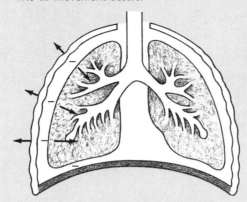

During inspiration
• Inspiratory muscles contract.
• Diaphragm descends.
• Negative alveolar pressure is maintained.
• Air moves into the lungs.

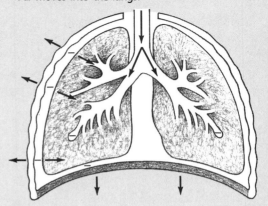

---

tory and expiratory movement of the lungs and chest wall. The lungs' tendency to recoil inward, balanced by the chest wall's tendency to spring outward, creates a subatmospheric pressure in the closed pleural cavity. This pressure, which is about 5 mm Hg below atmospheric pressure (−5 mm Hg), makes lung ventilation (gas volume movement) possible. (See *Understanding the mechanics of breathing*.)

Airflow is opposed by the following three forces of resistance, which can restrict ventilation and add to the work of breathing:
• elastic resistance—caused by the elastic structure of the lungs and the surface tension at the gas-liquid interface in the alveoli
• viscous resistance—exerted by the diaphragm and the abdominal contents. Simply lying flat, especially if the patient is pregnant or obese, can increase viscous resistance and the work of breathing.
• airflow resistance—or resistance to airflow

owing to the dynamics of the tracheobronchial tree. Laminar airflow, in which the air molecules flow in a streamlined manner, offers the least resistance. Random movement of gas molecules produces turbulence, which slows airflow. High flow rates through irregular airways, such as those with mucus present, can cause turbulent airflow. The smaller the airway, the greater the airflow resistance.

Neurologic control of ventilation

The respiratory center is located in the medulla and pons of the brain stem. The medulla regulates the rate and depth of respirations, whereas the pons acts as the pacemaker, regulating the rhythm of breathing.

Central chemoreceptors located in the anterior medulla respond to pH changes in the cerebrospinal fluid (CSF), stimulating the respi-

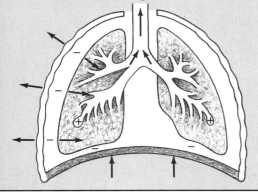

During expiration
- Inspiratory muscles relax, causing lungs to recoil to their resting size and position.
- Diaphragm ascends.
- Positive alveolar pressure is maintained.
- Air moves out of the lungs.

ratory rate as the pH decreases. The pH of the CSF corresponds directly to the CO_2 level in arterial blood. If the CO_2 level increases, the pH of CSF decreases, stimulating ventilation. Peripheral chemoreceptors, located in the aortic and carotid bodies, sense changes in O_2 tension and directly stimulate the central chemoreceptors to increase the rate and depth of respirations.

Gas exchange and transport

Diffusion is the exchange of gases—O_2 and CO_2—between the alveoli and the capillaries. In this process, O_2 diffuses through the alveolar epithelium, the epithelial basement membrane, the capillary basement membrane, and the capillary endothelial membrane. O_2 dissolves in the plasma and passes through the red blood cell (RBC) membrane, where it attaches to hemoglobin.

CO_2 diffuses from the alveolar capillary, where it has been brought from the tissues, into the alveoli. The CO_2 is then exhaled.

Health history

The patient's health history can yield vital clues about the cause of his respiratory problem, his level of functioning, and his health needs. During your history, be sure to note the patient's ability to follow the interview. Does he understand the questions you pose? Is he sleepy or restless? Patients with respiratory problems often have difficulty speaking, so ask questions that can be easily understood and answered, perhaps with one word or by a nod of the head.

If your patient is very tired and short of breath, try to make him more comfortable and allow him to rest. In some cases, you may have to postpone the interview until the patient is able to answer your questions fully.

Chief complaint

The most common chief complaints of the respiratory system include dyspnea, nonproductive cough, productive cough, and chest pain. (See *Quantifying dyspnea*, page 152.) To investigate these or any respiratory chief complaints, ask the patient relevant questions about such particulars as onset, duration, and severity. Also ask what precipitates the symptom, what makes it worse, and what makes it better. For more information on exploring the chief complaint, see Chapter 3.

After you've thoroughly explored the chief complaint, ask the patient about his medical history, family history, psychosocial history, and activities of daily living.

Medical history

Ask the patient if he's had any respiratory problems, such as asthma or tuberculosis. If so, determine which treatments he's received.

ASSESSMENT INSIGHT

Quantifying dyspnea

What one patient considers to be severe shortness of breath may seem mild to another. To make your assessment as objective as possible, ask your patient to briefly describe how various activities affect his dyspnea. Then document his response using this grading system.

Grade 1
Shortness of breath during mild exertion, such as running a short distance or climbing a flight of stairs

Grade 2
Shortness of breath while walking a short distance at a normal pace on level ground

Grade 3
Shortness of breath during a mild daily activity such as shaving or bathing

Grade 4
Shortness of breath while at rest

Grade 5
Shortness of breath when supine

Has the patient been exposed to anyone who has a respiratory disease? Certain respiratory disorders, such as influenza, pneumonia, and other infections, are highly contagious. Does he have allergies that flare up during particular seasons? If so, what causes them?

Does the patient use any treatments, such as over-the-counter drugs and inhalers? If so, he may have built up a tolerance to these drugs. Plus, they may interact with medications the doctor may want to prescribe. When did the patient last have a chest X-ray? A tuberculin skin test?

Family history

Determine whether any member of the patient's family has had emphysema, asthma, respiratory allergies, or tuberculosis. Some patients have familial predispositions to emphysema and allergies. If a family member has had tuberculosis, find out when the patient may have been exposed. This will help you determine the need for a tuberculin skin test.

Psychosocial history

Ask the patient what impact the disorder has had on him and on his family. Is he able to meet family responsibilities? If not, additional stress and family conflict may result, possibly exacerbating his respiratory problems.

Obtain an overview of the patient's family structure and support systems. How have family members and friends reacted to his illness? Does he have someone to rely on in time of need? A patient with chronic respiratory illness requires considerable help and may feel depressed and isolated.

Activities of daily living

Details about the patient's activities of daily living reveal how his respiratory problems affect his life-style. For instance, have his sleeping patterns changed because of breathing problems? Changes in sleep patterns could lead to fatigue, which, in a patient with chronic obstructive pulmonary disease (COPD), could make breathing even more tiring. Does stress at home or work affect his breathing? A patient with asthma may be able to identify an action-reaction cycle that includes stress and dyspnea.

Ask the patient about his current and previous occupations and possible exposure to air pollutants. Certain occupations, such as mining, chemical manufacturing, and working in a smoke-filled office, can expose a patient to respiratory irritants.

If the patient has a chronic respiratory problem, can he afford the medication, equipment, and oxygen required for his treatment? Noncompliance often results from insufficient funds, not a lack of interest or understanding.

Physical examination

Before starting your examination, position the patient so you'll have access to his posterior and anterior chest. If his condition permits, have him sit on the edge of the bed or examination table or on a chair, leaning slightly forward with his arms folded across his chest.

If this isn't possible, place him in semi-Fowler's position for the anterior chest examination. Then ask him to lean forward slightly and use the side rails or mattress for support while you quickly examine his posterior chest. If he can't lean forward, place him in a lateral position or ask another staff member to help him sit up.

Inspection

Quickly observe the patient's overall appearance for signs and symptoms of acute respiratory difficulty. Restlessness, anxiety, or a decreased level of consciousness may indicate hypoxemia (low blood O_2 levels) or hypercapnia (high CO_2 levels in the blood).

Continue your inspection by observing the patient's respiratory rate and pattern. Then examine his head, neck, and shoulders, and his chest, skin, and fingers.

Respiratory rate and pattern

Observe the patient at rest as he breathes naturally and effortlessly. To avoid altering his natural breathing pattern, don't make it obvious that you're counting his respirations. Count an adult's respirations for at least 1 minute. For an infant or a patient with periodic or irregular breathing, monitor the respirations for more than 1 minute to ensure accuracy. Note the duration of any periods of apnea. (The normal respiratory rate is 12 to 20 breaths/minute in adults and as much as 44 breaths/minute in infants.)

Assess the quality of respirations by observing the type and depth of breathing. Remember that men, children, and infants are usually diaphragmatic (abdominal) breathers, as are athletes and singers. Most women are intercostal (chest) breathers.

Head, neck, and shoulders

Examine the patient's mouth, noting the color of the mucous membranes. They should be pale pink to pink. Bluish or gray oral mucosa may indicate central cyanosis, resulting from prolonged hypoxia. Central cyanosis may appear in other highly vascular areas as well: the lips, the conjunctivae, the earlobes, and the tip of the nose.

Observe the neck and shoulders to determine whether the patient is using his accessory muscles—the sternocleidomastoid, scalene, and trapezius muscles—to breathe. Typically, the diaphragm and external intercostal muscles should easily maintain the breathing process. Hypertrophy of any of the accessory muscles may indicate frequent use, although it may be normal in a well-conditioned athlete. Use of accessory muscles as well as pursed-lip breathing, mouth breathing, and nasal flaring may indicate respiratory difficulty.

Chest

Examine the chest for wounds, bruises, scars, rib deformities, and masses. Then observe the shape of the thorax. In an adult, the transverse diameter (side to side) should be greater than the anteroposterior diameter (front to back).

Note the angle between the ribs and the sternum at the point immediately above the xiphoid process. This angle, called the costal angle, should be less than 90 degrees in an adult. If the patient's chest wall is chronically expanded because of intercostal muscle hypertrophy, the costal angle will be wider.

Inspect first the anterior chest and then the posterior chest, for symmetrical movement. Carefully observe the patient's quiet, deep breathing for equal expansion of the chest wall. Be alert for paradoxical movement—the abnormal collapse of part of the chest wall during inspiration, and the abnormal expansion of the same area during expiration. Such movement indicates a loss of normal chest wall function.

Skin and fingers

Since central cyanosis affects all body organs, inspect the patient's skin color to assess the degree of oxygenation. A dusky or bluish skin

Identifying clubbed fingers

Normally, the angle between the nail and the nail base is about 160 degrees, as shown in the first illustration. With clubbed fingers, the angle is greater than 180 degrees, as shown in the second illustration.

Normal fingers

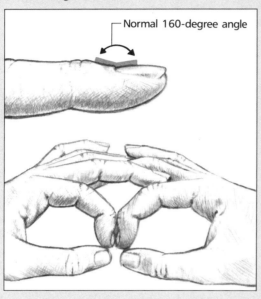

Normal 160-degree angle

Clubbed fingers

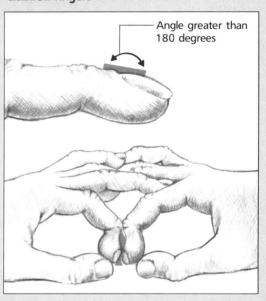

Angle greater than 180 degrees

color may indicate decreased O_2 levels in the arterial blood. For a patient with dark skin, inspect those areas where cyanotic changes would be most apparent: the oral mucous membranes and lips. Facial skin may be pale gray or yellowish brown in dark-skinned cyanotic patients. Check the nail beds in patients of all races.

Peripheral cyanosis results from vasoconstriction, vascular occlusion, or reduced cardiac output. Often seen in patients after exposure to the cold, peripheral cyanosis appears in the nail beds, nose, ears, and fingers. It doesn't affect mucous membranes.

While inspecting the skin, observe for finger clubbing, a sign of chronic tissue hypoxia. Typically, the angle between the fingernail and the point where the nail enters the skin is about 160 degrees. With clubbing, the angle

increases to 180 degrees or more. To confirm clubbing, ask the patient to place the first phalanx of each forefinger together. Normal, concave nail bases will create a small, diamond-shaped space. Clubbed fingers are convex at the nail bases and touch without leaving a space. (See *Identifying clubbed fingers.*)

Palpation

If possible, perform palpation immediately after your inspection. Using the palmar surface of your hands, including the base of your fingers, palpate the anterior and posterior chest. Assess skin temperature and turgor, identify thoracic structures, and evaluate tactile fremitus

(Text continues on page 159.)

Respiratory system and landmarks

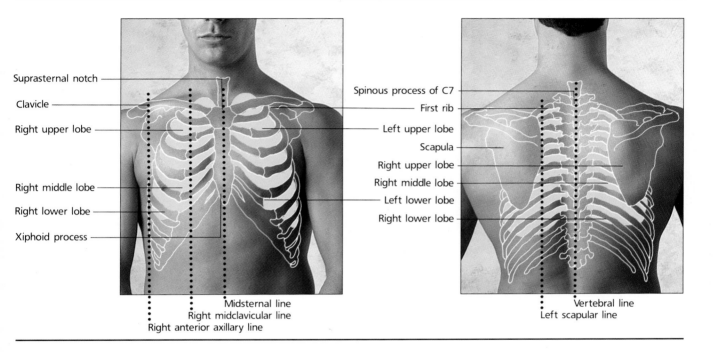

Suprasternal notch

Clavicle

Right upper lobe

Right middle lobe

Right lower lobe

Xiphoid process

Spinous process of C7

First rib

Left upper lobe

Scapula

Right upper lobe

Right middle lobe

Left lower lobe

Right lower lobe

Midsternal line
Right midclavicular line
Right anterior axillary line

Vertebral line
Left scapular line

Tactile fremitus

Palpating the
anterior chest over
the central airways

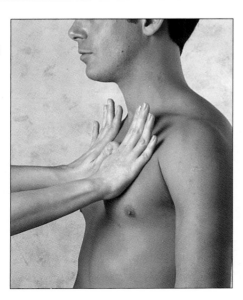

Palpating the
posterior chest over
the peripheral lung
fields

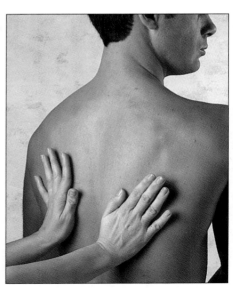

Diaphragmatic excursion

Percussing the posterior chest to locate the diaphragm on expiration

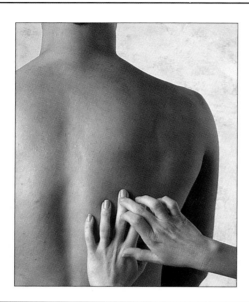

Measuring diaphragmatic excursion

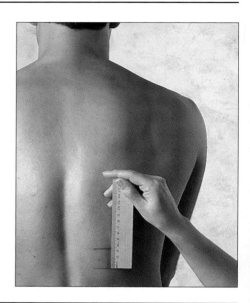

Respiratory excursion

Palpating the anterior chest for respiratory excursion

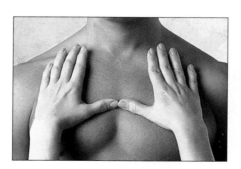
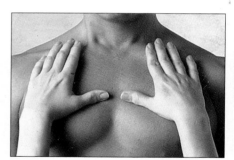

Palpating the posterior chest for respiratory excursion

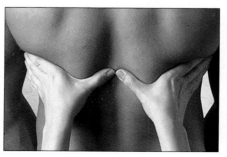
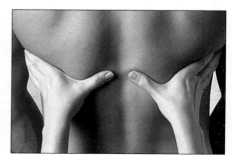

Normal percussion sounds

These photographs show you the areas of the chest where you'll normally hear dullness and resonance.

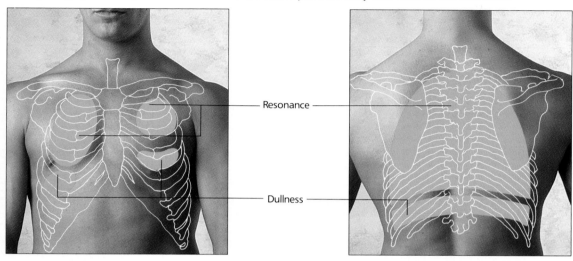

Resonance

Dullness

Normal breath sounds

These photographs show you the areas where you'll hear the four normal breath sounds.

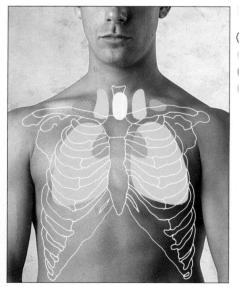

Key

○ Tracheal
Bronchial
Bronchovesicular
Vesicular

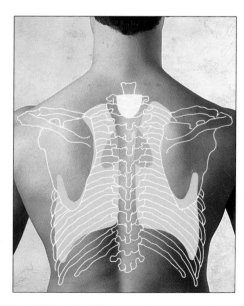

Adventitious breath sounds

These photographs show you common locations of four adventitious breath sounds—crackles, wheezes, rhonchi, and pleural friction rubs.

Crackles

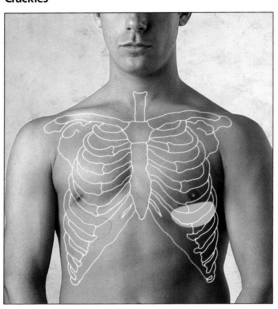

Wheezes

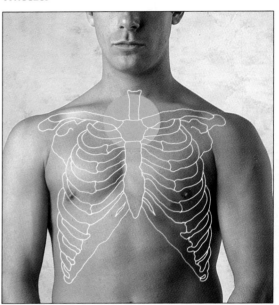

Rhonchi

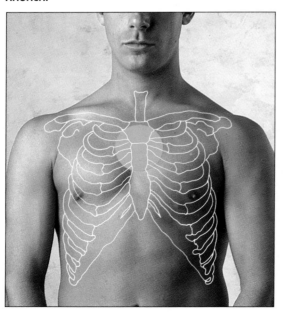

Pleural friction rubs

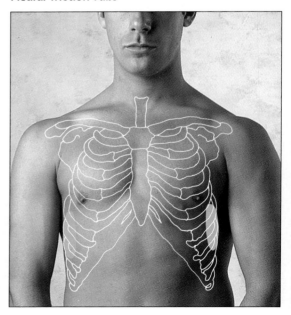

and respiratory excursion. Note any tenderness, swelling, or abnormalities, such as masses.

Skin
Begin by palpating the skin for temperature, moisture, turgor, tender areas, and masses. Cold, clammy skin results from increased sympathetic stimulation, which may be caused by hypoxia or circulatory failure. Warm, dry, or moist skin may indicate infection. Decreased turgor indicates dehydration, whereas edema suggests inadequate circulation that could involve the respiratory system.

Thoracic structures
Palpate bony structures, including the thoracic spine, scapulae, and sternum, noting any tenderness, swelling, or deformities. A normal spine feels straight from the cervical area through the beginning of the thoracic area. Normal scapulae are symmetrical, with well-developed surrounding musculature. A normal chest wall feels stable at the junctions of the ribs, spine, and sternum. Note any deviations that may interfere with ventilation. (See *Respiratory system and landmarks*, page 155.)

Gentle palpation shouldn't elicit pain. If it does, note the location, any radiation, and the severity. Note any other unusual findings, including skin irregularities and crepitus—a crackling feeling under the patient's skin that may indicate subcutaneous emphysema. Also, note any masses.

Tactile fremitus
To palpate for tactile fremitus (vibrations in the thorax), place your open palms against the upper portion of the anterior chest, making sure your fingers don't touch the chest. Avoid placing your palms over bony prominences or organs, such as the heart, by starting above the clavicles anteriorly. Then ask the patient to repeat "ninety-nine" or another resonant phrase while you systematically move your palms over the chest from the central airways to each lung's periphery and back. You should feel vibrations of equal intensity on both sides of the chest. Assess the posterior thorax in a similar manner. (See *Tactile fremitus*, page 155.)

Fremitus typically occurs in the upper chest close to the bronchi and feels strongest at the second intercostal space on either side of the sternum. Little or no fremitus should occur in the lower chest. The intensity of the vibrations varies according to the thickness and structure of the patient's chest wall as well as the patient's voice intensity and pitch.

Increased fremitus indicates consolidation, possibly from pneumonia. Decreased fremitus, which commonly occurs with COPD, indicates increased physiologic dead space (pulmonary space that doesn't participate in gas exchange).

Respiratory excursion
You'll assess respiratory excursion in three areas on the patient's anterior chest. To assess the first area, place your hands on the upper chest with your thumbs at the second intercostal spaces. Your thumbs should barely touch at the midline, and your palms and fingers should be flat on the chest wall. Don't apply pressure; this may alter the patient's inspiratory effort. As the patient inhales deeply, observe your thumbs. They should separate simultaneously and equally to a distance several centimeters from the sternum. Repeat the procedure with your thumbs at the fifth intercostal spaces and then again with your thumbs at the tenth intercostal spaces.

You'll assess respiratory excursion in two areas on the posterior chest. Stand behind the patient and place your thumbs at the infrascapular areas on either side of the spine at the level of the tenth rib. Grasp the lateral rib cage and rest your palms gently over the lateroposterior surface. As the patient inhales, the posterior chest should move upward and outward, and your thumbs should move apart. When the patient exhales, your thumbs should return to the midline and touch. Repeat the procedure, placing your thumbs lateral to the vertebral column in the interscapular area, with your fingers extending into the axillary area.

Unequal excursion may be caused by conditions that cause pain on deep inspiration or by underlying structural problems, such as fractures or masses. (See *Respiratory excursion*, page 156.)

Percussion and auscultation sequences

Follow the percussion and auscultation sequences shown here to distinguish between normal and abnormal sounds in the patient's lungs. Remember to compare sound variations from one side to the other as you proceed. Carefully describe any abnormal sounds you hear and include their locations.

Anterior sequence

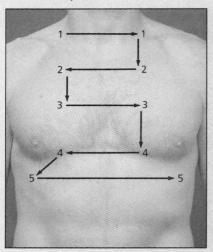

Lateral sequence

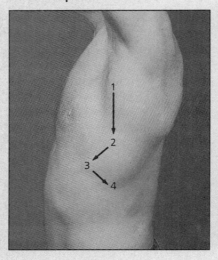

Posterior sequence

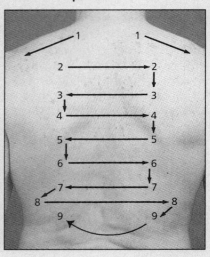

Percussion

Indirect percussion, the most frequently used percussion technique, allows you to assess structures 1¾" to 3" (4.4 to 7.6 cm) deep. You'll use indirect percussion to identify the boundaries of the lungs and to determine if they contain gas, liquid, or solid matter. You'll also use indirect percussion to determine diaphragmatic excursion — the distance that the diaphragm travels between inhalation and exhalation. To interpret your findings, you must be able to recognize five percussion sounds:
• resonance—a low-pitched, moderate to loud sound with a hollow quality
• tympany—a high-pitched loud sound with a drumlike quality
• dullness—a high-pitched, soft to moderate sound with a thudlike quality
• hyperresonance—a very low-pitched, loud sound with a booming quality

• flatness—a high-pitched, soft sound with an extremely dull quality.

Be sure to work systematically, percussing the anterior, lateral, and posterior chest over the intercostal spaces. (See *Percussion and auscultation sequences*.)

Anterior chest

Begin by percussing the lung apices (in the supraclavicular areas), comparing the right and left sides. Then percuss downward in 1¼" to 2" (3.2- to 5-cm) intervals.

You should hear resonance, which indicates normal lung tissue, until you reach the third or fourth intercostal space to the left of the sternum, where you'll hear a dull sound produced by the heart. This sound should continue as you percuss down toward the fifth intercostal space and laterally toward the midclavicular line. At the sixth intercostal space at the left midclavicular line, you'll hear resonance again.

As you percuss downward, you'll hear tympany over the stomach. (See *Normal percussion sounds,* page 157.)

On the right side, you should hear resonance, indicating normal lung tissue. Near the fifth to seventh intercostal spaces, you'll hear dullness, marking the superior border of the liver.

Lateral chest

To percuss the lateral chest, instruct the patient to raise his arms over his head. Percuss laterally, comparing the right and left sides as you proceed. These areas should also be resonant.

Posterior chest

Percuss the posterior chest, following the percussion sequence. Start percussing across the top of each shoulder, and move downward toward the patient's diaphragm at 1¼" to 2" (3.2- to 5-cm) intervals. The area from the shoulders to the level of the 10th thoracic vertebra should be resonant.

Diaphragmatic excursion

While percussing the patient's posterior chest, measure his diaphragmatic excursion. Instruct him to take a deep breath and hold it. Starting at the lower border of the right scapula, percuss down the posterior chest until you note dullness, indicating the location of the diaphragm. Mark this point. Instruct the patient to take a few normal breaths. Then, ask him to exhale completely and again hold his breath. Next, percuss up to the area of dullness. Mark this point, too. Repeat the entire procedure on the left side of the posterior chest.

Finally, using a tape measure or ruler, measure the distance between the two marks on each side of the posterior thorax to determine diaphragmatic excursion. Normal diaphragmatic excursion is 1¼" to 2¼" (3.2 to 5.7 cm). Failure of the diaphragm to contract adequately may indicate paralysis or muscle flattening, possibly caused by COPD. (See *Diaphragmatic excursion,* page 156.)

Auscultation

Lung auscultation helps you detect abnormal fluid or mucus as well as obstructed passages. You can also determine the condition of the alveoli and surrounding pleura.

Before you begin auscultation, note whether the patient has excess chest hair. If so, wet and mat it with a damp washcloth. That way, the hair won't cause sounds that can be confused with crackles.

Instruct the patient to take full, slow breaths through his mouth. (Nose breathing changes the pitch of the breath sounds.) Listen for one full inspiration and expiration before moving the stethoscope. Remember, a patient may try to accommodate you by breathing quickly and deeply with every movement of the stethoscope, which can cause hyperventilation. If your patient becomes light-headed or dizzy, stop auscultation and allow him to breathe normally for a few minutes.

Auscultation sequence

Using the diaphragm of the stethoscope, begin auscultating over the patient's trachea. Moving to the upper lobes, auscultate a point on one side of the anterior chest and then on the other side, following the same sequence you used for percussion.

To assess the middle lung lobes, auscultate laterally at the level of the fourth to sixth intercostal spaces, following the lateral auscultation sequence.

In the same way you auscultated your patient's anterior chest, auscultate his posterior chest, comparing sounds on both sides before moving to the next area.

Breath sounds

You'll hear four types of normal breath sounds: tracheal, bronchial, bronchovesicular, and vesicular. You'll hear tracheal breath sounds — harsh, discontinuous sounds — over the trachea. These sounds occur equally during inspiration and expiration. Bronchial breath sounds — high-pitched, discontinuous sounds that occur during expiration — can be heard over the manubrium. Bronchovesicular breath sounds — medium-pitched, continuous sounds that are equally audible during inspiration and expiration—occur over the upper third of the sternum anteriorly and in the interscapular area posteriorly. And vesicular breath sounds—low-pitched, continuous sounds that are prolonged during inspiration—can be heard over the peripheral lung fields. If you hear any of these four sounds in areas other than those described, you've detected an abnormal breath sound. Bronchial breath sounds over the peripheral lung fields, for instance, may indicate consolidation or atelectasis. (See *Normal breath sounds,* page 157.)

As you auscultate, classify normal and abnormal breath sounds according to their location, intensity (amplitude), characteristic sound, pitch (tone), and duration. Also identify the inspiratory and expiratory phases of normal and abnormal breath sounds, and then determine whether the sound occurs during inspiration, expiration, or both.

Vocal fremitus

Now assess your patient's vocal fremitus—the sounds produced by chest vibrations as he speaks. Instruct the patient to say "ninety-nine" as you systematically auscultate his chest. Normally, you should hear vocal fremitus as muffled, unclear sounds, loudest medially and softest in the lung periphery. If you hear "ninety-nine" distinctly (a finding known as bronchophony), suspect lung tissue consolidation.

To further evaluate vocal fremitus, ask the patient to repeat the sound "ee-ee" several times. If you hear it through the stethoscope as "ay-ay," accompanied by a nasal or bleating vocal tone, you've detected egophony, which indicates pleural effusion.

Abnormal findings

Abnormal respiratory findings usually fall into four categories: abnormal respiratory patterns, abnormal breath sounds, adventitious breath sounds, and thoracic deformities. As you perform your respiratory assessment, you may de-

tect one or more of the common abnormalities described below.

Abnormal respiratory patterns

The rate, rhythm, and depth of your patient's respirations provide important clues to his respiratory status and overall condition. Abnormal respiratory patterns include tachypnea, bradypnea, apnea, hyperpnea, Kussmaul's respirations, Cheyne-Stokes respirations, and Biot's respirations. (See *Recognizing abnormal respiratory patterns.*)

Tachypnea
A common sign of cardiopulmonary disorders, tachypnea is shallow breathing with an abnormally fast respiratory rate—20 or more breaths/minute. Generally, respirations increase by 4 breaths/minute for every 1° F rise in body temperature. Other causes of tachypnea include pleuritic chest pain, restrictive lung disease, respiratory distress, and an elevated diaphragm.

Bradypnea
Often preceding life-threatening apnea or respiratory arrest, bradypnea is a pattern of regular respirations with a rate of fewer than 10 breaths/minute in adults. This sign may result from such conditions as central nervous system depression, excessive sedation, and diabetic coma, which depress the brain's respiratory control centers.

Apnea
The cessation of spontaneous respiration, apnea may be periodic, as occurs during Cheyne-Stokes and Biot's respirations. More often, however, it's a life-threatening emergency that requires immediate intervention.

Hyperpnea
Characterized by rapid, deep breathing, hyperpnea (or hyperventilation) may result from anxiety, pain, metabolic acidosis, or exercise. In the comatose patient, this sign may indicate hypoxia or hypoglycemia.

Kussmaul's respirations

Usually associated with metabolic acidosis, Kussmaul's respirations are characterized by deep, rapid, sighing respirations without pauses.

Cheyne-Stokes respirations

The most common pattern of periodic breathing, Cheyne-Stokes is characterized by a period of rapid, deep respirations alternating with a shorter period of apnea. Possible causes include brain damage, congestive heart failure, and uremia. This pattern may be normal in children and in elderly people during sleep.

Biot's respirations

A late, ominous sign of neurologic deterioration, Biot's respirations are fast, deep breaths of equal volume interrupted by irregular periods of apnea. Possible causes include respiratory depression and brain damage.

Abnormal breath sounds

Because solid tissue transmits sound better than air or fluid, breath sounds (as well as spoken and whispered sounds) will be louder than normal over an area of consolidation. However, if pus, fluid, or air fills the pleural space, breath sounds will be quieter than normal. If a foreign body or secretions obstruct a bronchus, breath sounds will be diminished or absent over distal lung tissue.

Diminished breath sounds may indicate an obstructed airway, partial or total lung collapse, thickening of the pleurae, emphysema, or chronic lung disease.

Absent breath sounds typically indicate loss of ventilation power. Underlying causes may include laryngospasm, bronchospasm, pneumonectomy, phrenic nerve palsy, pneumothorax, hemothorax, or a malpositioned endotracheal tube.

Adventitious breath sounds

These sounds occur when air passes either through narrowed airways or through mois-

Recognizing abnormal respiratory patterns

Tachypnea
Shallow breathing with increased respiratory rate

Bradypnea
Decreased but regular respirations

Apnea
Absence of breathing; may be periodic

Hyperpnea
Deep respirations at normal rate

Kussmaul's respirations
Faster, deeper respirations without pauses; in adults, over 20 breaths/minute; breathing usually sounds labored, with deep breaths that resemble sighs

Cheyne-Stokes respirations
Respirations gradually becoming faster and deeper than normal and then slower, over a 30- to 170-second period; alternate with periods of apnea for 20 to 60 seconds

Biot's respirations
Faster, deeper respirations with abrupt pauses between them; each breath has same depth

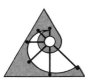

Interpreting wheezes

During auscultation, you're more likely to hear wheezing on expiration when the airways normally narrow. Hearing both inspiratory wheezes and expiratory wheezes usually indicates that your patient's condition is more severe.

However, if your patient's wheezing stops, you shouldn't assume that his condition has improved. This change could mean that the affected portion of the airway has narrowed so much that no air is passing through it.

---

ture, or when the membranes lining the chest cavity and the lungs become inflamed. Adventitious breath sounds include crackles, rhonchi, wheezes, and pleural friction rubs. Usually, these sounds indicate pulmonary disease. (See *Adventitious breath sounds,* page 158.)

Crackles
Resulting from air moving through fluid-filled airways, crackles are heard during both inspiration and expiration. They're discrete sounds that vary in pitch and intensity and can be classified as fine, medium, or coarse. (See *How crackles occur.*)

Fine crackles
Often called end-inspiratory crackles, fine crackles are high-pitched sounds heard near the end of inspiration. To simulate this sound, hold several strands of hair close to your ear and roll them between your fingers. Typically, you'll first detect fine crackles over the lung bases.

Fine crackles result from fluid in small airways or small atelectatic areas that expand when the patient breathes deeply. You may hear fine crackles in a patient who has either pulmonary edema or pneumonia. Usually, fine crackles won't clear when the patient breathes deeply or coughs.

Medium crackles
Lower-pitched and coarser than fine crackles, medium crackles result from fluid in slightly larger airways, such as the bronchioles. They occur during the middle or end of inspiration; thus, you may hear them called mid-inspiratory crackles. Medium crackles won't clear when the patient breathes deeply or coughs.

Coarse crackles
Resulting from a large amount of fluid or exudate in the large airways—including the primary and the secondary bronchi—coarse crackles produce a loud bubbling or gurgling sound on both inspiration and expiration. Coarse crackles indicate increasing pulmonary congestion and usually won't clear with deep breathing or coughing.

Rhonchi
When thick secretions partially obstruct airflow through the large airways, rhonchi develop. Loud, coarse, and low-pitched, these sounds resemble snoring. You'll hear rhonchi most often on expiration and sometimes on inspiration. A patient may be able to clear rhonchi by coughing up secretions.

Wheezes
Like rhonchi, wheezes occur on expiration and sometimes on inspiration. Continuous, high-pitched, musical squeaks, wheezes result when air moves rapidly through airways narrowed by asthma or infection—or when an airway is partially obstructed by a tumor or foreign body.

In a patient with mild asthma, you'll probably hear bilateral wheezes on expiration. If his condition worsens, you'll hear wheezes on both expiration and inspiration. Unilateral, isolated wheezing usually indicates a tumor or foreign body obstruction. (See *Interpreting wheezes.*)

Pleural friction rubs
As the name suggests, these adventitious breath sounds result when inflamed visceral and parietal pleurae rub together. The distinctive grating sound resembles the sound made by rubbing leather. Pleural friction rubs may be

caused by pleuritis, pneumonia, a tumor, or a pulmonary infarction extending into the pleural space. A small pleural effusion in a patient with cancer or one who is receiving hemodialysis may also cause a pleural friction rub.

Thoracic deformities

For an adult, the anteroposterior diameter of the thorax should be less than the transverse diameter. The normal ratio of these diameters is between 1:2 and 5:7. If you note an abnormal anteroposterior-transverse ratio or another deviation, the patient may have one of the following thoracic deformities: barrel chest, pigeon or chicken chest, funnel chest, or thoracic kyphoscoliosis. (See *Identifying chest deformities,* page 166.)

Barrel chest
In elderly adults, infants, and some patients with pulmonary disease, the chest may be rounded and barrel-shaped. Known as barrel chest, this configuration is characterized by a slight kyphosis of the thoracic spine, horizontal ribs, and a prominent sternal angle.

Pigeon chest
Also known as chicken chest and pectus carinatum, this chest configuration is characterized by a sternum that protrudes beyond the abdomen's frontal plane. The displaced sternum increases the chest's anteroposterior diameter.

Funnel chest
A patient with funnel chest (or pectus excavatum) will have a funnel-shaped depression in all or part of the sternum. This deformity may interfere with respiratory or cardiac function. If the deformity causes cardiac compression, you may detect murmurs.

Thoracic kyphoscoliosis
With this chest deformity, the spine curves to one side, and the vertebrae are rotated. Respiratory assessment may be more difficult.

PATHOPHYSIOLOGY

How crackles occur

Crackles occur when air passes through fluid-filled airways, causing collapsed alveoli to pop open as airway pressure equalizes. They can also occur when membranes lining the chest cavity and the lungs become inflamed. The illustrations below show a normal alveolus and two pathologic alveolar changes, which cause crackles.

Normal alveolus
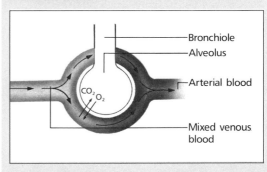

Edematous alveolus
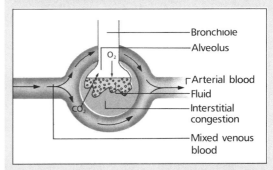

Inflamed alveolus
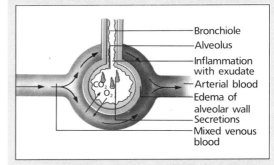

Identifying chest deformities

As you inspect your patient's chest, note any deviations in size and shape. The illustrations here show a normal adult chest and four chest deformities. The shape below each illustration represents the horizontal cross-sectional view. (A indicates anterior; P indicates posterior.)

Normal adult chest

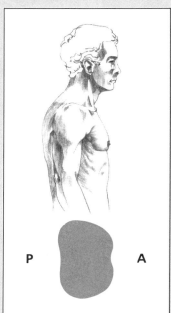

Barrel chest
Increased anteroposterior diameter

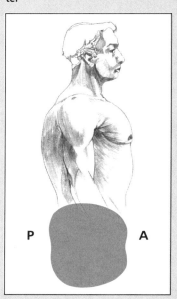

Pigeon chest
Anteriorly displaced sternum

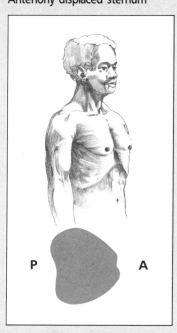

Funnel chest
Depressed lower sternum

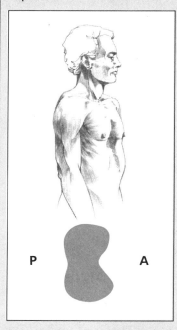

Thoracic kyphoscoliosis
Raised shoulder and scapula, thoracic convexity, and flared interspaces

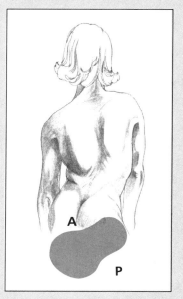

Interpreting arterial blood gas findings

NORMAL VALUES	ABNORMAL FINDINGS	POSSIBLE CAUSES OF ABNORMAL FINDINGS
pH: 7.35 to 7.42 **Pao$_2$**: 75 to 100 mm Hg **Paco$_2$**: 35 to 45 mm Hg **HCO$_3^-$**: 22 to 26 mEq/liter **Sao$_2$**: 94% to 100%	pH <7.35 and Paco$_2$ >45 mm Hg (respiratory acidosis)	Central nervous system depression from drugs, injury, or disease; asphyxia; hypoventilation caused by pulmonary, cardiac, musculoskeletal, or neuromuscular disease
	pH >7.42 and Paco$_2$ <35 mm Hg (respiratory alkalosis)	Hyperventilation from anxiety or pain; respiratory stimulation by drugs, disease, hypoxia, fever, or high room temperature
	pH <7.35 and HCO$_3^-$ <22 mEq/liter (metabolic acidosis)	HCO$_3^-$ depletion caused by renal disease, diarrhea, or small-bowel fistula; excess production of organic acids associated with hepatic disease, endocrine disorder, hypoxia, shock, or drug intoxication
	pH >7.42 and HCO$_3^-$ >26 mEq/liter (metabolic alkalosis)	Loss of hydrochloric acid from prolonged gastric suctioning; loss of potassium from increased renal excretion, as in diuretic therapy or steroid overdose; excessive alkali ingestion

Pertinent diagnostic tests

Several essential diagnostic tests can help in assessing a patient's respiratory problem. These include laboratory tests, such as arterial blood gas (ABG) analysis, total hemoglobin, and sputum analysis. Also, a wide range of pulmonary function tests can be used to aid in the diagnosis of pulmonary dysfunction. To visualize respiratory abnormalities, such tests as chest radiography, pulmonary angiography, ventilation-perfusion studies, and thoracic computed tomography (CT) scan may be ordered.

ABG analysis

This laboratory test evaluates gas exchange in the lungs by measuring the partial pressures of oxygen (Pao$_2$) and carbon dioxide (Paco$_2$) and the pH of arterial blood. The Pao$_2$ reading indicates how much O$_2$ the lungs deliver to the blood, and the Paco$_2$ reading shows how efficiently the lungs eliminate CO$_2$. The pH level indicates the acid-base level of the blood by measuring the hydrogen ion concentration.

ABG measurements also show the level of bicarbonate ions (HCO$_3^-$) and the oxygen saturation (Sao$_2$) of the blood. (See *Interpreting arterial blood gas findings*.)

Total hemoglobin

Hemoglobin enables RBCs to carry O$_2$ from the lungs and CO$_2$ from the tissues. This test measures the grams of hemoglobin found in a deciliter (g/dl) of whole blood and thus indirectly evaluates the blood's ability to carry O$_2$.

Normal values for men are 14 to 18 g/dl; for women, 12 to 16 g/dl; for children, 11 to 13 g/dl; and for neonates, 17 to 22 g/dl. An increased hemoglobin level may result from disorders such as polycythemia and COPD, or from environmental conditions such as living at a high altitude. A decreased hemoglobin level may be caused by anemia or overhydration.

Sputum analysis

Normal sputum is white and translucent. A color change from white to yellow or green indicates infection. Foul-smelling, green sputum may result from a *Pseudomonas* infection. Brown or rust-colored sputum may result from trauma caused by coughing or from underlying disease; red or blood-tinged sputum indicates fresh bleeding.

Interpreting pulmonary function tests

PULMONARY FUNCTION MEASUREMENT	METHOD OF CALCULATION	IMPLICATIONS
Tidal volume (VT): amount of air inhaled or exhaled during normal breathing	Determine the spirographic measurements for 10 breaths; then divide by 10.	Decreased VT may indicate restrictive disease and requires further tests, such as full pulmonary function studies or chest X-rays.
Minute volume (V̇E): total amount of air breathed per minute	Multiply VT by the respiratory rate.	Normal V̇E can occur in emphysema; decreased V̇E may indicate other diseases, such as pulmonary edema.
Inspiratory reserve volume (IRV): amount of air inspired after normal inspiration	Subtract VT from inspiratory capacity.	Abnormal IRV alone doesn't indicate respiratory dysfunction; IRV decreases during normal exercise.
Expiratory reserve volume (ERV): amount of air that can be exhaled after normal expiration	Use direct spirographic measurement.	ERV varies, even in healthy people.
Residual volume (RV): amount of air remaining in lungs after forced expiration	Subtract ERV from functional residual capacity.	RV >35% of total lung capacity after maximal expiratory effort may indicate obstructive disease.
Vital capacity (VC): total volume of air that can be exhaled after maximum inspiration	Use direct spirographic measurement; or add VT, IRV, and ERV.	Normal or increased VC with decreased flow rates may indicate reduction in functional pulmonary tissue. Decreased VC with normal or increased flow rates may indicate decreased respiratory effort, decreased thoracic expansion, or limited movement of diaphragm.
Inspiratory capacity (IC): total amount of air that can be inhaled after normal expiration	Use direct spirographic measurement, or add IRV and VT.	Decreased IC indicates restrictive disease.
Functional residual capacity (FRC): amount of air remaining in lungs after normal expiration	Use helium dilution technique measurement; or add ERV, VT, and IRV.	Increased FRC indicates overdistended lungs, which may result from obstructive disease.
Total lung capacity (TLC): total volume of the lungs at peak inspiration	Add VT, IRV, ERV, and RV; add FRC and IC; or add VC and RV.	Low TLC indicates restrictive disease; high TLC indicates obstructive disease.
Forced vital capacity (FVC): total amount of air that can be exhaled after maximum inspiration	Use direct spirographic measurements at 1-, 2-, and 3-second intervals.	Decreased FVC indicates flow resistance in respiratory system from obstructive disease, such as chronic bronchitis, emphysema, or asthma.
Forced expiratory volume (FEV): volume of air expired in the first (FEV$_1$), second (FEV$_2$), or third (FEV$_3$) second of FVC maneuver	Use direct spirographic measurement, and express value as percentage of FVC.	Decreased FEV$_1$ and increased FEV$_2$ and FEV$_3$ may indicate obstructive disease; decreased or normal FEV$_1$ may indicate restrictive disease.
Maximal mid-expiratory flow (MMEF): average flow rate during middle half of FVC; also called forced expiratory flow	Calculate from the flow rate and the time needed for expiration of middle 50% of FVC.	Low MMEF indicates obstructive disease.
Maximal voluntary ventilation (MVV): greatest volume of air breathed per unit of time; also called maximum breathing capacity	Use direct spirographic measurement.	Decreased MVV may indicate obstructive disease; normal or decreased MVV may indicate restrictive disease.

Analysis of a Gram-stained or cultured sputum specimen can help in diagnosing respiratory disorders, such as bronchitis, tuberculosis, lung abscess, or pneumonia; in identifying the cause of a pulmonary infection; and in identifying abnormal lung cells. If the doctor suspects a bacterial infection, he'll order a culture and sensitivity test to help him select an effective antibiotic. A negative culture suggests a viral infection.

Streptococcus pneumoniae suggests pneumonia; *Mycobacterium tuberculosis* suggests tuberculosis; and *Legionella pneumophila* suggests Legionnaires' disease.

Pulmonary function tests
Lung volume and capacity tests aid in diagnosing pulmonary dysfunction. These tests may be ordered to evaluate ventilatory function, determine the cause of dyspnea, assess the effectiveness of therapy (such as bronchodilators and steroids), differentiate between obstructive and restrictive diseases, and evaluate the extent of dysfunction. (See *Interpreting pulmonary function tests.*)

Chest radiography
By themselves, chest X-rays don't always provide definitive diagnostic information; for example, they may not reveal mild to moderate obstructive pulmonary disease. But they can show the location and size of a lesion and identify structural abnormalities that influence ventilation and diffusion.

Abnormal chest X-ray findings include tracheal deviation from the midline (possibly indicating tension pneumothorax or atelectasis); visible bronchi and lung fields (possibly indicating bronchial pneumonia or atelectasis); deviation and widening of the mediastinum due to an elevation or flattening of the diaphragm (possibly indicating pneumonia, pleurisy, acute bronchitis, atelectasis, asthma, emphysema, or pneumothorax); broken or misaligned ribs (indicating fractured sternum or ribs); and widening of the intercostal spaces between ribs (indicating emphysema).

Pulmonary angiography
Also called pulmonary arteriography, this test allows an examination of the pulmonary circulation. First, a catheter is inserted into the pulmonary artery or one of its branches. Then, a radioactive contrast dye is injected through the catheter, and a series of X-rays is taken to detect blood flow abnormalities in the lungs. Possible causes of such abnormalities include emboli or pulmonary infarction.

Ventilation-perfusion study
Like pulmonary angiography, a ventilation-perfusion study (also called a lung scan) requires the injection of a radioactive contrast dye. The scan is ordered to evaluate mismatching of ventilation and perfusion, to detect pulmonary emboli, and to evaluate pulmonary function.

Thoracic CT scan
This study provides a three-dimensional image of the lung and is used to assess abnormal configurations of the trachea and major bronchi and to define masses or lesions, such as tumors or abscesses.

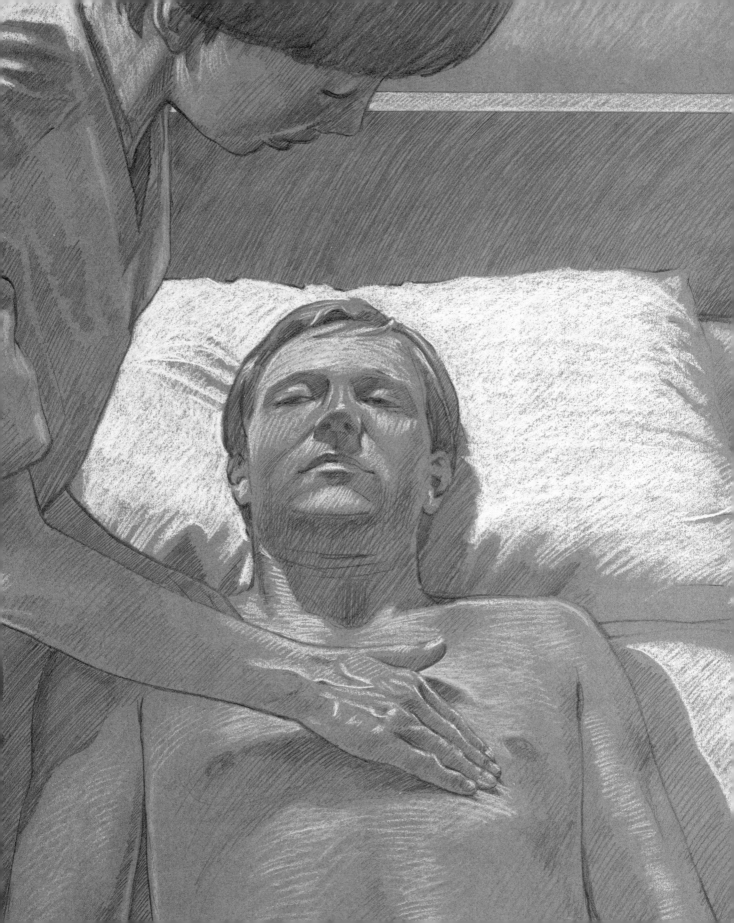

CHAPTER 8

Cardiovascular system

No body system wears out, breaks down, or otherwise malfunctions so often, in so many people, as the cardiovascular system. Cardiovascular disease, after all, affects people of all ages and can take many forms. It can be congenital or acquired, and it can develop suddenly or insidiously. (Atherosclerosis, for example, can be far advanced or even life-threatening before signs and symptoms appear.) And among hospitalized patients, cardiovascular disease causes the majority of serious complications, including pulmonary embolism, thrombophlebitis, congestive heart failure, shock, and cardiac arrhythmias.

Thus, mastering cardiovascular assessment is essential. But performing a complete cardiovascular system assessment is complex and requires special skills and knowledge. For instance, you must be adept at inspecting neck veins, palpating the precordium, and auscultating heart sounds and murmurs — advanced skills that require time and practice.

This chapter helps you acquire those advanced skills. It explores the complex cardiovascular system, its anatomy and physiology, and its relation to other body systems. It also describes the steps needed to obtain a thorough health history and perform a physical examination, and explains the significance of abnormal findings. Finally, the chapter discusses essential diagnostic tests that may be ordered to detect or evaluate cardiovascular dysfunction.

Anatomy and physiology

The cardiovascular system performs two basic functions: It delivers oxygenated blood to body tissues and removes waste substances through the action of the heart. The average person's heart beats 60 to 100 times/minute, pumping 4 to 6 liters of blood in that time.

Controlled by the autonomic nervous system, the heart pumps blood through the entire body. The vascular network that carries blood throughout the body consists of high-pressure arteries, which deliver the blood, and low-pressure veins, which return it to the heart. This complex network keeps the pumping heart filled with blood and maintains blood pressure.

Heart

A muscular organ, the heart accounts for about 0.5% of a person's total body weight and is about the size of a closed fist. It lies obliquely in the chest, with two-thirds located to the left of the sternum. The base of the heart (the superior portion) corresponds to the level of the third costal cartilage. The apex of the heart (the inferior portion) is normally located at the fifth left intercostal space at the midclavicular line.

Heart chambers
The heart contains four chambers—two atria and two ventricles—encircled by a thin outer sac called the pericardium. Located in the superior portion of the heart, the atria function

as receptacles for blood during ventricular contraction or systole. The larger ventricles lie below and receive blood from the atria and eject it into the pulmonary system and systemic circulation. (See *Reviewing the heart's structure*.)

Atria
The right atrium receives venous blood returning from the systemic circulation by way of the inferior and superior venae cavae. The left atrium receives oxygenated blood from the pulmonary system by way of the pulmonary veins (the only veins that carry oxygenated blood). During ventricular diastole, the atria allow the blood to pass into the corresponding right and left ventricles.

The atria consist of three layers of muscle tissue. The outer layer, called the epicardium, contains nerve fibers, coronary blood vessels, and large flattened cells called mesothelium. The middle layer, called the myocardium, is thick, muscular, and rich in nerve and sensory fibers. The endocardium is the smooth inner layer.

Ventricles
During ventricular diastole, the right ventricle receives unoxygenated blood from the right atrium by way of the tricuspid valve. The left ventricle receives oxygenated blood from the left atrium by way of the mitral valve.

During ventricular systole, the right ventricle ejects blood through the pulmonary valve into the pulmonary system by way of the pulmonary artery (the only artery to carry deoxygenated blood). The left ventricle expels blood through the aortic valve into the aorta and, eventually, the systemic circulation.

The ventricles contain the same three layers of muscle tissue as the atria. But the myocardium of the left ventricle is two to three times thicker than that of the right ventricle. The reason: Much higher pressure is required to eject blood into the systemic circulation than to eject blood into the pulmonary system.

Heart valves
The heart has four valves—the mitral, tricuspid, aortic, and pulmonary—which ensure that

ANATOMY

Reviewing the heart's structure

This cross-sectional view shows the heart's major structures.

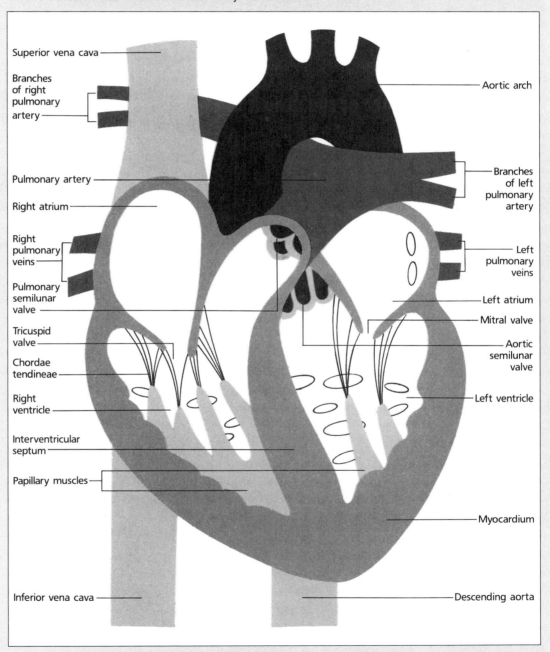

Superior vena cava

Branches of right pulmonary artery

Pulmonary artery

Right atrium

Right pulmonary veins

Pulmonary semilunar valve

Tricuspid valve

Chordae tendineae

Right ventricle

Interventricular septum

Papillary muscles

Inferior vena cava

Aortic arch

Branches of left pulmonary artery

Left pulmonary veins

Left atrium

Mitral valve

Aortic semilunar valve

Left ventricle

Myocardium

Descending aorta

Understanding the cardiac cycle

The cardiac cycle consists of five phases: isovolumetric ventricular contraction, ventricular ejection, isovolumetric relaxation, ventricular filling, and atrial systole. The small arrows in the illustrations indicate the direction of blood flow.

Isovolumetric ventricular contraction
In response to ventricular depolarization, tension in the ventricles increases. The rise in ventricular pressure leads to closure of the mitral and tricuspid valves. The pulmonary and aortic valves stay closed during this entire phase. So, for a short time, all four valves are closed.

Ventricular ejection
Ventricular pressure soon exceeds aortic and pulmonary arterial pressure. The aortic and pulmonary valves open, and the ventricles eject blood.

Isovolumetric relaxation
This phase occurs when ventricular pressure falls below pressure in the aorta and pulmonary artery. The drop in pressure causes the aortic and pulmonary valves to close. Again, all four valves are closed. Atrial diastole occurs as blood fills the atria.

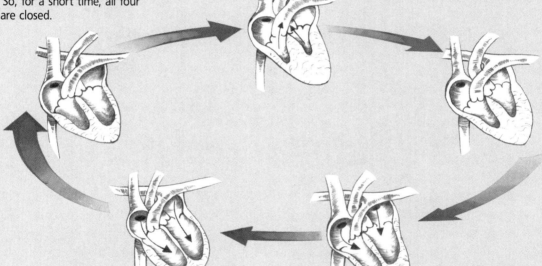

Atrial systole
This last phase coincides with late ventricular diastole when the atria contract in response to atrial depolarization. Known as the atrial kick, this phase supplies the ventricles with the remaining 20% of blood.

Ventricular filling
During this phase, atrial pressure exceeds ventricular pressure. This triggers the opening of the mitral and tricuspid valves, allowing passive blood flow into the ventricles. About 80% of ventricular filling takes place during this phase.

blood moves in the right direction without backflow (or regurgitation). Each valve consists of cusps (or leaflets) that open with pressure from downstream and close with pressure from upstream.

The two atrioventricular valves are the tricuspid valve, which normally has three leaflets, and the mitral valve, which normally has two. The tricuspid valve separates the right atrium from the right ventricle; the mitral valve separates the left atrium from the left ventricle.

Both atrioventricular valves are attached to the chambers by a complex of interconnected structures. The papillary muscles, which arise from the ventricular wall, are connected to the valve leaflets by the chordae tendineae, a series of fibrous cords that cause the valve leaflets to close during ventricular systole.

The two semilunar valves are the pulmonary valve, which separates the right ventricle from the pulmonary artery, and the aortic valve, which separates the left ventricle from the aorta. These valves have three cusps that open during ventricular systole, allowing blood to pass into the pulmonary system and the systemic circulation. During ventricular diastole, the valve cusps close, preventing regurgitation of blood into the ventricles.

Normal heart sounds

When the heart valves close, they produce two normal heart sounds, known as the first heart sound (S_1) and the second heart sound (S_2). S_1 occurs at the beginning of ventricular systole when rising pressure in the ventricles forces the two atrioventricular valves shut. This sound is commonly referred to as the *lub* of the *lub-dub* sound made by the first two heart sounds.

S_2 occurs at the beginning of ventricular diastole when ventricular pressure falls below the pressure in the aorta and the pulmonary artery, and the aortic and pulmonary valves snap shut. The sound is known as the *dub* of *lub-dub.*

Cardiac cycle

This cycle is the period from the beginning of one heartbeat to the beginning of the next. Each complete cycle consists of two parts: contraction or systole and relaxation or diastole. The cycle's duration varies with heart rate. When the heart rate is 72 to 75 beats/minute, one cardiac cycle occurs every 0.8 second. This short interval accommodates the complex sequence of events from ventricular systole to the end of diastole. (See *Understanding the cardiac cycle.*)

Heart's blood supply

Myocardial tissue contains a vast network of vascular structures that deliver oxygen and nutrients to and remove metabolic end products from heart cells. Coronary arteries and their branches supply the heart with oxygenated blood. Cardiac veins make up the heart's venous system, which removes oxygen-depleted blood.

Coronary arteries

The four prominent coronary arteries include the left main artery, left anterior descending artery, circumflex artery, and right coronary artery.

Short and thick, the left main coronary artery originates at the aorta and supplies all of the blood flow to the left ventricle. It branches to form the left anterior descending and the circumflex arteries.

The left anterior descending artery transverses the anterior surface along the interventricular sulcus of the left ventricle. Its many diagonal and septal branches supply blood to the ventricular myocardium, the ventricular septum, the bundle branches, and the papillary muscles located in the anterolateral section of the left ventricle.

Encircling the left ventricle and terminating at its posterior surface, the circumflex artery supplies blood to the left atrium and the posterolateral surface of the left ventricle. A small number of people have an additional coronary artery called the ramus between the left anterior descending and the circumflex arteries.

The right coronary artery also originates at the aorta but descends along the right atrioventricular groove. This artery and its many branches deliver blood to the right atrium, right ventricle, sinoatrial (SA) and atrioventricular (AV) nodes, posterior ventricular septum, and posterior papillary muscle of the left ventricle.

The coronary arteries and their branches weave throughout the ventricular myocardium, dividing to form a capillary network that provides cells with oxygen and nutrients.

Heart's conduction system

In the intrinsic conduction system of the heart, each electrical impulse travels from the sinoatrial (SA) node via internodal pathways to the myocardial muscle cells of the atria, producing atrial contraction. The impulse slows momentarily as it passes through the atrioventricular (AV) node to the bundle of His. Then it travels down the left and right bundle branches to the Purkinje fibers, which stimulate ventricular contraction.

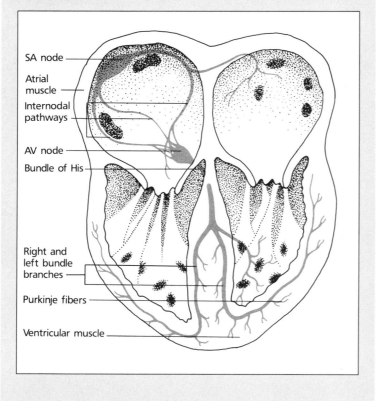

SA node
Atrial muscle
Internodal pathways
AV node
Bundle of His
Right and left bundle branches
Purkinje fibers
Ventricular muscle

Cardiac veins
The heart's venous system includes the coronary sinus and its tributaries, the anterior cardiac veins, and the thebesian veins. The coronary sinus and its connecting coronary veins make up the largest venous network. They drain the left ventricular tissue and empty into the right atrium. The anterior cardiac veins drain the right ventricular tissue and also empty into the right atrium. The thebesian veins drain the right and left atria.

Conduction system
The heart's conduction system includes the SA and AV nodes, atrial internodal conducting pathways, bundle of His, right and left bundle branches, and Purkinje fibers. (See *Heart's conduction system.*)

The SA node, called the heart's pacemaker, initiates electrical impulses at a rate of 60 to 100 beats/minute under resting conditions. These impulses move from the lateral wall of the right atrium through the atria to the AV node by way of three internodal pathways—anterior, middle, and posterior—and culminate in atrial contraction.

The AV node conducts the electrical impulses from the atria to the ventricles. As it does, it delays the progress of the electrical current. This allows time for the ventricles to fill completely before diastole takes place. If the SA node misfires, the AV node can also generate electrical impulses at a rate of 40 to 60 beats/minute.

After the electrical current passes into the bundle of His, it spreads into the right and left bundle branches. The single, slender right bundle branch conducts current down the right ventricular septum into the right ventricular tissue. The anterior fascicle of the left bundle branch conducts current into the superior-anterior-lateral left ventricular tissue, whereas the shorter, thicker posterior fascicle conducts current into the inferior-posterior-lateral left ventricular tissue. (A smaller middle fascicle of the left bundle branch has also been identified.) The network of Purkinje fibers brings the electrical current to its destination in the ventricular myocardium.

Cardiac innervation
As with other organs, the heart is influenced by the autonomic nervous system. Sympathetic nerve fibers are located throughout the myocardium, and parasympathetic nerve fibers are located in the atria, SA node, and AV node.

During activity, or when the fight-or-flight reaction is triggered, sympathetic nerve fibers release norepinephrine, which increases the heart rate as well as the force of ventricular contraction.

When the body is at rest, the heart is controlled by the parasympathetic nervous system through the stimulation of the vagus nerve and the release of acetylcholine. Activation of this system decreases the heart rate and the force of ventricular contraction.

Chemoreceptors located in the carotid and aortic bodies are sensitive to oxygen, carbon dioxide, and pH changes within the blood. These changes stimulate the vasomotor center in the medulla and alter heart and respiratory rates accordingly.

Stretch receptors also influence heart rate by responding to changes in blood pressure and volume. Venous return stretches the receptors, thereby stimulating the vasomotor center in the medulla and, in turn, increasing heart rate and cardiac output.

Peripheral vascular system

Thick-walled arteries carry blood from the heart, distributing it to all parts of the body. With thinner walls but larger diameters than their companion arteries, veins return blood to the heart through the superior and inferior venae cavae. The capillaries—high-resistance, thin-walled vessels consisting of one endothelial layer—connect the smallest arteries (arterioles) with the smallest veins (venules).

Maximum blood pressure (systolic pressure) occurs during peak ventricular ejection; minimum pressure (diastolic pressure) occurs just before ventricular contraction. (See *Reviewing the vascular system,* page 178.)

Arteries
The largest artery, the aorta, is the systemic circuit's trunk. The aorta and its branches are elastic arteries—so called because their middle layers contain many elastic fibers. The distributing arteries, which carry blood to the organs, have more smooth muscle in their middle layers and are called muscular arteries.

The pulmonary artery and its branches constitute a low-pressure system that transports blood to the lungs for reoxygenation.

Veins
The venous system consists of deep veins, which accompany companion arteries, and superficial veins, which lie in the superficial fascia under the skin. The veins are low-resistance vessels that carry blood from the tissues to the heart and can adjust their own diameter to compensate for blood volume variations.

Capillaries
About 5% of the total circulating blood is always flowing through the capillary beds. The work of the capillaries is the ultimate function of the entire cardiovascular system: to exchange nutrients and metabolic end products. In effect, the rest of the system—the heart and vessels—functions solely to bring blood into and out of the body's several thousand capillaries.

Peripheral pulses
The pulsation that can be felt in any artery results from the difference between systolic and diastolic pressures (called pulse pressure). The easiest arteries to palpate are the radial, carotid, femoral, popliteal, posterior tibial, dorsalis pedis, ulnar, and temporal.

Health history

Use the health history interview to obtain precise details about the patient's chief complaint, medical history, family history, psychosocial history, and activities of daily living. As you analyze the patient's problem, remember that age, sex, and race are all essential considerations in identifying patients at risk for cardiovascular disorders. For example, coronary artery disease (CAD) most commonly affects white men between ages 40 and 60; hypertension occurs most often in blacks. Women are also vulnerable to heart disease, especially postmenopausal women and those with diabetes mellitus. And elderly people have an increased incidence of cardiovascular disease.

During the interview, watch the patient's facial expressions, body positioning, and hand

Reviewing the vascular system

The illustration below shows the major veins and arteries of the vascular system.

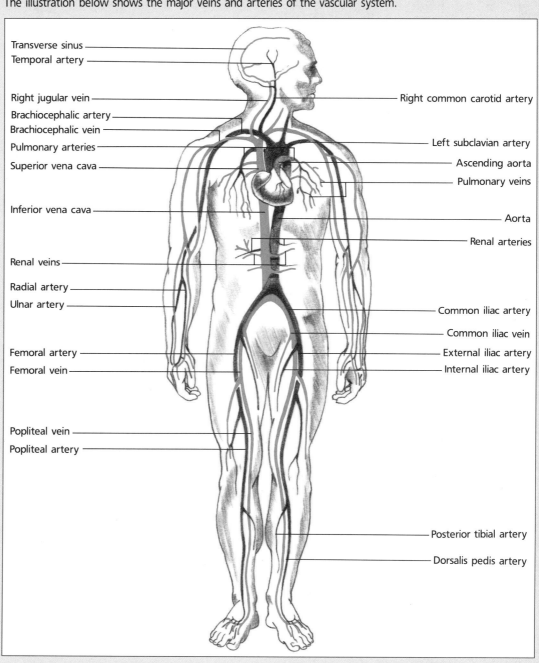

Transverse sinus

Temporal artery

Right jugular vein

Brachiocephalic artery

Brachiocephalic vein

Pulmonary arteries

Superior vena cava

Inferior vena cava

Renal veins

Radial artery

Ulnar artery

Femoral artery

Femoral vein

Popliteal vein

Popliteal artery

Right common carotid artery

Left subclavian artery

Ascending aorta

Pulmonary veins

Aorta

Renal arteries

Common iliac artery

Common iliac vein

External iliac artery

Internal iliac artery

Posterior tibial artery

Dorsalis pedis artery

movements for clues to his condition. If he's in acute distress, you won't have time to obtain a complete history. Instead, focus the interview with a series of pointed questions about the patient's chief complaint. Later, when the patient's condition permits, you can complete the health history.

Chief complaint

The most common chief complaints of the cardiovascular system include chest pain, dyspnea, fatigue and weakness, irregular heartbeat, and peripheral changes (especially dry skin and extremity pain). In some patients, chest pain may radiate to other parts of the body, including the jaw, back, left arm, right arm, elbows, little fingers, teeth, and scrotum. (See *Understanding chest pain*, page 180.)

To investigate these or any cardiovascular chief complaints, ask your patient relevant questions about such particulars as onset, duration, and severity. Also ask what precipitates the symptom, what makes it worse, and what makes it better. For more information on exploring the chief complaint, see Chapter 3.

Medical history

Determine whether the patient has a history of diabetes, hypertension, or heart disease. If so, at what age did he develop this condition? How was it diagnosed and treated?

Ask about previous surgeries and invasive procedures, including percutaneous transluminal coronary angioplasty, coronary artery bypass graft surgery, and valve surgery. Has the patient experienced any complications related to the disease or its treatment? Assess the patient's understanding of his condition to determine the need for further teaching. Obtain a medication history.

If your patient is a woman, obtain a menstrual history. Has she had a hysterectomy? Has she ever been pregnant? If so, was the pregnancy complicated by hypertension? Ask about any past or current use of oral contraceptives or hormone replacement therapy.

Women who take oral contraceptives are at higher risk for developing hypertension or myocardial infarction (MI); the risk increases with prolonged use of these contraceptives and smoking.

Family history

Note any family history of cardiovascular disorders, especially hypertension, angina, MI, valve disease, pulmonary edema, heart failure, palpitations, or hyperlipidemia. Have any family members died suddenly because of a cardiovascular problem? At what age did the disorder or sudden death occur? Having a blood relative with heart disease, especially before age 55, greatly increases a patient's risk for developing heart disease. Also find out about the family member's treatment regimen and quality of life — factors that can greatly influence the patient's attitude toward his own condition and its treatment.

Note any family history of diabetes mellitus, which causes atherosclerotic changes. If applicable, find out about the family member's age at onset, treatment regimen, and any associated complications, such as vision changes, kidney problems, cerebrovascular accident, or cardiac dysfunction. Did the family member die of this problem? If so, at what age?

Psychosocial history

Explore the patient's personality traits and lifestyle. Although difficult to prove or define precisely, a positive correlation between a type A personality and CAD seems to exist.

Determine the patient's stress level. If he believes that he's under stress, what does he consider to be the cause? Is his occupation emotionally or physically demanding? Does he have any domestic or financial problems? Do his family and friends provide adequate emotional support? Ask about any stress-related symptoms, aggravating factors, and relief measures (especially the use of prescription drugs, such as sedatives).

Have the patient's sleeping habits changed?

Understanding chest pain

Does your patient complain of chest pain? To accurately assess his cardiac status, find out what type of chest pain he's having. Use the chart below as a guide.

CHARACTERISTICS	LOCATION	AGGRAVATING FACTORS	ALLEVIATING FACTORS	CAUSE
Cardiovascular origin				
Aching, squeezing, pressure, heaviness, burning; usually subsides within 10 minutes	Substernal; may radiate to jaw, neck, arms, and back	Eating, physical effort, smoking, cold weather, stress, anger, hunger, lying down	Rest, nitroglycerin (*Note:* Unstable angina appears even at rest.)	Angina pectoris
Pressure, burning, aching, tightness; may be accompanied by shortness of breath, diaphoresis, weakness, anxiety, or nausea; sudden onset; lasts ½ to 2 hours	Across chest; may radiate to jaw, neck, arms, and back	Exertion, anxiety	Pain relieved by narcotic analgesics, such as morphine sulfate	Acute myocardial infarction
Sharp and continuous; may be accompanied by friction rub; sudden onset	Substernal; may radiate to neck, left arm	Deep breathing, supine position	Sitting up, leaning forward, anti-inflammatory agents	Pericarditis
Excruciating, tearing; may be accompanied by blood pressure difference between right and left arm; sudden onset	Retrosternal, upper abdominal, or epigastric; may radiate to back, neck, shoulders	None	Analgesics	Dissecting aortic aneurysm
Pulmonary origin				
Sudden, stabbing; may be accompanied by cyanosis, dyspnea, or cough with hemoptysis	Over lung area	Inspiration	Analgesics	Pulmonary embolus
Sudden; severe; may be accompanied by dyspnea, increased pulse rate, decreased breath sounds, or deviated trachea	Lateral thorax	Normal respiration	Analgesics, chest tube	Pneumothorax
GI origin				
Dull, pressurelike, squeezing	Substernal, epigastric	Food, cold liquids, exercise	Nitroglycerin, calcium channel blockers	Esophageal spasm
Sharp, severe	Lower chest or upper abdomen	Eating a heavy meal, bending, lying down	Antacids, walking, semi-Fowler's position	Hiatal hernia
Burning feeling after eating; may be accompanied by hematemesis or tarry stools; sudden onset; usually subsides within 15 to 20 minutes	Epigastric	Lack of food or highly acidic foods	Food, antacids	Peptic ulcer
Gripping, sharp; nausea and vomiting may also be present	Right epigastric or abdominal areas; may radiate to shoulders	Eating fatty foods, lying down	Rest and analgesics, surgery	Cholecystitis
Musculoskeletal origin				
Sharp; may be tender to the touch; gradual or sudden onset; continuous or intermittent pain	Anywhere in chest	Movement, palpation	Time, analgesics, heat applications	Chest wall syndrome
Psychological origin				
Dull or stabbing pain, usually accompanied by hyperventilation or breathlessness; sudden onset; may last less than a minute or for several days	Anywhere in chest	Increased respiratory rate; stress or anxiety	Slowing of respiratory rate, stress relief	Acute anxiety

Does he wake up short of breath, gasping, or coughing? Has he experienced fatigue, irritability, decreased attention span, or personality changes? Does he use illicit drugs?

Activities of daily living

Assess your patient's activity level. How many times a week does he engage in aerobic activity? Exercise strengthens the heart and benefits overall cardiovascular conditioning. Does illness, injury, or another factor prevent him from exercising? How does he feel during and after exercise? How long does it take before he tires? Does rest relieve the fatigue? Has his exercise program changed over the past 5 to 10 years? If so, why and how?

If your patient is elderly, ask how he feels after physical activity. Does he get light-headed or unsteady when he changes positions? Has he noticed any difficulty with breathing? The heart's ability to respond to physical and emotional stress may decrease markedly with age. Usually, aging also contributes to arterial and venous insufficiency as the strength and elasticity of blood vessels decrease. These factors contribute to the increased incidence of cardiovascular disease in elderly people.

Find out if the patient uses tobacco. If he smokes cigarettes, how long has he smoked and how much does he smoke? Record this data in pack years. Does he use filters? Has he ever stopped smoking? If so, what motivated him to stop and what techniques helped him to quit? Smoking is a significant risk factor for peripheral vascular disease.

A brief history of the patient's eating habits, particularly his intake of carbohydrates and fats, may determine his potential for CAD. A high-sodium diet can contribute to the development of edema and may be associated with the development of hypertension. Ask the patient to describe his diet, including his use, if any, of dietary supplements, alcohol, and caffeinated foods and beverages. A high caffeine intake can lead to hypertension and cardiac arrhythmias. Does he know his current levels of total cholesterol, high-density lipoprotein (HDL) cholesterol, low-density lipoprotein (LDL) cholesterol, and triglycerides? What have these levels been in the past?

Physical examination

When you assess your patient's cardiovascular system, you'll examine not only his chest but also his head and neck, skin, and extremities. After inspecting the patient for overt signs of cardiac risk factors and recording his vital signs, you'll examine him from head to toe, using inspection, palpation, percussion, and auscultation.

Inspection

During your general inspection, record your initial impressions of the patient's body type, posture, gait, and movement, as well as his overall health and basic hygiene. Be alert for clues about the patient's cardiovascular status. For example, head jerking (Musset's sign) may indicate severe aortic insufficiency. Also, note observable cardiac risk factors, such as cigarette smoking, obesity, and fatty tissue deposits (xanthomas). Observe facial expressions for signs of pain or anxiety. During conversation, assess mental status, particularly the appropriateness of responses and the clarity of speech. Determine his apparent mood. Is he cooperative or withdrawn, fearful, or depressed?

Head
To help determine the adequacy of cardiac output, assess the skin color of the patient's face, mouth, and earlobes. Note any deep creases or folds in the earlobes (McCarthy's sign), which may indicate CAD. Check the condition of the mucous membranes; moistness indicates adequate hydration.

Note the color of the conjunctivae (normally pink) and the sclerae (normally white). Look for an opaque ring around the cornea (corneal arcus) and yellow fatty nodules on the eyelids (xanthelasma).

Estimating CVP

To estimate central venous pressure (CVP), place the patient in semi-Fowler's position under a gooseneck lamp and determine the height from the right atrium to the highest level of visible pulsation in the jugular vein.

To locate the right atrium, first palpate the clavicles where they join the sternum (the suprasternal notch). Place your first two fingers on the suprasternal notch and slide them down the sternum

until you feel a bony protuberance. This is the angle of Louis. The right atrium lies about 2" (5 cm) below this point.

Then, measure the vertical distance between the highest level of visible pulsation and the angle of Louis. Add 2" to this figure to estimate the total distance between the highest level of visible pulsation and the right atrium.

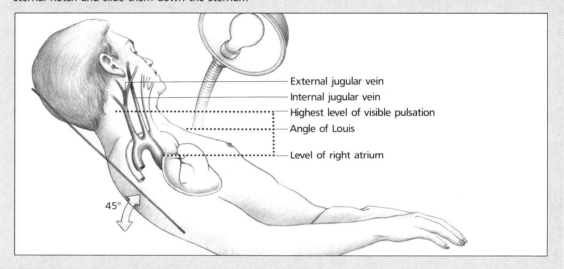

External jugular vein
Internal jugular vein
Highest level of visible pulsation
Angle of Louis
Level of right atrium

45°

Neck

Your inspection of the neck focuses on the jugular vein and the carotid artery. First, inspect jugular vein pulsations. Place the patient in semi-Fowler's position. (In this position, his neck veins shouldn't be prominent if his heart function is normal.) Turn his head slightly away from you to relax the sternocleidomastoid muscle so it doesn't obstruct your view of the veins. Next, arrange the lighting to cast small shadows along the neck. Then, observe the pulsations of the internal jugular vein. Noting the force of these pulsations helps you to indirectly evaluate the amount of pressure in the right atrium.

You can estimate a patient's central venous pressure (CVP) indirectly by determining the height from the right atrium to the highest

level of visible pulsation in the jugular vein. First, note the highest level of visible pulsation. Next, locate the angle of Louis, or sternal notch. To do this, palpate the clavicles where they join the sternum (the suprasternal notch). Place your first two fingers on the suprasternal notch and slide them down the sternum until you feel a bony protuberance. This is the angle of Louis. The right atrium lies about 2" (5 cm) below this point.

To estimate CVP, measure the vertical distance between the highest level of visible pulsation and the angle of Louis. Normally, this distance is less than 1⅛" (2.9 cm). Add 2" to this figure to estimate the total distance between the highest level of visible pulsation and the right atrium. A total distance that exceeds

Jugular vein pulsations

The waveform at right shows jugular vein pulsations, as seen on a hemodynamic monitor. Each waveform has five components, called waves: three positive, or ascending, waves (*a*, *c*, and *v*) and two negative, or descending, waves (*x* and *y*).

The *a* wave, the first ascending wave, occurs when a small amount of blood regurgitates into the superior vena cava during right atrial contraction. If atrial contraction doesn't occur, the *a* wave won't appear. A patient with atrial fibrillation, for example, lacks visible *a* waves because his atria don't contract in an organized manner. Accentuated *a* waves occur when the closed tricuspid valve prevents atrial blood from draining into the right ventricle. The blood then regurgitates into the venous system, producing a giant *a* wave. Other causes of giant *a* waves include arrhythmias, atrial wall stiffness, right ventricular infarction, right atrial infarction, and right ventricular failure.

The *c* wave is a small positive wave that corresponds with ventricular contraction. It occurs on the *a* wave's downstroke.

After atrial contraction and tricuspid valve closure, the right atrium refills with blood. Venous pressure then decreases and the *x* descent appears.

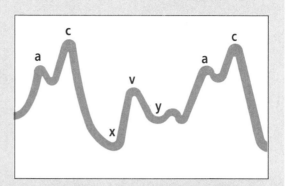

The third positive wave, the *v* wave, appears as blood fills the right atrium during atrial diastole.

The *y* descent appears next, as the tricuspid valve opens and blood streams into the right ventricle. Decreased volume and pressure in the right atrium make the blood column in the jugular vein fall, producing the *y* descent.

Diminished *c*-wave amplitude results from decreased right ventricular contractile force secondary to muscle damage. Tricuspid insufficiency can cause an accentuated *cv* wave combination or an absent *x* descent.

4″ (10 cm) may indicate elevated CVP and right ventricular failure. (See *Estimating CVP.*)

If the patient has a central venous line connected to a hemodynamic monitoring system, you can observe jugular vein pulsations to obtain information about the dynamics of the right side of the heart. As you assess, use the carotid pulse or heart sounds to time the venous pulsations with the cardiac cycle. (See *Jugular vein pulsations.*)

Finally, inspect the carotid arteries, noting whether the pulsations are weak (hypokinetic) or strong and bounding (hyperkinetic).

Chest
Begin inspecting the patient's chest by quickly identifying anatomic landmarks. The critical landmarks for cardiovascular assessment are the suprasternal notch and the xiphoid process. (See *Identifying cardiac landmarks,* page 184.) Other important landmarks include the midsternal line, the midclavicular line, and the anterior axillary, midaxillary, and posterior axillary lines.

Inspect the patient's entire thorax for shape, size, symmetry, obvious pulsations, and retractions. Look for an apical impulse, or point of maximal impulse (PMI), normally located in the fifth intercostal space at about the midclavicular line. You can see the PMI as a pulsation produced by the thrust of the contracting left ventricle against the chest wall. The apical impulse reflects cardiac size, especially left ventricular size and location, and is evident in about half the normal adult population. Because it occurs almost simultaneously with the

Identifying cardiac landmarks

These photographs show the locations of critical landmarks for cardiovascular assessment.

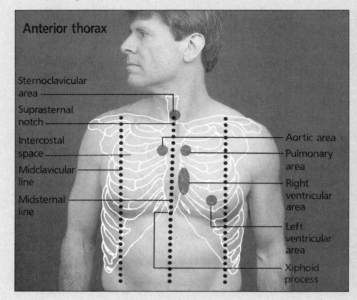

Anterior thorax

Sternoclavicular area
Suprasternal notch
Intercostal space
Midclavicular line
Midsternal line

Aortic area
Pulmonary area
Right ventricular area
Left ventricular area
Xiphoid process

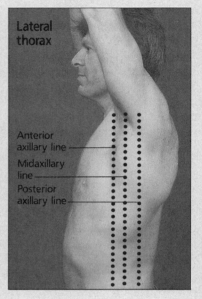

Lateral thorax

Anterior axillary line
Midaxillary line
Posterior axillary line

---

carotid pulse, palpating this pulse can help you identify it.

Also check for abnormal respiratory movements, such as the use of accessory shoulder and neck muscles, intercostal bulging or retraction, and tachypnea (greater than 20 breaths/ minute in an adult).

Skin
Assess the patient's skin color and condition. Is his skin pale or cyanotic? Does it feel warm and dry, or cool and clammy?

Also inspect the patient's skin texture. In a patient with chronic poor circulation, the skin appears thick, waxy, fragile, and shiny.

Extremities
To evaluate the peripheral circulation, observe the hair distribution on the patient's arms and legs.

Inspect the fingers for clubbing, a common sign of hypoxia caused by congenital heart de-

fects or pulmonary disorders. Note the condition of the fingertips and nails. Are the fingertips enlarged? Are the nail bases spongy and swollen?

Also check the hands and feet for Osler's nodes (tender erythematous lesions on the finger and toe pads, palms, or soles) and Janeway's spots (nontender hemorrhagic lesions on the palms and soles). These findings may indicate infective endocarditis.

Inspect the patient's hands, arms, legs, ankles, and feet for edema. (If the patient has been confined to bed, also check for edema in his buttocks and sacral area. Remember, edema occurs in the most dependent body parts.)

Palpation

Next, you'll use palpation to evaluate the patient's arterial pulses. Then you'll palpate appropriate areas over the precordium. After assessing the patient's skin turgor, you'll check for edema.

Arterial pulses

Lightly palpate the patient's peripheral pulses, using the pads of your index and middle fingers. Note pulse volume or amplitude and symmetry.

To estimate pulse volume or amplitude, palpate the blood vessel during ventricular systole. Characterize your patient's pulse volume using this scale:

+4 Significantly elevated
+3 Moderately elevated
+2 Normal
+1 Normal but weak
 0 Absent.

To determine symmetry, palpate contralateral pulses simultaneously and note any inequality. Proceed systematically, moving from the head (temporal, facial) to the arms (brachial, radial, ulnar) to the legs (femoral, popliteal, posterior tibial, and dorsalis pedis). Palpate gently, or you may obliterate the pulses, especially those in the legs, which are farthest from the heart and therefore have the lowest pressure. (See *Palpating arterial pulses*, page 186.)

If the patient has an arterial line, identify any pulse abnormalities by comparing the peripheral pulse wave with the normal pulse wave.

With the patient in semi-Fowler's position and his head turned toward you, palpate each carotid pulse for rate, rhythm, equality, contour, and amplitude. To locate the carotid artery, feel the trachea and roll your fingers laterally into the groove between it and the sternocleidomastoid muscle. Don't exert too much pressure or massage this area; doing so may induce bradycardia. Also, palpate only one carotid artery at a time; palpating the carotid arteries simultaneously can trigger cerebral ischemia.

Chest

Using the pads of your fingers, start at the sternoclavicular area and move methodically to the aortic, pulmonary, right ventricular, apical, and epigastric areas. At the sternoclavicular

area, you may feel the pulsation of the aortic arch, especially in a thin patient or one with an average build. At the epigastric area, you may palpate the abdominal aorta pulsation in a thin patient.

Use your fingertips and the ball of your hand to palpate the apical impulse at the fifth intercostal space at the left midclavicular line. The apical impulse correlates with the S_1 and carotid pulsation. To be sure you're feeling it, you can use your other hand to palpate the patient's carotid artery. Note the amplitude, size, intensity, location, and duration of the apical impulse. Normally, you'll feel a soft, gentle pulsation in an area about ½" to ¾" (1.3 to 2 cm) in diameter.

Skin turgor and edema

Evaluate the patient's skin turgor by grasping and raising the skin between two fingers and releasing it. Normally, the skin should snap back into place. If the patient is elderly, pinch the skin over the clavicle, sternum, or forehead.

Next, palpate the patient's extremities for edema. If you detect this abnormality, note the location and extent. Also note whether it's pitting or nonpitting and whether it's unilateral or bilateral. If the patient has pitting edema, assess the degree of pitting. (See *Evaluating edema*, page 187.)

Percussion

In cardiovascular assessment, percussion has limited value because inspection, palpation, and chest X-rays more accurately determine heart size and borders. Plus, many patients with cardiovascular problems also have related lung problems, which reduce the accuracy of precordial percussion.

To locate the left border of the heart, begin percussing at the left anterior axillary line at the fifth intercostal space, and move toward the sternum. The sound will change from resonance to dullness at the left border of the heart, usually near the PMI. If the sound extends to the left of the midclavicular line, the heart may be enlarged. The right border of the

Palpating arterial pulses

To palpate the arterial pulses, apply pressure with your index and middle fingers. The following illustrations show where to position your fingers when palpating the various pulses.

Carotid pulse
Lightly place your fingers just medial to the trachea and below the jaw angle.

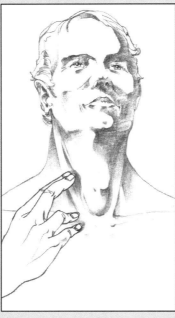

Femoral pulse
Press relatively hard at a point inferior to the inguinal ligament. For an obese patient, palpate in the crease of the groin halfway between the pubic bone and the hip bone.

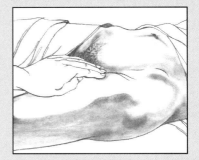

Popliteal pulse
Press firmly against the popliteal fossa at the back of the knee.

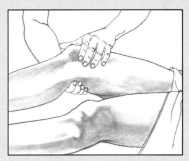

Brachial pulse
Position your fingers medial to the biceps tendon.

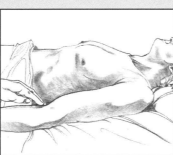

Posterior tibial pulse
Apply pressure behind and slightly below the malleolus of the ankle.

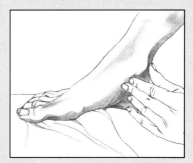

Radial pulse
Apply gentle pressure to the medial and ventral side of the wrist just below the thumb.

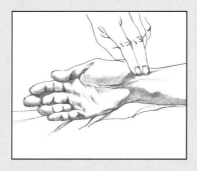

Dorsalis pedis pulse
Place your fingers on the medial dorsum of the foot while the patient points the toes down. In this site, the pulse is difficult to palpate and may seem to be absent in some healthy patients.

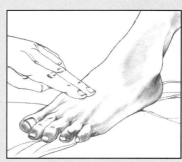

heart can't be percussed because it lies underneath the sternum.

Auscultation

Auscultating over the central and peripheral arteries for vascular sounds and over the precordium for heart sounds remains the most useful examination technique for learning about cardiac function. The bell of the stethoscope works best for auscultating the carotid, femoral, and popliteal arteries and the abdominal aorta. When auscultating heart sounds, you'll use the diaphragm of the stethoscope to detect high-pitched sounds and the bell to detect low-pitched sounds and murmurs.

Acquiring expertise in identifying heart sounds and murmurs takes a great deal of practice. You'll find that the amount of tissue between the source of the sound and the outer chest wall can affect the sounds you can hear. Fat, muscle, and air tend to reduce sound transmission. So if a patient is obese or has a muscular chest wall, the sounds may seem more distant and difficult to hear.

Be sure to follow the same sequence each time you auscultate.

Vascular sounds
To assess the carotid arteries, ask the patient to hold his breath while you auscultate with the bell of the stethoscope on both sides of the trachea. To evaluate the femoral and popliteal arteries, place the bell of the stethoscope over the pulse sites that you palpated earlier. Finally, auscultate the abdominal aorta by listening at the epigastric area. Normally, auscultation should detect no vascular sounds. (You may hear bowel sounds when auscultating the abdominal aorta.)

Heart sounds
Before auscultating for heart sounds, be sure that the room is as quiet as possible. Select a stethoscope with a bell that's the appropriate size for the patient's chest. (If necessary, choose a pediatric bell for a thin adult.) The earpieces of the stethoscope should fit snugly

Evaluating edema

When you detect edema, determine the degree, using a scale of +1 to +4. Press your fingertip firmly for 5 to 10 seconds over a bony surface, such as the subcutaneous tissue over the patient's tibia, fibula, sacrum, or sternum. Then, note the depth of the imprint your fingertip leaves on the skin. A slight imprint indicates +1 edema. If the imprint is deep and the skin is slow to return to its baseline shape, the edema is a +4.

With severe edema, the skin swells so much that fluid can't be displaced. Called brawny edema, this condition resists pitting but makes the skin appear distended.

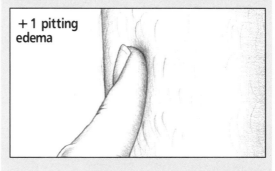

+1 pitting edema

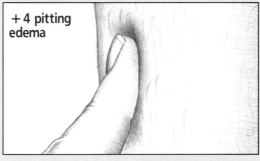

+4 pitting edema

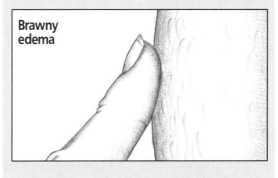

Brawny edema

Positioning the patient for chest auscultation

If heart sounds are faint or undetectable, try listening to them with the patient seated and leaning forward, or lying on his left side. Repositioning the patient may enhance the sounds or make them seem louder by bringing the heart closer to the surface of the chest.

Forward-leaning position

This position is best for hearing high-pitched sounds related to semilunar valve problems, such as aortic and pulmonary valve murmurs. To auscultate these sounds, place the diaphragm of the stethoscope over the aortic and pulmonary areas in the right and left second intercostal spaces.

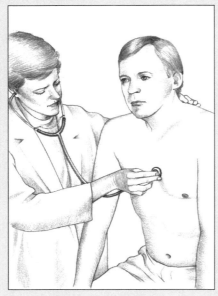

Left-lateral recumbent position

This position is best for hearing low-pitched sounds related to atrioventricular valve problems, such as mitral valve murmurs and extra heart sounds. To auscultate these sounds, place the bell of the stethoscope over the apical area.

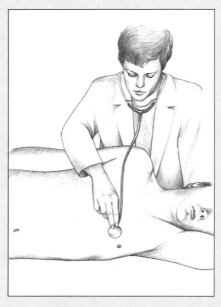

and the tubing should be about 12″ (30 cm) long.

Explain the procedure to the patient, and instruct him to breathe normally, inhaling through his nose and exhaling through his mouth. Warm the stethoscope chest piece by rubbing it between your hands.

Don't try to auscultate through clothing or other barriers; doing so will muffle sounds or make them inaudible. Drape the patient appropriately to limit the area exposed for auscultation.

Have the patient lie supine. If you're right-handed, stand at his right side so you can manipulate the stethoscope with your dominant hand and assist him as needed with your non-dominant hand. (See *Positioning the patient for chest auscultation*.)

S_1 and S_2

To auscultate heart sounds, listen carefully at the aortic, pulmonary, tricuspid, and mitral areas. (See *Listening for heart sounds*.) At each area, try to hear both normal heart sounds, S_1 and S_2, using the diaphragm of the stethoscope. Always identify S_1 and S_2 first because you can only recognize abnormal sounds by comparing them with normal sounds.

Begin at the aortic area (second intercostal space, right sternal border), where S_2 is loudest. Then move the stethoscope across to the pulmonary area (second intercostal space, left sternal border). From there, inch the stethoscope down the left sternal border to the tricuspid area (fifth intercostal space, left sternal border). Finally, move to the mitral area (fifth intercostal space, midclavicular line), where S_1 is loudest.

If you have difficulty distinguishing S_1 from S_2, try palpating the carotid artery as you auscultate. S_1 occurs at almost the same time as the beat of the carotid pulse.

When you auscultate normal heart sounds, you may hear a splitting of S_1 and S_2. That's because events in the left side of the heart occur just before those in the right side. So the mitral valve closes before the tricuspid valve, causing a split of S_1, and the aortic valve closes before the pulmonary valve, splitting S_2. You'll hear the S_1 split best at the tricuspid area,

Listening for heart sounds

To auscultate your patient's heart sounds, place the diaphragm of the stethoscope at the aortic, pulmonary, tricuspid, and mitral areas.

Aortic area

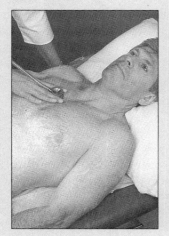

Pulmonary area

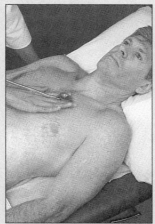

Tricuspid area

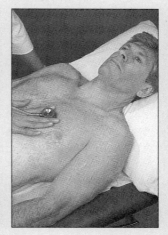

Mitral area

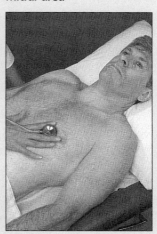

whereas you'll hear the S_2 split best at the pulmonary area at the end of expiration. Typically, a split S_2 is easier to hear than a split S_1 because the sound of the tricuspid valve closure tends to be faint.

S_3 and S_4

Now auscultate at each of the four areas, using the bell of the stethoscope. As you do, you may hear S_3 or S_4, normal variants in children and young adults but considered abnormal in others. Unlike the first two heart sounds, S_3 and S_4 are low-pitched. To hear them best, have the patient lie supine or on his left side.

You'll hear S_3 in early diastole, right after S_2. (It may sound like *lub-dub-dee.*) Called a ventricular gallop because of its triple sound, S_3 results from early rapid ventricular filling. Right and left ventricular S_3 sounds may occur either individually or together. A left ventricular S_3 is best heard at the apex, whereas a right ventricular S_3 may be heard best at either the xiphoid process or the lower left sternal border.

You'll hear S_4 late in diastole or presystole, just before S_1. (It may sound like *dee-lub-dub.*) Also called atrial gallop, S_4 results from increased resistance to ventricular filling after atrial contraction.

Pericardial friction rubs

As you auscultate, be alert for a pericardial friction rub, an extra heart sound that resembles squeaking leather, which may occur at any time during the cardiac cycle. Although you may hear these sounds anywhere on the chest, usually you'll hear them best at the third intercostal space, left sternal border.

Heart murmurs

Listen too for heart murmurs, which result from either turbulent blood flow produced by valvular or septal wall abnormalities or increased blood flow. Note the murmur's timing in the cardiac cycle as well as its quality, pitch, location, radiation, intensity, and configuration.

Determine timing by noting whether the murmur occurs during the systolic phase or the diastolic phase. A midsystolic murmur is also called an ejection murmur; a murmur heard throughout the systolic phase is called a pansystolic or holosystolic murmur. Describe the quality or sound of the murmur: Is it blowing, harsh, musical, or rumbling? Identify the pitch or frequency of the murmur as high, medium, or low. Note the location where you hear the murmur best. Is it the aortic, pulmonary, tricuspid, or mitral area? Also, note any radiation to other body structures. For example, pulmonary murmurs may radiate to the left side of the neck, whereas mitral murmurs may radiate to the axilla.

Use this rating system to describe the intensity of the murmur:
• Grade 1 — barely audible
• Grade 2 — audible but quiet, soft
• Grade 3 — moderately loud, without a thrust or thrill
• Grade 4 — loud, with a thrill
• Grade 5 — very loud, with a thrust or thrill
• Grade 6 — heard before the stethoscope comes in contact with the chest.

Also, establish the murmur's configuration, which represents the murmur much as it would appear on a phonocardiogram. This shows the approximate relation of the murmur to the normal heart sounds in timing and intensity. Crescendo indicates that the murmur begins softly and grows louder. Decrescendo indicates the opposite. Crescendo-decrescendo is a combination of the two patterns. And plateau indicates that the murmur is fairly constant, not appreciably altering in intensity.

Abnormal findings

After completing the health history and physical examination, you're ready to evaluate your findings. These findings may suggest a particular diagnosis or indicate a need for specific diagnostic tests.

Abnormal inspection findings

Inspection of the patient's head, neck, chest, skin, and extremities may reveal important clues about his cardiovascular status. You also may detect findings that reflect associated problems. For example, nasal flaring may indicate respiratory difficulty and anxiety, which may accompany cardiovascular disorders.

Head
When inspecting the patient's eyes, you may note bluish conjunctivae (a late sign of cyanosis and shock), white-centered petechiae of the conjunctivae (possibly indicating infective endocarditis), or bluish sclerae (suggesting aortic regurgitation and Marfan's syndrome). In a young adult, an opaque ring around the cornea, or corneal arcus, may suggest CAD; in a middle-aged adult, this sign could indicate high cholesterol. Yellow fatty deposits, or xanthelasma, found on the eyelids may indicate hyperlipidemia. And, although exophthalmos and staring most commonly stem from hyperthyroidism, they may also signal advanced congestive heart failure (CHF).

Neck
Stemming from increased right atrial pressure, jugular vein distention reflects a rise in fluid volume caused by dysfunction in the right side of the heart.

Abnormal findings revealed by hemodynamic monitoring may include increased wave amplitude (possibly indicating tricuspid stenosis, right ventricular infarction, right atrial enlargement, high-grade atrioventricular blocks, ventricular tachycardia, or other conditions that impede the transfer of blood from the right atrium to the right ventricle). Decreased x-wave activity may indicate tricuspid insufficiency.

A weak carotid artery pulsation may stem from diminished cardiac output. Strong or bounding pulsations usually occur in high cardiac output states, such as hypoxia, anemia, and anxiety.

Chest

Increased cardiac output or an aortic aneurysm may produce pulsations in the aortic area. Elevated pulmonary pressure from left ventricular failure may cause an abnormal pulsation in the pulmonary area. A patient with a thin chest, anemia, increased cardiac output, or anxiety may have slight pulsations to the right and left of the sternum in the precordial area.

Displacement of the apical impulse sometimes indicates left ventricular enlargement, which may result from CHF or systemic hypertension. An epigastric pulsation sometimes reflects early CHF or an aortic aneurysm.

Skin

Cyanosis or pallor may indicate poor cardiac output and tissue perfusion. Central cyanosis is found in the warm areas of the body, such as the conjunctivae and mucous membranes; peripheral cyanosis occurs in the cooler body areas, such as the earlobes, outer surface of the lips, nail beds, and nose.

Conditions resulting in decreased cardiac output and perfusion will cause the skin to become cool or cold. Conversely, conditions that cause fever or hyperdynamic cardiac output may make the skin warm or even hot.

Extremities

Patchy hair distribution on the legs may indicate peripheral vascular disease. An absence of normal body hair on the arms and legs may indicate diminished arterial blood flow to these areas.

Finger clubbing often indicates long-standing hypoxic disease. In early clubbing, the normal 160-degree angle between the nail and the nail base approximates 180 degrees. As clubbing progresses, this angle widens and the base of the nail becomes visibly swollen. In late clubbing, the angle where the nail meets the now-convex nail base extends more than halfway up the nail.

Edema can stem from CHF or venous insufficiency, which may be caused by varicosities or thrombophlebitis. Chronic right ventricular failure may cause ascites, which leads to generalized edema and abdominal distention. Venous compression in a specific area may result in localized edema along the path of the compressed vessel.

Abnormal palpation findings

Among the abnormalities you may detect during palpation are bilateral differences in pulse amplitude; a weak, bounding, or irregular pulse; abnormal pulsations; thrills; and heaves. These findings reveal important information about the patient's cardiac output, vascular resistance, arterial pressure, and valvular function.

Arterial pulses

Weak pulses indicate low cardiac output or increased peripheral vascular resistance, as occurs in arterial atherosclerotic disease. Weak pedal pulses are common in elderly patients. A strong bounding pulse occurs in patients with hypertension and in high cardiac output states, such as exercise, pregnancy, anemia, and thyrotoxicosis. (See *Identifying arterial pulse abnormalities,* pages 192 and 193.)

Chest

A more forceful and longer apical impulse (lasting longer than one-third of the cardiac cycle) may indicate increased cardiac output. A pulsation in the aortic, pulmonary, or right ventricular area can result from chamber enlargement or valvular disease. A pulsation in the sternoclavicular or epigastric area suggests an aortic aneurysm.

A palpable thrill (fine vibration) indicates blood flow turbulence, usually related to valvular dysfunction. A heave (a strong outward thrust during systole) along the left sternal border may indicate right ventricular hypertrophy. Over the left ventricular area, a heave suggests a ventricular aneurysm.

Skin

A patient with cool, moist skin may have sympathetic peripheral vasoconstriction caused by decreased cardiac output. Taut, shiny skin that can't be grasped and raised may reveal ascites or marked edema. Decreased skin turgor may indicate dehydration from fluid challenges or potent diuretic therapy.

Identifying arterial pulse abnormalities

To identify arterial pulse abnormalities, compare your patient's peripheral pulse wave with the normal pulse wave, which is shown at right.

Then review the remaining six waveforms, which are associated with cardiovascular disorders. They include weak and bounding pulse and pulsus alternans, paradoxus, bigeminus, and biferiens.

Normal pulse

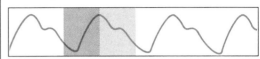

A normal pulse has two components: systole and diastole. Indicated by the initial upstroke, systole (shown in gray) signifies the arterial pressure during ventricular contraction. Diastole (shown in green), the downstroke, indicates the arterial pressure during ventricular relaxation when the heart fills.

Weak pulse

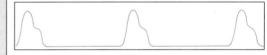

The contour of this waveform demonstrates a slower upstroke and downstroke with a slightly rounded, extended peak. The amplitude is decreased. Some possible causes of this waveform include increased peripheral vascular resistance, such as occurs in cold weather or severe congestive heart failure; and decreased stroke volume, such as occurs in hypovolemia or aortic stenosis.

Bounding pulse

The contour of the bounding pulse is opposite that of the weak pulse. It has a sharp upstroke and downstroke with a pointed peak. The amplitude is elevated. Possible causes include increased stroke volume, as in aortic regurgitation; increased stiffness of arterial walls, as in atherosclerosis or normal aging; exercise; anxiety; fever; and hypertension.

Generalized edema may occur with right ventricular failure; dependent edema may indicate left ventricular failure.

Abnormal auscultation findings

The abnormalities that you hear during auscultation are among the most significant indicators of cardiovascular disease. Vascular sounds, abnormal heart sounds, and heart murmurs provide specific clues that help pinpoint a diagnosis.

Vascular sounds

A bruit heard during arterial auscultation may indicate occlusive arterial disease or an arteriovenous fistula. Various high cardiac output conditions, such as anemia, hyperthyroidism, or pheochromocytoma, may also cause bruits.

Heart sounds

Abnormal heart sounds you may hear during chest auscultation include three types of pathologic split S_2, S_3 (ventricular gallop), S_4 (atrial gallop), summation gallop, opening snap, ejection click, pericardial friction rub, and heart murmurs.

Pulsus alternans

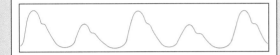

This condition is represented by an alternating pattern of a weak pulse followed by a stronger pulse. The time interval between each wave is equal. This pulse wave is commonly associated with severe left ventricular failure.

Pulsus bigeminus

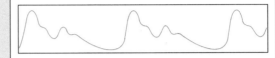

This pattern is similar to the pulsus alternans but the weaker wave occurs early, making the time intervals irregular. Premature atrial and ventricular contractions may cause this pattern because the heart has less ventricular filling time. These premature contractions may stem from heart failure or hypoxia.

Pulsus paradoxus

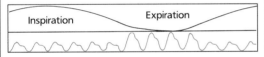

With this pattern, increases and decreases in amplitude are associated with the respiratory cycle, and marked decreases occur during inspiration. Pulsus paradoxus may be associated with conditions such as pericardial tamponade, constrictive pericarditis, advanced heart failure, and severe lung disease.

Pulsus biferiens

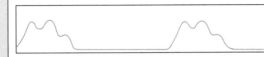

This pattern shows an initial upstroke, a downstroke, and a second upstroke during systole. Aortic stenosis, regurgitation, or insufficiency may cause this pattern.

Pathologic split S_2

There are three types of pathologic split S_2: wide split, fixed split, and paradoxical split. The *wide split S_2*, indicative of pulmonary stenosis or right bundle-branch block, is heard on both inspiration and expiration, but the split sound is wider on inspiration. The *fixed split S_2* is present during both inspiration and expiration. The length of the split is equal in both these phases of respiration. Atrial septal defects and right ventricular failure may cause fixed S_2 splitting. Left bundle-branch block may cause a *paradoxical split S_2*. The split sound is present on expiration but not on inspiration.

The intensity of the split S_2 provides key diagnostic information. A louder aortic component of the split may indicate systemic hypertension or aortic dilation. A softer aortic component may signal aortic stenosis. A louder pulmonary component may be associated with pulmonary hypertension, but it may also be normal in a patient with a thin chest wall. A softer pulmonary component suggests pulmonary stenosis.

Third heart sound

Heard in early diastole, a ventricular gallop (S_3) results from vibrations during rapid ventricular

PATHOPHYSIOLOGY

Three causes of murmurs

Heart murmurs may result from high blood flow through a normal valve, decreased blood flow through a stenotic valve, or backflow at an insufficient valve. The illustrations at the right show these three causes of murmurs.

High blood flow

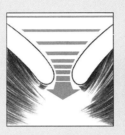

Decreased blood flow

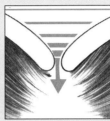

Backflow of blood

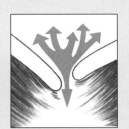

filling and signals CHF. Movements that increase venous return may strengthen S_3. The sound usually disappears when the rapid-filling disorder resolves.

S_3 may also be associated with acute MI, pulmonary edema, ventricular or atrial septal defect, and either mitral or aortic insufficiency.

Fourth heart sound
Atrial gallop, or S_4, may be a sign of cardiovascular problems, such as hypertension, aortic stenosis, mitral regurgitation, acute MI, systemic or pulmonary hypertension, and CAD.

Summation gallop
In adults with severe myocardial disease and tachycardia, you may hear the cumulative effect of S_3 and S_4. This abnormality is known as a summation gallop.

Opening snap
Forcible falling of valve leaflets into a ventricle may produce a plopping, snapping sound. In mitral stenosis, the valve leaflets may snap into the left ventricle early in diastole. The resulting opening snap—a short, high-frequency sound—is best heard halfway between the mitral and pulmonary areas at the fourth intercostal space. In tricuspid stenosis or atrial septal defect, you may hear the snap at the left sternal border.

Ejection click
Often associated with stenotic aortic or pulmonary valves, the high-pitched ejection click may also be associated with hypertension and a dilated aorta or pulmonary artery. In aortic stenosis, the click doesn't change with respiration and is best heard at the apex. Conversely, in pulmonary stenosis, the click is best heard during expiration at the upper left sternal border.

Pericardial friction rub
A grating, raspy sound, a pericardial friction rub may stem from inflammation of the pericardial sac, which causes the parietal and visceral surfaces to rub together.

Heart murmurs
Three mechanisms cause murmurs: increased blood flow through a normal valve, impeded flow through a narrowed valve, and backflow due to an incompetent valve leaflet. (See *Three causes of murmurs.*)

Systolic murmurs occur during ventricular systole and may result from turbulent blood flow through a stenotic aortic or pulmonary valve, regurgitant flow through an incompetent mitral or tricuspid valve, or flow through a ventricular septal defect. Diastolic murmurs occur during ventricular diastole and may result from turbulent flow through a stenotic mitral or tricuspid valve or regurgitant flow through an incompetent aortic or pulmonary valve.

The timing of the murmur helps you identify the cause. For instance, an early systolic murmur reflects a direct blood flow between the right and left ventricles and may indicate a small ventricular septal defect. Usually, the shunt is from left to right because of the higher pressure in the left ventricle.

A midsystolic murmur accompanied by a palpable thrill at the pulmonary area, a split S_2, and an ejection click suggests pulmonary stenosis. Characterized by a crescendo-decrescendo pattern, the murmur varies with respiration. It's best heard at the pulmonary area and radiates to the left shoulder.

A midsystolic murmur that radiates to the neck and apex may stem from aortic stenosis. Associated findings may include a palpable thrill at the aortic area, a softened S_2, and an ejection click. The murmur is harsh with a crescendo-decrescendo pattern.

Midsystolic murmurs can also result from an accelerated flow of blood through the heart valves caused by such conditions as fever, fluid overload, exercise, anemia, thyrotoxicosis, and heart block. A late systolic murmur associated with an ejection click may indicate mitral valve prolapse.

A murmur heard through the entire systolic period (called a pansystolic or holosystolic murmur) may reflect a significant ventricular septal defect. A loud, high-pitched pansystolic murmur in the mitral area that radiates toward the left axilla may stem from mitral regurgitation. Associated findings may include a decreased S_1 and an apical thrill. A high-pitched, blowing pansystolic murmur that radiates to the right of the sternum and is accentuated by inspiration over the tricuspid area suggests tricuspid regurgitation.

Suspect pulmonary regurgitation if you hear an early diastolic murmur that increases with respiration and is harsh, short, rough, and soft-pitched with a decrescendo pattern. An early diastolic murmur that is best heard over the aortic area and may radiate to the left sternal border may stem from aortic regurgitation. This high-pitched, blowing decrescendo murmur is often heard in conjunction with S_3

and may be caused by rheumatic fever, congenital heart disease, endocarditis, Marfan's syndrome, or aortic root dissection.

Middiastolic to late diastolic murmurs are low-pitched and rumbling. These murmurs may indicate mitral or tricuspid stenosis or mitral regurgitation.

Pertinent diagnostic tests

Various studies—including laboratory tests, electrocardiography (ECG), radiography, echocardiography, cardiac nuclear imaging procedures, and invasive procedures—may prove useful when assessing a patient with cardiovascular problems. Some tests, such as cardiac catheterization, evaluate cardiovascular function. Others, such as cardiac enzyme and isoenzyme tests, help pinpoint a diagnosis of heart disease. Still others, such as a stress ECG, can be used to determine the effectiveness of treatment for existing disorders, such as CAD.

Laboratory tests

Common laboratory tests used to evaluate a patient's cardiovascular status include cardiac enzyme tests, lipid studies, and electrolyte studies.

Cardiac enzyme tests. An analysis of cardiac enzyme and isoenzyme levels can aid in the diagnosis of an MI. Commonly used tests include total creatine phosphokinase (CPK), CPK-MM in skeletal muscles, CPK-MB in the heart muscle, CPK-BB in the brain and in nerve tissue, total lactate dehydrogenase, lactate dehydrogenase 1, and lactate dehydrogenase 2.

Lipid studies. Measurements of total cholesterol, LDL cholesterol, HDL cholesterol, and triglyceride levels help detect cardiovascular disease.

Electrolyte studies. Magnesium, calcium, potassium, and sodium levels can help identify causes of certain cardiac conduction abnormalities. For example, a prolonged QT interval may result from hypocalcemia, whereas a shortened QT interval may be caused by hypercalcemia.

Electrocardiography

The following tests yield important diagnostic information about the patient's cardiovascular status: 12-lead ECG, stress ECG, Holter monitoring, signal-averaged ECG, and esophageal pill electrode ECG.

12-lead ECG. This test provides 12 views of the heart's electrical activity. It aids in diagnosing such disorders as myocardial ischemia, injury, and infarction; heart blocks; hypertrophy; electrolyte abnormalities; and drug toxicity.

Stress ECG. This test uses the 12-lead ECG to record the heart's electrical activity during and after exercise (usually on a treadmill). Blood pressure readings are correlated with ECG findings during and after the test. If a patient is suspected of having CAD, the test may indicate underlying ischemia even though the patient doesn't have any symptoms. The test may also be used to assess pulmonary function and exercise-induced arrhythmias and to evaluate the effectiveness of drug therapy for CAD.

Holter monitoring. Used to record the heart's electrical activity over a 24-hour period, Holter monitoring identifies arrhythmias as they occur during the patient's normal day. Holter monitoring may be used when a patient has symptoms of an unknown origin, such as syncope, light-headedness, palpitations, or chest discomfort.

Signal-averaged ECG. With standard 12-lead ECG techniques, very low amplitudes are difficult to evaluate. But signal-averaged ECG can decrease and filter extraneous noise that may conceal late potentials associated with sustained ventricular tachycardia and sudden death. The test may be useful for patients who have significantly decreased left ventricular function, dilated cardiomyopathy, or syncope of unknown origin.

Esophageal pill electrode ECG. Used to diagnose wide-complex electrical tachycardias of unknown origin, this test requires the patient to swallow a small gelatinous pill with a bipolar electrode. When the pill descends about 18″ (45 cm) past the teeth, a three-channel ECG with an amplifier records the heart's electrical rhythm.

Cardiac nuclear imaging

Among the nuclear imaging procedures commonly ordered to evaluate cardiac function are thallium scanning, technetium Tc 99m pyrophosphate scanning, and multiple-gated acquisition (MUGA) scanning.

Thallium scanning. Also called cold-spot imaging, this test uses thallium-201, a radioactive analogue of potassium, to evaluate myocardial blood flow. Typically, healthy myocardial cells take up thallium. Myocardial ischemia or necrosis, however, causes diminished uptake of thallium.

Technetium Tc 99m pyrophosphate scanning. Also called hot-spot imaging, technetium Tc 99m scanning reveals damaged myocardial tissue as hot spots (areas in which radioisotopes accumulate), especially in the right ventricle and the posterior section of the left ventricle. The test also detects ventricular aneurysms, contusions, and damage from electric current.

MUGA scanning. MUGA scanning is used to evaluate left ventricular function, to detect aneurysms of the left ventricle and other myocardial wall-motion abnormalities, and to detect intracardiac shunting. The test is also known as radiographic ventriculography, wall-motion study, and gated blood pool imaging.

Invasive procedures

The following invasive diagnostic procedures may be ordered to assess cardiovascular function: cardiac catheterization, aortography, electrophysiologic studies, digital subtraction angiography, angiography by videodilution, and venography.

Cardiac catheterization. This procedure permits the examiner to view the coronary arteries and to determine heart size and valvular integrity.

Aortography. With this test, the examiner injects a contrast medium to enhance radiographic visualization of the aorta.

Electrophysiologic studies. These studies use electrical stimulation of the myocardial tissue to identify electrical accessory pathways. They're also used to determine a differential diagnosis of tachycardias, the origin of ectopy, and the effectiveness of drug therapy in controlling ectopy.

Digital subtraction angiography. For this test, a contrast dye is injected and then computer-enhanced fluoroscopic imaging is used to view vascular structures, especially the carotid arteries and renal vasculature.

Angiography by videodilution. After a catheter is placed in a selected section of an artery, this test evaluates the flow of arterial blood.

Venography. This invasive procedure provides information about abnormal conditions found in the venous structures of the arms and legs. It can help analyze anatomic structure and patency.

Miscellaneous tests

Other tests that may be used to evaluate cardiovascular function include radiography, echocardiography, magnetic resonance imaging (MRI), plethysmography, phonocardiography, vectorcardiography, positron emission tomography, and cardiokymography.

Radiography. The chest X-ray is a standard diagnostic tool used to assess heart size, the presence of pericardial and pleural effusion, and the status of pulmonary infiltration and edema.

Echocardiography. This ultrasonic test provides two-dimensional and cross-sectional views of cardiac structures, such as the valves, septum, and heart chambers. Echocardiography is widely used to evaluate valvular disease; cardiac function; heart wall size, thickness, and motion; and pericardial effusion.

Transesophageal echocardiography allows for closer, more direct viewing of the heart structures and is used when conventional echocardiography can't provide the necessary information. For this test, the examiner inserts a gastroscope with an ultrasonic device to obtain the ultrasonic views of the heart.

Magnetic resonance imaging. Commonly referred to as MRI, this test visualizes the anatomic structures of the heart from a three-dimensional perspective. It's especially useful in assessing valvular and coronary arterial structure, detecting effusion and tumors, and identifying the presence of injured tissue, congenital defects, and aneurysms.

Plethysmography. This test measures the volume and flow of blood in the patient's extremities.

Phonocardiography. Used to supplement echocardiography, this test records heart sounds phonographically. Phonocardiography is most useful when evaluating the timing of abnormal heart sounds and murmurs.

Vectorcardiography. This test provides a three-dimensional illustration of the flow of ventricular electrical activity. It yields additional information about electrical ventricular conduction defects, can detect an MI when multiple conduction defects are present, and reveals ventricular enlargement.

Positron emission tomography. This test can identify changes in normal physiologic function caused by an MI.

Cardiokymography. Used in conjunction with the stress ECG, cardiokymography provides an electromagnetic evaluation of the state of the heart's contractility.

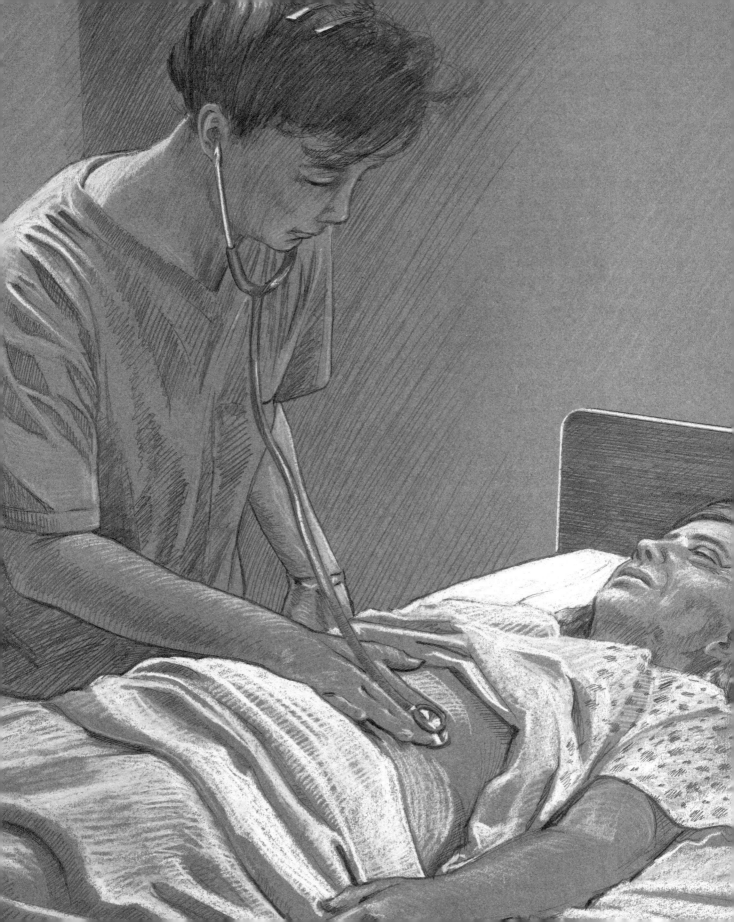

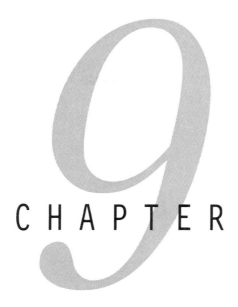

CHAPTER

Gastrointestinal system

The gastrointestinal (GI) system performs the essential functions of ingestion, digestion, and elimination. Any interruption of these functions can quickly affect a patient's well-being. Obviously, GI problems can disrupt a patient's nutritional status. They can have other serious consequences too. Vomiting and diarrhea, for instance, can trigger an acid-base imbalance.

To identify the cause of such GI disturbances, you need to perform a thorough, accurate nursing assessment. After presenting a review of GI anatomy and physiology, this chapter explains how to perform a skilled GI assessment. The chapter gives you guidelines for taking a health history and describes the techniques you'll use to examine your patient's GI system. After these sections on the actual assessment, you'll find a review of the abnormal findings you'll most often encounter. The last section of the chapter covers the diagnostic tests commonly used in evaluating patients' GI symptoms.

Anatomy and physiology

The GI system consists of two major components: the alimentary canal and the accessory GI organs. The alimentary canal—a hollow, muscular tube—begins in the mouth and ends in the anus. Also called the GI tract, the alimentary canal includes the pharynx, esophagus, stomach, small intestine, and large intestine. Accessory organs of the GI system include the liver, gallbladder and bile ducts, and pancreas.

The major functions of the alimentary canal and accessory organs are digestion and elimination. Digestion breaks down food and fluid into simple chemicals that the bloodstream can absorb and transport throughout the body. Elimination gets rid of the body's waste products by excreting feces. (See *Reviewing the GI system*.)

Alimentary canal

The alimentary canal consists of muscle tissue alternating with nerve tissue and blood vessels. The circular and longitudinal fibers of the canal cause a series of muscle contractions called peristalsis, which propels food through the canal. Along the 25' (6-m) length of the canal, the GI glands and accessory organs break down ingested food into useful components and eliminate unabsorbed residues.

Mouth
The digestive process begins with chewing, salivating, and swallowing. Unlike other sites of GI activity, your patient's mouth is completely visible, so you can see exactly where these processes take place.

The hard and soft palates form the roof of the mouth, or buccal cavity, and the tongue forms the floor. The cheeks and lips complete the structure. An adult normally has 32 teeth, which he uses to chew. The tongue assists in chewing and swallowing as well as in tasting.

Along with the mucous glands in the mouth, three pairs of glands produce saliva: the parotid, the submandibular, and the sublingual. As a result of chewing and mixing with saliva, food is broken down into digestible form. The salivary enzyme amylase begins starch digestion by hydrolyzing starch to maltose. Salivation can be stimulated by the sight, taste, smell, and even the thought of food.

Pharynx
The pharynx, or throat, secretes mucus and assists in the act of swallowing. When food reaches the back of the mouth, the epiglottis, a lid of fibrocartilage, closes over the larynx and the soft palate rises to close off the nasal cavity.

Esophagus
A muscular tube, the esophagus moves food from the pharynx to the stomach. When swallowing occurs, the upper esophageal sphincter relaxes, and the bolus of food slides into the esophagus. Peristaltic contraction of the esophagus propels the food toward the stomach.

The gastroesophageal sphincter at the lower end of the esophagus, which is normally closed to prevent gastric reflux, opens during swallowing, belching, and vomiting.

Stomach
This curved organ lies obliquely in the left upper quadrant (LUQ) of the abdomen. (See *Reviewing the abdominal quadrants*, page 202.) The cardiac sphincter guards the entrance to the stomach, and the pyloric sphincter guards the exit.

The stomach has three major functions: storing food, mixing food with gastric juices, and slowly passing chyme—the watery food bolus mixed with digestive juices—into the small intestine for continued digestion and absorption. Protein digestion begins in the stomach, and small amounts of water, glucose, alcohol, and electrolytes are absorbed there. An average meal remains in the stomach for 3 to 4 hours. Accordion-like folds in the stomach wall called rugae allow the stomach to distend to accommodate entire meals of food and fluid.

Small intestine
The small intestine completes the digestive process by absorbing the end products of diges-

ANATOMY

Reviewing the GI system

Use this illustration to review the GI system's major anatomic structures.

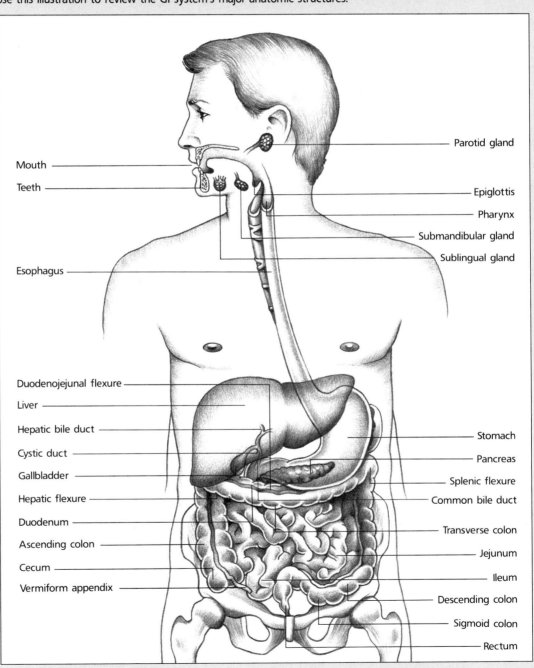

Mouth

Teeth

Esophagus

Duodenojejunal flexure

Liver

Hepatic bile duct

Cystic duct

Gallbladder

Hepatic flexure

Duodenum

Ascending colon

Cecum

Vermiform appendix

Parotid gland

Epiglottis

Pharynx

Submandibular gland

Sublingual gland

Stomach

Pancreas

Splenic flexure

Common bile duct

Transverse colon

Jejunum

Ileum

Descending colon

Sigmoid colon

Rectum

Reviewing the abdominal quadrants

To help visualize the location of your patient's abdominal organs, mentally divide his abdomen into regions. The simplest method for doing this, the quadrant method, uses two imaginary lines crossing perpendicularly at the umbilicus.

Right upper quadrant
Liver and gallbladder
Pylorus
Duodenum
Head of pancreas
Hepatic flexure of colon
Portions of ascending and transverse
   colon

Left upper quadrant
Left liver lobe
Stomach
Body of pancreas
Splenic flexure of colon
Portions of transverse and descending
   colon

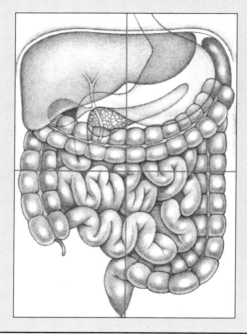

Right lower quadrant
Cecum and appendix
Portion of ascending colon
Lower portion of right kidney
Bladder (if distended)

Left lower quadrant
Sigmoid colon
Portion of descending colon
Lower portion of left kidney
Bladder (if distended)

tion. Carbohydrates are hydrolyzed to mono-saccharides, fats to glycerol and fatty acids, and proteins to amino acids. Glands in the small intestine, enzymes from the pancreas, and bile from the liver provide the secretions responsible for digestion.

A long, coiled tube that extends from the pylorus to the ileocecal valve, the small intestine has a serous outer coat formed by the peritoneum. Millions of small, fingerlike projections called villi greatly increase the surface area available for absorption. The villi secrete mucus from their goblet cells, and their enzymes digest food as it's absorbed.

Segmental contractions move the chyme short distances, allowing it to mix with many digestive enzymes. Peristalsis propels the contents through the small intestine over periods varying from 3 to 10 hours.

The small intestine also reacts to nervous stimulation. The vagus nerve stimulates motility and secretion, the sympathetic system inhibits motility, and the sensory fibers of the sympathetic system relay pain.

Large intestine

The large intestine consists of the cecum and appendix; the ascending, transverse, descending, and sigmoid portions of the colon; the rectum; and the anal canal. The two key functions of the large intestine are to absorb water and electrolytes and to form feces.

Food entering the stomach and duodenum initiates gastrocolic and duodenocolic reflexes, causing peristalsis in the colon. The parasympathetic nervous system innervates the large intestine, stimulating the secretion of a protective mucus and the contraction of the strong muscular layer. The sympathetic nervous system inhibits both secretion and motility.

The colon harbors microorganisms used for putrefying proteins not digested or absorbed in the small intestine. Ammonia, a by-product of this decomposition process, is carried to the liver and converted to urea. Bacterial synthesis of vitamin K and some B vitamins also occurs in the colon, and these bacteria produce flatus.

The rectum, a short segment of the large intestine, ends at the anal canal, which is held closed by the anal sphincter. Defecation through this canal involves both involuntary and voluntary control. Feces in the rectum stimulate sensory nerve endings, producing an impulse to defecate. But voluntary control can keep the anal sphincter closed to suppress defecation.

Accessory GI organs

Although not parts of the alimentary canal, three organs—the liver, gallbladder, and pancreas—play critical roles in the digestive process. Certain vascular structures, including the abdominal aorta and the gastric and splenic veins, also contribute to digestion.

Liver

Located in the right upper quadrant (RUQ), the liver is the largest organ in the body. It has two major lobes—the right lobe and the smaller left lobe—which are divided by the falciform ligament. About two-thirds of the liver lies to the right of the midline.

The liver plays a major role in carbohydrate metabolism. It also detoxifies various plasma toxins and synthesizes plasma proteins, nonessential amino acids, and vitamin A. Plus, the liver stores essential nutrients, including iron and vitamins D, K, and B_{12}, and converts ammonia to urea for excretion.

The liver also secretes bile—a greenish liquid composed of water, electrolytes, and phospholipids that helps break down fat and absorb fatty acids, cholesterol, and other lipids. Bile also helps prevent jaundice by causing the liver to excrete conjugated bilirubin, an end product of hemoglobin degradation.

Gallbladder

The gallbladder lies below the right lobe of the liver. This small, pear-shaped organ stores bile until it's discharged into the biliary ductal system, which empties into the duodenum.

Pancreas

The pancreas lies horizontally in the upper abdomen behind the stomach with its tail touching the spleen. The head of the pancreas is attached to the duodenum.

The pancreas has both endocrine and exocrine functions. As an endocrine gland, it releases insulin and glycogen into the circulation. As an exocrine gland, it produces pancreatic juice that travels to the duodenum for use in digestion.

Vascular structures

The abdominal aorta supplies blood to the alimentary canal. The aorta enters the abdomen at the level of the 12th thoracic vertebra, divides into the common iliac arteries, and continues to branch into the many arteries throughout the length of the canal.

Absorbed nutrients are carried away from the alimentary canal by way of the gastric and splenic veins and other veins that drain into the portal vein of the liver. The blood circulates through the liver, exits by way of the hepatic vein, and empties into the inferior vena cava.

Health history

Because GI symptoms may cause your patient substantial pain or discomfort, you'll need to move quickly through the stages of your assessment. But no matter how urgent or painful your patient's GI complaint may be, always take a health history. Even a few minutes of questioning can help you make important associations between the patient's health practices and his current GI problem.

The health history should consist of an exploration of the patient's chief complaint and pertinent questions about his medical history, family history, psychosocial history, and activities of daily living.

Chief complaint

Pain, heartburn, nausea, vomiting, and altered bowel habits are among the most common chief complaints of the GI system. To investigate these or any chief complaints, ask your patient relevant questions about such particulars as onset, duration, and severity. Also, ask what precipitates the symptom, what makes it worse, and what makes it better. For more information on exploring the chief complaint, see Chapter 3.

Medical history

Determine whether your patient has ever had a GI problem before. Use a checklist of common GI symptoms to help jog his memory about disorders of the mouth, throat, abdomen, and rectum. Make sure you ask about long-term GI conditions, such as chronic ulcerative colitis, which can predispose him to colorectal cancer.

Ask about other major disorders as well. Neurologic disorders such as a cerebrovascular accident or peripheral nerve damage can impair movement of the tongue, mouth, and throat. Other major disorders (such as chronic obstructive pulmonary disease, hypothyroidism, and diabetes mellitus) can cause constipation or other bowel problems.

Does your patient have any allergies? Allergic reactions to foods or medications may lead to various GI symptoms.

If he has traveled recently, where did he go and for how long? Diarrhea, a parasitic infection, or hepatitis may result from drinking contaminated water or eating contaminated food.

Ask your patient about any surgery or treatment he has had, including oral surgery. Find out why he had the surgery or treatment and how well he recovered.

Ask if he's taking any prescription drugs or over-the-counter drugs. Specifically, ask if he's using any drugs for GI problems, or if he has in the past. Many medications affect GI function.

Ask too if he uses vitamins, mineral supplements, laxatives, mineral oil, aspirin or other analgesics, or herbal remedies. Any of these can trigger GI problems. A patient taking aspirin for its positive cardiovascular effects should keep the dose small; large amounts of aspirin can cause GI bleeding.

Family history

Ask your patient about the health history of his immediate family members. What diseases have they had? Ask too about the causes of death. Ask specifically about Crohn's disease, ulcerative colitis, colon cancer, gallbladder disease, alcoholism, and stomach ulcers.

Psychosocial history

Your patient's occupation, family life, and emotional state all affect his risk of developing GI disorders. Financial pressures too can contribute to GI symptoms. Ask your patient to describe how his chief complaint is affecting him. Then ask him specifically about his occupation and his family situation. A patient in a high-stress job, for example, faces a greater risk of developing a duodenal ulcer than someone in a relaxed work environment. And when an unemployed patient tells you he can't afford food for his children, he's probably not getting adequate nutrition himself.

Emotional crises or significant losses can put patients at risk for many GI symptoms, including pain, nausea, and anorexia. For example, an elderly widower now cooking for himself faces a significant risk of anorexia.

Your patient's self-image also can affect his susceptibility to GI problems. Ask him if he's satisfied with his current weight. Has obesity or anorexia ever been a problem? Also ask if he feels generally fit and healthy and if he's sexually active.

Activities of daily living

How your patient cares for himself on a daily basis directly affects his GI system. So ask him about his diet, exercise patterns, and use of tobacco and alcohol.

To investigate your patient's diet, ask what he's eaten in the past 24 hours and if this represents a typical day. Does he usually have a good appetite, and has his appetite changed recently? Find out who buys and prepares the food in your patient's household. Does he follow a special diet or avoid certain foods? Also ask if he regularly drinks coffee, tea, or other caffeine products.

Ask your patient if he exercises regularly, or if he has recently started or stopped an exercise program. Does exercise make his current GI complaint better or worse?

Ask your patient if he smokes or drinks and if so, how much. Smoking can aggravate an ulcer and predispose a patient to oral and lung cancers. Consuming excessive amounts of alcohol may irritate the stomach lining and can precipitate hepatic and pancreatic diseases. Because alcohol provides calories, but no essential nutrients, chronic alcohol abuse can lead to malnutrition.

Also determine whether the patient goes to the dentist regularly. If he wears dentures, have him describe how he cleans them. Ill-fitting dentures may cause gingival or palatal irritation.

Physical examination

Start your examination by assessing the patient's nutritional status. Then conduct a thorough examination of his mouth, and assess his abdomen, liver, and rectum. During your assessment, explain the examination techniques you'll be using, and tell the patient that some of them may cause discomfort.

Before starting your examination, make sure the room is private, quiet, warm, and well lighted.

Nutritional status

First, measure and weigh your patient and compare your findings with the normal values on a standardized chart. Next, observe him for clues to his nutritional status, keeping in mind the information you collected during the health history. Does he appear well nourished, obese, or emaciated?

Unless your patient has an urgent complaint, take the time to perform anthropometric arm measurements. These measurements provide information about the caloric reserves in subcutaneous fat and indicate skeletal muscle mass. First, locate and mark the midpoint of his upper arm. Then measure his skin-fold thickness with calipers, measure his midarm circumference with a tape measure, and calculate his midarm muscle circumference. (See *Taking anthropometric arm measurements,* page 206.)

Mouth

Begin by inspecting the patient's mouth and jaw for asymmetry and swelling. Can he move his mouth freely? Check his bite and note whether he has a malocclusion.

Inspect the patient's lips, noting any abnormal color or texture. Also look for lesions. Palpate the outer and inner lips, checking for lesions, nodules, and fissures.

Using a penlight, inspect the patient's teeth and gums. Does he have obvious dental caries? Note any broken, missing, or displaced teeth as well as any dental appliances. Check the gums for recession, redness, pallor, hypertrophy, ulcers, and bleeding and palpate them for tenderness.

Does the patient's tongue deviate to one side? Note any tremors, redness, swelling, ulcers, or lesions. Does the tongue have an abnormal coating?

Using a tongue blade and bright light, inspect the mucosa. Next, examine the hard and soft palates. You may want to use a mirror to inspect the hard palate. Check for redness, lesions, patches, petechiae, and pallor.

Finally, examine the patient's pharynx. Look

Taking anthropometric arm measurements

Follow these steps to determine triceps skin-fold thickness, midarm circumference, and midarm muscle circumference.

Triceps skin-fold thickness

Determine the triceps skin-fold thickness by grasping the patient's skin between the thumb and forefinger about 1 cm above the midpoint, as shown below. Hold the calipers at the midpoint and squeeze for about 3 seconds. Record the measurement registered on the handle gauge to the nearest 0.5 mm. Take two more readings; then average all three to compensate for any error.

Midarm circumference and midarm muscle circumference

At the midpoint, measure the midarm circumference, as shown here. Then calculate midarm muscle circumference by multiplying the triceps skin-fold thickness (in centimeters) by 3.143 and subtracting the result from the midarm circumference.

Record all three measurements as percentages of the standard measurements by using the following formula:

$$\frac{\text{Actual measurement}}{\text{Standard measurement}} \times 100$$

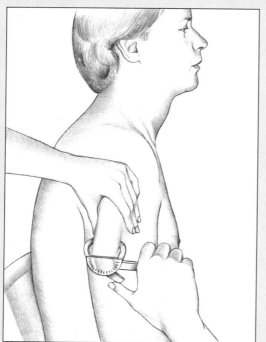

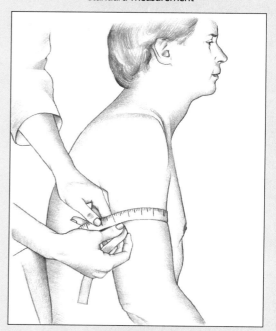

Compare the patient's percentage measurement with the standard. A measurement less than 90% of the standard indicates caloric deprivation; a measurement over 90% indicates adequate or more than adequate energy reserves.

MEASUREMENT	STANDARD	90%
Triceps skin-fold thickness	*Men:* 12.5 mm *Women:* 16.5 mm	*Men:* 11.3 mm *Women:* 14.9 mm
Midarm circumference	*Men:* 29.3 cm *Women:* 28.5 cm	*Men:* 26.4 cm *Women:* 25.7 cm
Midarm muscle circumference	*Men:* 25.3 cm *Women:* 23.2 cm	*Men:* 22.8 cm *Women:* 20.9 cm

for uvular deviation, tonsillar abnormalities, lesions, ulcers, plaques, and exudate. Note any unusual breath odors.

Abdomen

When you examine your patient's abdomen, you'll alter the usual sequence of the four assessment techniques. Because percussion and palpation can affect bowel activity and thus bowel sounds, you should always auscultate before percussing and palpating. If your patient has abdominal pain, assess the painful area last.

Make sure your patient has voided before the abdominal examination. Prepare him for the examination by placing him in the supine position. A pillow behind his head and another behind his knees will help him relax the abdominal muscles.

Inspection

Begin by inspecting the patient's entire abdomen. Note its general contour and symmetry as well as any abnormalities of the skin or umbilicus. Document any visible pulsations.

A normal abdomen is slightly rounded or convex with symmetrical, slightly curved borders, but contours vary depending on body type. A slender patient may have a flat or slightly concave abdomen, whereas an obese patient's abdomen will protrude.

Ask your patient to breathe deeply, and inspect his abdomen. If it appears distended, make a mental note to check for ascites when percussing and palpating later on. Irregular contours or asymmetrical distention will also require further assessment later.

If your patient's abdomen is distended, measure the girth with a tape held at the level of the umbilicus. Mark the abdomen with a felt-tip pen to ensure that subsequent readings accurately reflect changes.

Then, observe with your eyes at the level of the patient's abdomen. His skin should be smooth and unbroken, with varying amounts of hair. Note any discoloration, striae (lines or stretch marks), rashes, lesions, dilated veins, or scars.

Auscultating for vascular sounds

After listening to your patient's bowel sounds, use the bell of your stethoscope to auscultate for vascular sounds at the sites shown in this illustration.

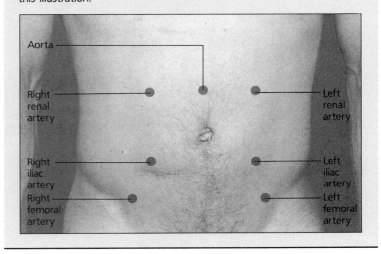

Ordinarily, you won't be able to see any abdominal movements except in very thin patients. Some slight, wavelike motion may be visible, but if you see strong contractions crossing the abdomen, report them; they may signal a bowel obstruction. If you detect aortic pulsations in the epigastric region, note their rate, intensity, and exact location. Never palpate a visible midline pulsation; it may indicate an abdominal aneurysm.

Your patient's umbilicus should be concave and positioned at the midline. An everted navel is a normal variation. If the umbilicus protrudes when your patient raises his head and shoulders, he may have an umbilical hernia.

Auscultation

After inspecting your patient's abdomen, you're ready to auscultate for bowel sounds, vascular sounds, and friction rubs. You should establish a regular sequence that you use every time you listen for bowel sounds. For instance, start in the RUQ and move clockwise. By using the same sequence every time, you'll ensure a thorough assessment.

Distinguishing between spleen and kidney enlargement

Typically, if you ask the patient to take a deep breath and then you percuss along the 9th and 10th left intercostal spaces, you'll hear tympany produced by colonic or gastric air. If you hear dullness instead, the patient's spleen may be enlarged. If you hear resonance, his left kidney may be enlarged.

Place the diaphragm of the stethoscope on the RUQ and listen for sounds of air and fluid moving through the bowel. Note the character and frequency of the sounds you hear. If you don't hear bowel sounds right away, be sure to listen for at least 2 minutes.

Normal bowel sounds are best described as soft bubbling or gurgling noises with no discernible pattern. They may last from less than 1 second to several seconds and may occur about 5 to 34 times each minute.

After you hear bowel sounds in the RUQ, move on to the other quadrants. If you don't hear any bowel sounds in a particular quadrant, the patient may have paralytic ileus. Or his bladder may be so full that it obscures the sounds. After 2 minutes of silence, try gently pressing on the abdomen or flicking your finger against it. Then auscultate again. Typically, this light pressure will provoke bowel sounds.

Next, auscultate your patient's abdomen for vascular sounds, using the bell of your stethoscope. Auscultate in the epigastric and umbilical regions to detect venous hums. Listen in the epigastric region and in each of the quadrants for bruits from the major abdominal arteries. Normally, you won't hear vascular sounds. (See *Auscultating for vascular sounds,* page 207.) Finally, place the diaphragm of the stethoscope over the liver and spleen and listen for friction rubs.

Percussion

You'll use percussion to check the size and location of your patient's abdominal organs and to detect excessive amounts of fluid and air in the abdomen. Don't use percussion (or palpation) on a patient who may have an abdominal aortic aneurysm or a patient who has had an abdominal organ transplant. Percuss cautiously in a patient who may have appendicitis.

As with auscultation, start in the RUQ and move clockwise. If your patient has abdominal pain, however, percuss the painful quadrant last.

Lightly percuss over the abdomen, identifying areas of tympany and dullness. You'll hear tympany when you percuss over a patient's air-filled stomach or intestine. You'll hear dullness over the liver and spleen and over a feces-filled intestine and urine-filled bladder. As you percuss, note where the abdominal sounds change from tympany to dullness. (See *Abdominal percussion sounds.*)

If the patient has a distended abdomen, assess him for ascites. With the patient supine, note if his flanks bulge, an indication of ascites. Then with him still supine, percuss for areas of tympany and dullness. You'll detect tympany over the upper abdomen because the bowel rises with the patient in this position. You'll detect dullness in the dependent parts of the abdomen. Check for shifting ascites by having the patient turn to the side and percussing again. If ascites is present, you'll note tympany in the superior portion of the abdomen and dullness in the dependent portion. To detect advanced ascites, place your palm and forearm along the patient's right flank. Next, tap the left flank with your other hand. If a large accumulation of fluid is present, a fluid wave will ripple across the abdomen and cause the patient's right flank to hit against your hand.

A normal spleen may produce a small area of dullness in the left midaxillary line at about the level of the 10th rib. However, in most patients, you won't be able to hear it because the tympany produced by colonic or gastric air will obscure it. To assess for splenic enlargement, ask the patient to inhale deeply. Then percuss along the 9th and 10th left intercostal spaces. A change from tympany to dullness as you percuss may indicate splenic enlargement. (See *Distinguishing between spleen and kidney enlargement.*)

Palpation

You'll use a combination of light and deep palpation and ballottement to assess your patient's abdomen. Again, start with the RUQ and move clockwise. However, if the patient complains of pain in one quadrant, palpate that one last. As you palpate, check for organ location, masses, muscle resistance, and areas of tenderness.

Begin with light palpation. If the patient finds palpation uncomfortable or if he's ticklish, have him put his hand on yours. This simple technique should relax him. If the patient complains of tenderness before you even touch him, try a different technique: Place the stethoscope on his abdomen as if you're going to auscultate, but instead use it to lightly palpate. Note whether the patient complains of pain.

Usually, you'll have to use deep palpation to evaluate abdominal masses. If you detect such a mass, note the location, size, shape, and consistency. Also note whether the mass is tender and whether it's fixed or mobile. Feel too for pulsations.

Be careful not to mistake a normal finding for a mass during abdominal palpation. The uterus, which you may palpate in the lower abdomen at the midline; the sacral promontory, which you may feel below the umbilicus in a thin patient; and a feces-filled colon, which you may palpate in the left lower quadrant, all can be mistaken for masses.

Usually, you won't be able to palpate the spleen. But unless you think it's ruptured, you should try to palpate it. Have the patient lie supine as you stand on his right side. Then support his posterior left lower rib cage with your left hand and have him take a deep breath. Use your other hand to press up and in toward the spleen. If you're able to feel the spleen, it's probably enlarged. (See *Palpating the spleen.*)

When a patient complains of pain or tenderness, you may try to elicit rebound tenderness, a sign of peritoneal irritation. Have the

Abdominal percussion sounds

When you percuss the abdomen, you'll normally hear dull and tympanic percussion sounds over the areas shown here.

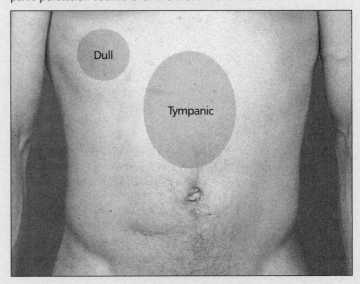

Palpating the spleen

With your patient in the supine position, stand on her right side. Then use your left hand to support her posterior left lower rib cage, and ask her to take a deep breath. With your right hand on the abdomen, press up and in toward the spleen, as shown.

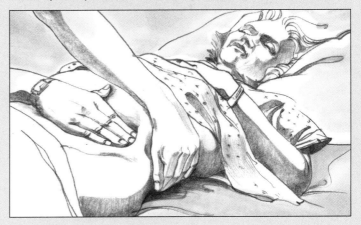

Eliciting rebound tenderness

Press your fingertips deeply and gently into the patient's abdomen at McBurney's point, as shown.

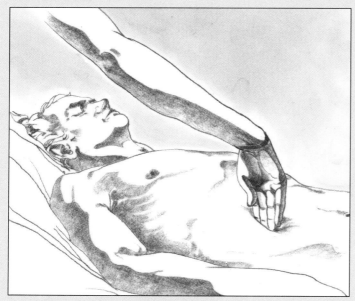

Then quickly withdraw your fingertips. If the patient feels pain when the tissue springs back, you've detected rebound tenderness.

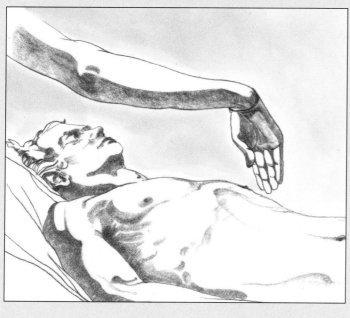

patient lie supine with his knees flexed. Next, locate McBurney's point (about one-third the distance between the right anterior superior iliac spine and the umbilicus). Press your fingertips slowly and deeply into this area; then release the pressure in a swift, smooth motion. If the patient complains of pain when the tissue springs back, you've elicited rebound tenderness.

This maneuver is controversial and considered unnecessary by many practitioners. If you use it, wait until the end of the examination because the resulting pain and muscle spasm can interfere with any further physical assessment. To lessen the risk of rupturing an inflamed appendix, don't repeat this maneuver. (See *Eliciting rebound tenderness*.)

Use light ballottement to detect areas of muscle resistance or guarding that may have been missed on deep palpation. Ballottement can also detect the movement or bounce of a freely movable mass.

Liver

To estimate the size of the liver, begin percussing the abdomen along the right midclavicular line below the level of the umbilicus. Move upward until the percussion sounds change from tympany to dullness. Typically, this occurs at or slightly below the costal margin. Mark this point with a felt-tip pen.

Next, starting above the nipple, percuss downward along the right midclavicular line until the percussion sounds change from normal lung resonance to dullness. Usually, this occurs between the fifth and seventh intercostal spaces. Again, mark the point where you hear the change. You can estimate the size of your patient's liver by measuring the distance between the two marks. (See *Percussing the liver*.)

Now, try to palpate the liver. Keep in mind that you won't be able to feel a normal-size liver in most patients. However, you may feel it in an extremely thin patient. And you may feel it in a patient with emphysema because his low diaphragm may displace the liver downward, making it easily palpable below the costal margin.

To palpate, place one hand on the patient's back at the approximate height of the liver. Place the other hand below your lower mark on the abdomen. Ask your patient to inhale deeply as you point your fingers toward the right costal margin and press gently. Try to feel the liver's edge as the diaphragm pushes it down to meet your fingertips. If the liver is palpable, its border should be smooth, rounded, firm, and nontender.

If you can't palpate the liver, you may want to try hooking it. Stand on your patient's right side near his shoulder. Place your hands side by side below the lower mark you've made. Then instruct the patient to inhale deeply and press your fingers inward and upward, attempting to feel the liver with the fingertips of both hands. (See *Palpating and hooking the liver*, page 212.)

If you suspect inflammation, hepatitis, or hepatomegaly, use fist percussion, or blunt percussion, to detect tenderness. You should attempt to palpate the liver before using fist percussion. Stop percussing if the patient complains of pain or discomfort. Tenderness on the right side during fist percussion suggests inflammation.

Rectum

With patients over age 40, perform a rectal examination as a routine part of a complete assessment. You should also perform a rectal examination on a patient with rectal discomfort or altered bowel habits and on a male patient with altered voiding patterns.

Many patients find the rectal examination embarrassing and uncomfortable. Examining the rectum last gives you time to establish a rapport with your patient and gives him a chance to relax. Before you begin, explain what you're going to do, and make sure the room is quiet and private. Before positioning your patient, open the packet for testing occult blood, and place your gloves and water-soluble lubricant within reach.

Percussing the liver

To estimate liver size, percuss along the right midclavicular line, moving upward from below the level of the umbilicus, as shown. Then percuss along the right midclavicular line, moving downward from above the level of the nipple.

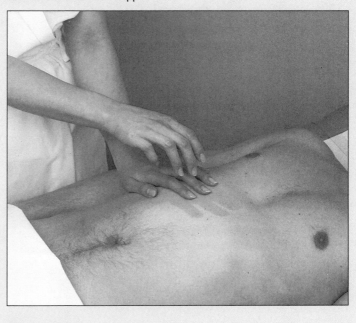

If your patient is in bed or on an examination table, help him to the knee-chest position. Place a frail, elderly patient or a pregnant patient in a modified Sims' position. You can have an ambulatory patient stand and bend forward over the examination table with his toes pointed inward.

Inspection
Spread the buttocks to expose the anus and surrounding area. Normally, the skin should be intact and have a somewhat darker pigmentation. Look for fissures, discharge, inflammation, lesions, scars, rectal prolapse, and external hemorrhoids. Skin tags often occur in patients with inflammatory bowel disease.

Ask the patient to strain as though he's going to defecate. The increased pressure may

Palpating and hooking the liver

These illustrations show you the correct hand positions for palpating and hooking the liver.

Liver palpation
Place one hand on the patient's back at the level of the liver and place the other hand below the area of liver dullness, as shown. As the patient inhales deeply, press gently.

Liver hooking
Standing near the patient's right shoulder, place your hands below the area of liver dullness, as shown. As the patient inhales deeply, press your fingers inward and upward.

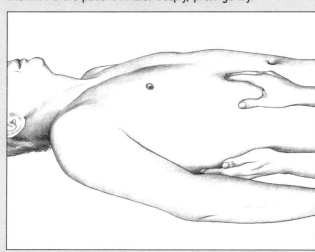

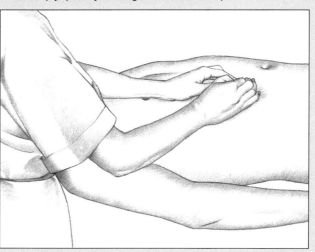

reveal internal hemorrhoids, fissures, polyps, or rectal prolapse.

Palpation
Put on a clean glove and lubricate your gloved index finger. Now, instruct your patient to strain again as you palpate the external rectum. Note any anal outpouchings, bulges, nodules, or tenderness.

Tell your patient that you'll be inserting your finger a short distance into the rectum and that it will feel similar to the pressure of defecation. Ask him to breathe through his mouth and relax. As the anal sphincter relaxes, gently insert your finger toward the umbilicus about 2½" to 4" (6 to 10 cm). If the sphincter doesn't relax, don't force your finger past the constricted anus. Rest your fingertip lightly on the sphincter and try again when the patient relaxes. (See *Palpating the rectum*.)

Rotate your inserted finger first clockwise and then counterclockwise, palpating the internal rectum for nodules, tenderness, irregularities, and fecal impaction. Typically, the rectal wall will feel smooth and soft. In a woman, you can sometimes palpate the posterior uterus through the anterior rectal wall. In a man, you'll palpate the prostate gland through the anterior rectal wall. The prostate should feel firm and smooth. For more information on palpating the prostate, see Chapter 10.

With your finger fully inserted, ask the patient to bear down again. This may cause lesions higher in the rectum to move down to where you can feel them. Ask the patient to tighten the anal muscles around your finger. In a patient with a normal sphincter, you'll feel circumferential tightening. After withdrawing your finger, inspect it for blood, mucus, and stool. Note the color of any stool, and test it for occult blood.

Abnormal findings

A patient's GI disorder will affect one or more of the GI system's basic functions: ingestion, digestion, and elimination. Ingestion disorders affect the mouth and esophagus. Most disorders of digestion affect the stomach, small intestine, liver, gallbladder, or pancreas. Elimination disorders include exocrine gland malfunction and intestinal problems. The most common findings of these GI disorders include dysphagia, nausea and vomiting, skin color changes, distention and protrusion, abdominal pulsations, abnormal abdominal sounds, ascites, abdominal pain, constipation, and diarrhea.

Dysphagia

Dysphagia may result from an obstruction, such as a tumor or stricture, or from a neurologic disease that affects the upper esophagus. But most often, dysphagia results from achalasia, a condition caused by impaired motor activity of the lower esophagogastric junction. Nausea and vomiting may accompany achalasia. Because most patients with dysphagia have trouble eating, you may also note a progressive weight loss.

Nausea and vomiting

Usually occurring together, nausea and vomiting affect both ingestion and digestion. A number of problems both inside and outside of the GI tract can cause nausea and vomiting. Myocardial infarctions and vestibular and neurologic disturbances can cause them. So can gastric and peritoneal irritations, appendicitis, cholecystitis, and acute pancreatitis.

Skin color changes

A bluish umbilicus (Cullen's sign) indicates intra-abdominal hemorrhage. Areas of redness may indicate inflammation. Retroperitoneal bruising on the flanks (Turner's sign) indicates retroperitoneal hemorrhage.

Abdominal striae are common after pregnancy or a significant weight loss. But sometimes they can indicate an abdominal tumor or another GI disorder. Cushing's syndrome characteristically causes purplish striae. Keep in

Palpating the rectum

Use these illustrations to review the correct way to palpate the rectum.

Gently insert your finger toward the umbilicus, as shown.

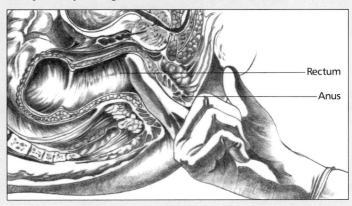

Rectum

Anus

To palpate as much of the rectal surface as possible, rotate your finger clockwise and then counterclockwise.

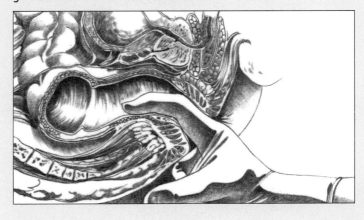

mind that striae appear pink or blue when they're new and become white or silver over time.

Dilated, tortuous, and visible abdominal veins may indicate an inferior vena cava obstruction. Cutaneous angiomas may indicate liver disease.

Distention and protrusion

Abdominal distention can result from the presence of feces, fluid, gas, or a tumor. If your patient has an umbilical hernia, you'll see a protrusion when he raises his head and shoulders from the supine position. You can detect an incisional hernia in the same way.

Abdominal pulsations

Strong visible waves of peristalsis, especially when accompanied by distention and cramping, often indicate intestinal obstruction.

Abnormal abdominal sounds

Hyperactive bowel sounds—rapid, high-pitched, loud, and gurgling sounds—indicate increased intestinal motility. These sounds may result from many causes, including laxative use, gastroenteritis, and a life-threatening intestinal obstruction.

Hypoactive bowel sounds, or bowel sounds that occur with less than normal frequency, may be caused by recent surgery involving the bowel. Or they may result from a full colon. An absence of bowel sounds can result from paralytic ileus.

Friction rubs auscultated in the epigastric region over the liver and spleen may indicate a splenic infarct or hepatic tumor. Abdominal bruits (or purring sounds) may indicate an aneurysm or partial arterial obstruction. A venous hum over the abdomen may result from cirrhosis of the liver. (See *Interpreting abnormal abdominal sounds.*)

Ascites

An accumulation of fluid in the abdomen, ascites is often accompanied by distention; tight, glistening skin; and umbilical protrusion.

Abdominal pain

Pain in the abdomen can result from many GI disorders, including an ulcer, intestinal obstruction, appendicitis, cholecystitis, peritonitis, and other inflammatory disturbances.

If your patient has gnawing, burning abdominal pain and abdominal tenderness, he may have a duodenal ulcer. The pain will be steady, typically occurring in the midepigastric area 2 to 4 hours after meals. It may be so intense that it wakens the patient. Food or antacids may provide relief.

Rebound tenderness during abdominal palpation may indicate peritonitis or appendicitis. Appendicitis may also be accompanied by increased abdominal wall resistance and guarding. Not all patients with appendicitis will have classically localized pain, and some older adults will have less abdominal rigidity—an important sign of peritoneal inflammation—than younger adults.

Constipation

Occurring frequently in hospitalized or bedridden patients, constipation can result from immobility, a sedentary life-style, or medications. It can also indicate a diet low in fiber.

If your patient's constipation is accompanied by a dull, generalized abdominal ache or feeling of fullness and hyperactive bowel sounds, it may be caused by irritable bowel syndrome. Other signs of irritable bowel syndrome include nausea without vomiting, mucus in the stools, and a slightly distended abdomen. A patient with a complete intestinal obstruction won't pass stools or flatus, and you won't be able to detect bowel sounds below the obstruction.

Diarrhea

A common GI sign, diarrhea can occur alone or with other GI signs and symptoms. If it's accompanied by abdominal tenderness, anorexia, cramping, and hyperactive bowel sounds, the patient may have Crohn's disease. Diarrhea accompanied by cramping, fever, and vomiting may be caused by a toxin. Despite the cause, a patient with diarrhea may suffer a significant loss of fluid and electrolytes.

Pertinent diagnostic tests

Based on your assessment findings, further diagnostic tests may be ordered to identify the source of your patient's GI problem. Tests that may be used include blood studies, urinalysis,

Interpreting abnormal abdominal sounds

SOUND AND DESCRIPTION	LOCATION	POSSIBLE CAUSE
Abnormal bowel sounds • Hyperactive sounds (unrelated to hunger)	• Any quadrant	• Diarrhea or early intestinal obstruction
• Hypoactive, then absent sounds	• Any quadrant	• Paralytic ileus or peritonitis
• High-pitched tinkling sounds	• Any quadrant	• Intestinal fluid and air under tension in a dilated bowel
• High-pitched rushing sounds coinciding with abdominal cramps	• Any quadrant	• Intestinal obstruction
Systolic bruits • Vascular blowing sounds resembling cardiac murmurs	• Over abdominal aorta	• Partial arterial obstruction or turbulent blood flow
	• Over renal artery	• Renal artery stenosis
	• Over iliac artery	• Hepatomegaly
Venous hum • Continuous, medium-pitched tone created by blood flow in a large, engorged vascular organ, such as the liver	• Epigastric and umbilical regions	• Increased collateral circulation between portal and systemic venous systems, as in hepatic cirrhosis
Friction rub • Harsh, grating sound like two pieces of sandpaper rubbing together	• Over liver and spleen	• Inflammation of the peritoneal surface of liver, as from a tumor

stool analysis, radiography, endoscopy, ultrasonography, computed tomography (CT) scan, and nuclear imaging. Depending on the circumstances, one or several tests may be ordered.

Blood studies
Certain blood studies can provide valuable clues about the cause of your patient's GI symptoms. Commonly used blood studies include alkaline phosphatase; gamma glutamyl transpeptidase; bilirubin; cholesterol; serum aspartate aminotransferase (AST), formerly SGOT; serum alanine aminotransferase (ALT), formerly SGPT; lactate dehydrogenase; prothrombin time; ammonia; amylase; and lipase.

Alkaline phosphatase. This test assesses the level of alkaline phosphatase activity in the bones, intestine, and liver and biliary systems.

Elevated levels may indicate cholestasis; biliary obstruction; liver metastasis; viral, drug-induced, or chronic hepatitis; or space-occupying hepatic lesions.

Gamma glutamyl transpeptidase. The gamma glutamyl transpeptidase test measures this enzyme's activity in the renal tubules, liver, biliary tract epithelium, and pancreas. Elevated levels are common in patients with acute liver disease—especially from chronic alcohol abuse. Patients with obstructive jaundice, liver metastasis, or acute pancreatitis may also have high levels of this enzyme.

Bilirubin. This test measures the conjugation and excretion of bilirubin by the liver. High levels of bilirubin are common in hepatitis and other liver diseases.

Cholesterol. Cholesterol tests measure the metabolism of the liver and the synthesis of cholesterol, a bile acid precursor. Cholesterol levels may rise with incipient hepatitis, lipid disorders, pancreatitis, and cholestasis resulting from biliary disease or chronic alcohol abuse.

AST and ALT. These tests measure the cytoplasmic enzymes that leak into the plasma after cell damage. Elevated levels may indicate acute viral or drug-induced hepatitis, biliary obstruction or cirrhosis, pancreatitis, or liver metastasis.

Lactate dehydrogenase. The lactate dehydrogenase test measures the total enzyme level in the blood as well as the levels of five distinct isoenzymes. The test may help identify hepatitis, cirrhosis, and hepatic congestion.

Prothrombin time. This test measures clotting time to determine prothrombin and fibrinogen activity. Vitamin K deficiency or liver disease can cause an increased prothrombin time.

Ammonia. Measuring blood ammonia levels helps to evaluate the liver's ability to detoxify ammonia. High levels of ammonia are common in acute hepatic necrosis, hepatic encephalopathy, and cirrhosis.

Amylase. This measurement of amylase, a pancreatic enzyme active in the digestion of starch and glycogen, can indicate pancreatic damage. Amylase is markedly elevated in acute pancreatitis, and moderately elevated in obstruction of the common bile duct and pancreatic injury or cancer.

Lipase. This test measures the level of lipase, a pancreatic enzyme that is active in fat digestion. High levels of lipase may occur with acute pancreatitis; intestinal, pancreatic, or biliary duct obstruction; and a pancreatic tumor.

Urinalysis
Routine urinalysis can reveal a range of GI disorders, including liver or gallbladder disease.

Brownish yellow urine almost always indicates the presence of bilirubin, as found in hepatitis or other liver diseases. High levels of bilirubin also make the urine appear foamy.

Ketonuria can be detected in the urine when metabolic demands are acutely increased because of diarrhea, excessive vomiting, or starvation.

Elevated levels of urobilinogen suggest liver or gallbladder disease, or increased red blood cell destruction.

Stool analysis
Routine stool analysis may help detect bleeding or liver or GI disorders by identifying abnormalities in stool consistency, content, odor, and color.

Narrow, ribbonlike stools indicate a spastic or irritable bowel or a partial bowel or rectal obstruction. Hard stools often occur as a result of diet or medication. Soft, malformed stools may indicate a spastic bowel or viral infection. Soft stools mixed with blood or mucus may indicate bacterial infection; soft stools mixed with blood or pus, colitis.

Yellow or green stools indicate prolonged diarrhea. Black stools suggest GI bleeding or excessive iron intake. Tan or white stools signal liver or gallbladder duct blockage, cancer, or hepatitis. Red stools may indicate colon or rectal bleeding or the ingestion of certain foods, such as beets and kidney beans.

Normal stools contain 10% to 20% fat. Stools that appear pasty or greasy may indicate intestinal malabsorption or pancreatic disease.

Radiography
Radiographic tests of the GI system include routine abdominal X-rays, barium swallow, upper GI series, small-bowel series and enema, and barium enema. These tests may be used to detect intestinal blockage, intestinal wall tears, tumors, ulcers, strictures, and several other abnormalities.

Abdominal X-ray. Also called flat plate of the abdomen or kidney-ureter-bladder (KUB) radiography, abdominal X-ray can detect tumors, renal calculi, and abnormal gas collections. On the film, air appears black, fat looks gray, and bone looks white.

Barium swallow. A barium swallow is used to examine the pharynx and esophagus for strictures, ulcers, tumors, polyps, diverticula, hiatal hernia, esophageal webs, and motility disorders. Achalasia can sometimes be detected with a barium swallow.

Upper GI series. In this procedure, the passage of barium is traced from the patient's esophagus to his stomach. Usually combined with a small-bowel series, an upper GI series is most commonly used to diagnose gastric and duodenal ulcers. It can also detect gastritis, cancer, hiatal hernia, diverticula, strictures, and motility disorders.

Small-bowel series and enema. In this test, the examiner fluoroscopically observes the barium passing through the small intestine, distending it. The procedure can detect sprue, obstruction, motility disorders, malabsorption syndrome, Hodgkin's disease, lymphosarcoma, ischemia, bleeding, and inflammation.

Barium enema. In this procedure, barium is administered in an enema. The barium enema is most often used to detect lower intestinal disorders, such as colorectal cancer, polyps, and diverticula. But it can also be used to view the large intestine.

Endoscopy
With these procedures, an examiner can view the esophagus, stomach, and intestines through a flexible fiber-optic endoscope. Endoscopy can help in diagnosing inflammatory, ulcerative, and infectious diseases as well as neoplasms and other mucosal lesions. Endoscopy may also be used to perform biopsies.

Usually more accurate than barium studies, endoscopy is also easier to perform than angiography or explorative surgery.

Ultrasonography
This procedure uses a focused beam of high-frequency sound waves to create echoes, which then appear as spikes and dots on an oscilloscope. Although the intestines, which are gas filled, can't be seen with ultrasonography,

the process can differentiate between obstructive and nonobstructive jaundice. The procedure is also used to detect cholelithiasis, cholecystitis, metastasis, hematomas, tumors, abscesses, and cysts.

CT scan
In CT scanning, the action of multiple X-ray beams are translated into three-dimensional images by an oscilloscope. As in ultrasonography, CT images can distinguish between obstructive and nonobstructive jaundice. CT scanning can identify abscesses, cysts, hematomas, and tumors, and it can diagnose and evaluate pancreatitis. The procedure can also be used with a contrast medium.

Nuclear imaging
In nuclear imaging, the patient either swallows a radiopaque substance or he's injected with one. Tests include gastric-emptying studies and liver-spleen scanning. The latter provides the best method of detecting hepatocellular and fecal disease and hepatic metastasis. It can also help in diagnosing hepatomegaly, splenomegaly, and abnormal hematomas.

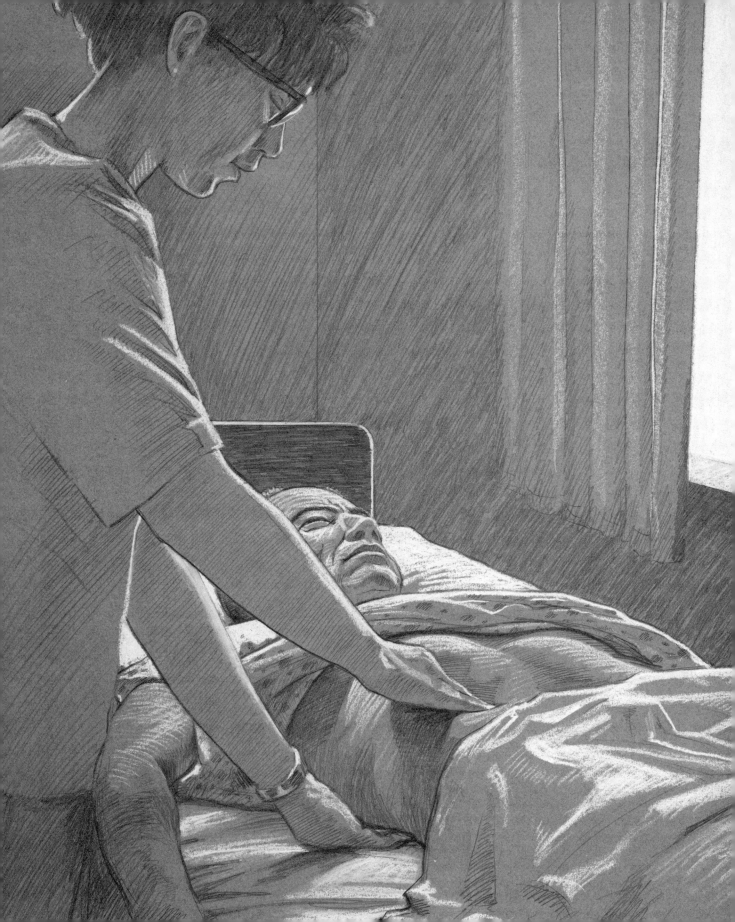

CHAPTER

Urinary and reproductive systems

A disorder of the urinary or reproductive system can have far-reaching consequences. Besides affecting the system itself, such a disorder can trigger problems in other body systems. Plus, it can affect the patient's quality of life and sense of well-being.

Despite these implications, a patient may be reluctant to discuss such problems with you or to have intimate areas of his body examined. So you face the challenge of performing assessments that are not only skilled but also sensitive. That means you must be aware of your patient's concerns as well as your own feelings about sexuality. Remember, if you appear comfortable discussing the patient's problem, your patient will be encouraged to talk openly too.

In this chapter, you'll find three sections covering the urinary system, the male reproductive system, and the female reproductive system. Each section presents a review of anatomy and physiology before explaining the health history and physical examination. The sections end with a discussion of common abnormal findings and pertinent diagnostic tests.

Urinary system

As you assess the urinary system, keep in mind that other body systems depend on it to maintain homeostasis by regulating fluid and electrolyte balance. Also remember that the urinary system depends on other systems—including the cardiovascular and neurologic—to perform this essential function.

Because of this interdependence, a disorder in another system can affect the urinary system. And a urinary system problem may produce signs and symptoms in other body systems.

Anatomy and physiology

The urinary system consists of the kidneys, ureters, bladder, and urethra. The essential functions of the system—such as forming urine and maintaining homeostasis—take place in the highly vascular kidneys. (See *Reviewing the urinary system*.)

Kidneys
The bean-shaped kidneys are about 4½" to 5" (11 to 13 cm) long and 2½" (6 cm) wide. Located retroperitoneally on either side of the lumbar vertebrae, they lie behind the abdominal organs and in front of the muscles attached to the vertebral column. The perineal fat layer also protects them. Crowded by the liver, the right kidney extends slightly lower than the left.

Each kidney consists of a cortex (outer portion) and a medulla (inner portion). An indentation at the center of the kidney, called the hilus, is the point where the renal artery and vein, lymphatic vessels, and nerves enter. The renal pelvis, an extension of the ureter, is also located in this region.

The medulla contains the renal pyramids, which hold most of the nephrons, the func-

tional units of the kidney. Each kidney contains roughly 1 million nephrons. Inside each nephron is a glomerulus, which is composed of capillaries; Bowman's capsule, which supports and surrounds the glomerulus; the proximal, distal, and collecting tubules; and the loop of Henle. Portions of the pyramids empty into the internal calyces, which carry urine to the renal pelvis.

Through glomerular filtration, tubular reabsorption, and secretion, the kidneys regulate fluid and electrolyte balance. They also rid the body of waste products by excreting urine.

Ureters
The ureters are about 10" to 12" (25 to 30 cm) long. The left ureter is slightly longer than the right because of the left kidney's higher position in the abdomen. The diameter of each ureter varies from ⅛" to ¼" (0.3 to 0.6 cm), with the narrowest portion at the ureteropelvic junction.

Located along the posterior abdominal wall, the ureters enter the bladder anteromedially. They carry formed urine from the renal pelvis, through the hilus, and into the bladder by peristaltic contractions that occur one to five times per minute.

Bladder
Located in the pelvis, the bladder is a hollow, spherical, muscular organ that serves as a container for urine collection. When empty, the bladder lies behind the pubic bones; when full, it's displaced under the peritoneal cavity. Bladder capacity ranges from 500 to l,000 ml (17 to 33 oz) in healthy adults and is usually less in children and elderly people. Located low on the bladder's posterior wall, the ureteral and urethral openings form the trigone, a triangular area.

Urination results from both involuntary and voluntary processes. The involuntary process begins when urine distends the bladder. The parasympathetic nervous system then causes the bladder to contract and the ureter's internal sphincter to relax. Next, the cerebrum stimulates the external sphincter, producing voluntary relaxation and contraction.

ANATOMY

Reviewing the urinary system

The illustration at right shows you the structures of the urinary system. The illustration below shows a cross section of the kidney.

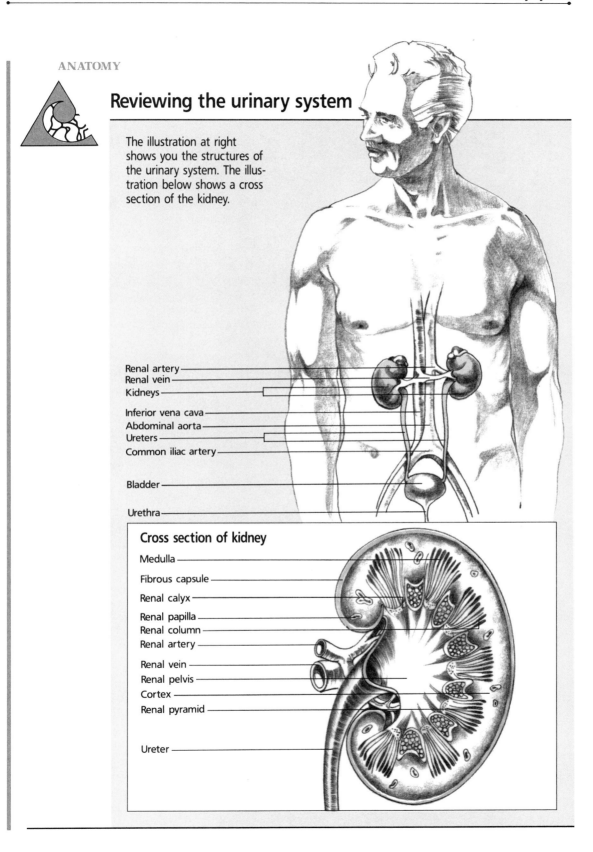

Renal artery
Renal vein
Kidneys

Inferior vena cava
Abdominal aorta
Ureters
Common iliac artery

Bladder

Urethra

Cross section of kidney

Medulla

Fibrous capsule

Renal calyx

Renal papilla
Renal column
Renal artery

Renal vein
Renal pelvis
Cortex
Renal pyramid

Ureter

Assessing urine appearance

The appearance of your patient's urine can provide important clues about his general health and the source of his genitourinary problem. So during the health history, ask him if he's noticed any changes from the normal straw color. If he has, use this list to help interpret the changes he reports.
• *Cloudy* —anxiety, chronic renal disease, diabetes insipidus, diuretic therapy, excessive fluid intake
• *Dark yellow or amber (concentrated urine)* —acute febrile disease, inadequate fluids, severe diarrhea or vomiting
• *Blue-green* —methylene blue ingestion
• *Green-brown* —bile duct obstruction
• *Dark brown or black* —acute glomerulonephritis, drugs (such as nitrofurantoin and chlorpromazine)
• *Orange-red or orange-brown* —drugs (such as phenazopyridine), obstructive jaundice, urobilinuria
• *Red or red-brown* —drugs (such as phenazopyridine), hemorrhage, porphyria

Urethra

A small duct, the urethra carries urine outside the body from the bladder. In women, the urethra is only 1″ to 2″ (2.5 to 5 cm) long, with its external opening (urethral meatus) anterior to the vaginal opening. In men, the urethra is much longer—about 8″ (20 cm)—because it must pass through the erectile tissue of the penis. The male urethra carries semen as well as urine.

Urine formation and output

Urine formation results from three processes that take place in the nephrons: glomerular filtration, tubular mineralocorticoid reabsorption, and tubular secretion. The composition of excreted urine depends on the substances that are reabsorbed and secreted in the nephrons.

In a healthy person, total daily urine output averages between 720 and 2,400 ml (24 and 81 oz). Output increases with increased fluid intake because the body rids itself of excess fluid. Output decreases with fluid deprivation or excessive sodium intake because the body conserves water to maintain normal fluid concentrations.

Hormone regulation

Hormones help regulate tubular reabsorption and secretion of solutes and water. Antidiuretic hormone (ADH) acts in the distal tubule and collection ducts to increase water reabsorption and urine concentration. A deficiency of ADH decreases water reabsorption, resulting in dilute urine.

The kidneys play an important role in blood pressure and fluid volume control by secreting the enzyme renin. Renin secretion is stimulated by the concentration of sodium in the renal tubules. Renin converts angiotensinogen to angiotensin I, which in turn is converted to angiotensin II in the lungs. Angiotensin II, a potent vasoconstrictor, stimulates the adrenal cortex to release aldosterone.

Elevation in aldosterone levels triggers sodium reabsorption from the distal tubules and collecting ducts. Water and sodium move passively into the blood for reabsorption. Blood volume and pressure are increased, which in turn increases glomerular function.

The kidneys also secrete erythropoietin in response to hypoxemia. Erythropoietin stimulates the bone marrow to increase red blood cell (RBC) production. This explains why patients with chronic renal failure are anemic: The kidneys are unable to secrete erythropoietin and fewer RBCs are produced. However, in high altitudes, many people adjust to chronic hypoxemia because the kidneys overrespond and secrete more erythropoietin. This increases RBC production (polycythemia).

Health history

Because the patient may feel uncomfortable discussing urinary problems, be sure to conduct the interview in private and without interruptions. Encourage open communication by phrasing questions clearly and tactfully. Resist the urge to rush or omit important facts because the patient seems embarrassed.

Also be sure to ask the patient about his general health because urinary problems can result from or cause problems in other parts of the body.

Chief complaint

The most common chief complaints of the urinary system include output changes (polyuria, oliguria, anuria), voiding pattern changes (hesitancy, frequency, urgency, nocturia, incontinence), urine color changes, and pain (suprapubic pain, flank pain, dysuria). (See *Assessing urine appearance*.)

To investigate these or any other urinary complaints, ask your patient relevant questions about such particulars as onset, duration, and severity of symptoms. Also ask what precipitates the symptom, what makes it worse, and what makes it better. For more information on exploring chief complaints, see Chapter 3.

Medical history

Ask if the patient has ever had a kidney or bladder infection. If so, was he hospitalized? Has he ever had kidney or bladder calculi? How were they treated? Has he ever had a kidney or bladder injury? Trauma can alter the structure and function of the kidneys and bladder. Ask too if he has ever been catheterized.

Does the patient have diabetes or high blood pressure? Patients with diabetes have an increased risk of urinary tract infections. Both diabetes and hypertension can lead to nephropathy; however, symptoms of diabetic nephropathy — edema, azotemia, and hypertension — may not appear until 10 to 15 years after the onset of the disease.

Determine whether the patient has any allergies. Allergic reactions can cause tubular damage. A severe anaphylactic reaction can produce temporary renal failure and permanent tubular necrosis.

Does the patient take any prescribed or over-the-counter drugs? Some drugs can affect the appearance of urine or alter urinary function.

Ask the female patient when she had her last menstrual period and whether she could be pregnant.

Assessing fluid status

To assess your patient's fluid status, weigh him at the same time every day on the same scale. Make sure he's wearing the same type of clothing too. A significant weight gain or loss within 24 to 48 hours indicates a change in fluid status, not in body mass.

You also need to measure and compare the patient's daily intake and output and note any output changes. When measuring output, be sure to consider insensible loss from perspiration and exhalation, as well as loss from vomiting, diarrhea, fever, and drainage from wounds or chest tubes. Normal hourly output is 30 to 100 ml (1 to 3 oz); normal 24-hour output, 720 to 2,400 ml (24 to 81 oz).

Family history

Ask if anyone in the patient's family has ever been treated for renal problems. Certain disorders, such as polycystic kidney disease and nephritis, can be transmitted genetically. Ask too if anyone has ever been treated for kidney or bladder calculi. Does anyone have hypertension, diabetes, gout, or coronary artery disease? These hereditary disorders can alter kidney function.

Activities of daily living

Find out the patient's occupation. Certain occupations put workers at risk for urinary problems. For example, jackhammer operators may develop renal ptosis. Does the patient have access to a restroom at work? Does he have sufficient time to use the restroom? Workers who must hold their urine for long periods may develop urinary stasis or infection.

Ask if the patient is on a low-sodium or fluid-restricted diet. Limiting sodium or fluids can affect urine output. Is he on a reducing diet? Prolonged liquid-protein diets have been associated with kidney dysfunction.

Find out if the patient's sleep patterns have changed. Staying awake at night and sleeping during the day is a sign of renal failure. Also determine whether leg cramps keep him awake at night. Such cramps may be an early symptom of renal failure.

Physical examination

Start your examination by taking the patient's vital signs, including measuring blood pressure in both arms. Also weigh him to assess his fluid status. Weight is an extremely valuable measurement for patients with urinary disorders or renal failure, especially those receiving dialysis. (See *Assessing fluid status,* page 223.)

Next, perform a general assessment followed by a specific assessment of the urinary system that includes inspection, auscultation, percussion, and palpation.

General assessment

Assess the patient's mental status by observing his behavior. Renal dysfunction can cause poor concentration, loss of memory, and disorientation. Progressive, chronic renal failure can cause lethargy, confusion, disorientation, stupor, convulsions, and coma.

Also inspect the patient's skin, noting its overall appearance and color. Pale skin may suggest a low hemoglobin concentration, as occurs in end-stage renal disease. Yellow-tan skin may result from retained urochrome pigment. Also note any scratches or dryness.

Look for uremic frost — snowlike crystals that form on the skin when the nonfunctioning kidneys cannot excrete urea and other metabolic wastes. Because of the widespread availability of dialysis, you'll see this only in patients with late-stage renal failure.

Then check the mouth and mucous membranes. A dry mouth can indicate recent, mild dehydration, but parched, cracked lips with markedly dry mucous membranes suggest severe dehydration. Also look for sunken eyes, a sign of dehydration.

Also inspect the extremities for edema, which occurs from the buildup of extra sodium or water in the interstitial spaces. Observe the abdomen for ascites.

Inspection

As part of your examination, inspect the patient's abdomen and urethral meatus carefully. First, have him urinate and then help him to lie comfortably in the supine position with his arms at his sides. Next, drape the patient, exposing only his abdomen from the xiphoid process to the symphysis pubis.

When the patient is supine, the abdomen should be smooth, flat or concave, and symmetrical. The skin should be free of lesions, bruises, discolorations, and prominent veins. Be alert for signs of ascites: distention with tight, glistening skin and striae (silvery streaks caused by rapidly developing skin tension). Ascites may accompany nephrotic syndrome, which is characterized by edema, increased urine protein levels, and decreased serum albumin levels. To confirm ascites, use the fluid wave test, as described in Chapter 9.

Put on gloves before examining the urethral meatus. If you're examining a man, have him remain supine. Drape him, exposing only his penis. Then compress the tip of the glans to open the urethral meatus. Note the location of the meatus. It should be located in the center of the glans. Check for swelling or discharge, signs of urethral infection, and for ulcerations, which can signal a sexually transmitted disease (STD).

Help a woman patient into the dorsal lithotomy position and drape her, exposing only the area to be assessed. Then spread the labia and look for the urethral meatus. It should be a pink, irregular, slitlike opening located at the midline just above the vagina. Check for swelling and discharge, signs of urethral infection; presence of a cystocele; and ulcerations, a sign of an STD. (See *Examining the urethral meatus.*)

Auscultation

To auscultate the renal arteries, have the patient exhale deeply as you press the bell of the stethoscope lightly against his skin at the midline between the upper abdominal quadrants. As you auscultate, move the stethoscope to the left; then return to the midline and move to the right. A whooshing sound indicates a

Examining the urethral meatus

To inspect a man's urethral meatus, compress the tip of the glans, as shown.

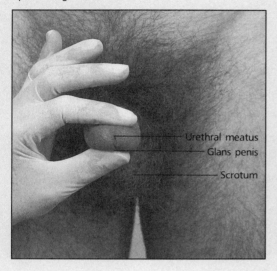

Urethral meatus
Glans penis
Scrotum

To inspect a woman's urethral meatus, spread the labia, as shown.

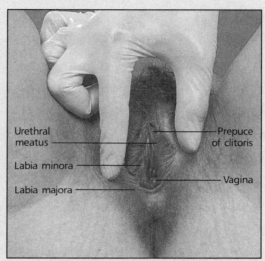

Urethral meatus
Labia minora
Labia majora
Prepuce of clitoris
Vagina

systolic bruit, which could signal renal artery stenosis in a patient with hypertension.

Percussion

Percuss the kidneys to elicit pain or tenderness, and percuss the bladder to elicit percussion sounds. Before you start, be sure to tell the patient what you're going to do. Otherwise, he may be startled, and you could mistake his reaction for a feeling of acute tenderness.

To assess the kidneys using the indirect fist percussion method, have the patient sit up. Then place the ball of one hand over the costovertebral angle and strike it with the ulnar surface of your other fist. Use just enough force to cause a painless, but perceptible, thud. (See *Performing fist percussion,* page 226.)

To use the direct method, strike the costovertebral angle directly with your fist, without putting your other hand down first. Be sure to percuss both sides of the body to assess both kidneys. Pain or tenderness suggests a kidney infection.

Before percussing the bladder, have the patient urinate. Then tell him to lie supine. Begin about 2″ (5 cm) above the symphysis pubis and percuss toward and over the bladder. You should hear tympany over the bladder. A dull sound can indicate retained urine in the bladder caused by bladder dysfunction or infection.

Palpation

Next, palpate the patient's kidneys and bladder. For kidney palpation, have the patient lie supine. To assess his left kidney, stand on his right side. Reach across him with your left arm, placing your hand under his left flank to elevate it and displace the kidney anteriorly. Ask him to take a deep breath, and use your right palm to deeply palpate the left upper quadrant. As an alternative, you can stand on the patient's left side, and use your right hand to lift his left flank and your left hand to palpate.

To examine the right kidney, stand on the patient's right side. Elevate his right flank with your left hand, and palpate deeply with your right hand.

Performing fist percussion

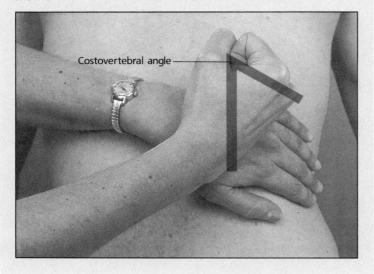

To use indirect fist percussion, place one hand at the costovertebral angle and strike it with the ulnar surface of your other hand, as shown.

Costovertebral angle

Normal kidneys usually aren't palpable in an adult. However, if the patient is very thin, you may be able to feel the lower end of the right kidney as a smooth, round mass that drops on inspiration. And in an elderly patient, you may be able to palpate both kidneys because of decreased muscle tone and elasticity. (See *Palpating the kidneys*.)

To locate the edge of the bladder, use deep palpation at the midline about 1" to 2" (2.5 to 5 cm) above the symphysis pubis. Continue palpating downward and assess for any masses or tenderness. Unless the bladder is distended with urine, it's usually not palpable. You'll feel a full bladder as a tense, smooth, round mass.

Abnormal findings

Your assessment may uncover the following abnormalities of the urinary system: polyuria, hematuria, urinary frequency, urinary urgency, urinary hesitancy, nocturia, urinary incontinence, and dysuria.

Polyuria

A fairly common finding, polyuria is the production and excretion of more than 2,500 ml (85 oz) of urine daily. It usually results from diabetes insipidus or diabetes mellitus or the use of a diuretic. Polyuria can also result from psychological, neurologic, renal, or urologic disorders (such as pyelonephritis or postobstructive uropathy). Patients with polyuria are at risk for developing hypovolemia.

Hematuria

A patient with hematuria may have brown or bright red urine. The timing of hematuria suggests the location of the underlying problem. Bleeding at the start of urination is caused by a disorder of the urethra, whereas bleeding at the end of urination signifies a disorder of the bladder neck, posterior urethra, or prostate. When bleeding occurs throughout urination, the disorder is located above the bladder neck. Hematuria may also result from other causes, including GI, prostatic, vaginal, and coagulation disorders.

Urinary frequency

An increased urge to urinate commonly results from decreased bladder capacity. This classic symptom of urinary tract infection (UTI) also occurs with other urologic disorders, such as benign prostatic hyperplasia (BPH) and urethral stricture, as well as with neurologic disorders, such as a spinal cord lesion. Pressure on the bladder from pregnancy or from a tumor of the prostate or uterus can also cause urinary frequency.

Urinary urgency

The sudden urge to urinate is often accompanied by bladder pain and is a classic symptom of UTI. Even small amounts of urine in the bladder can cause pain because inflammation decreases bladder capacity. Repeated, frequent urination produces little urine. Urgency without bladder pain may be a symptom of an upper motor neuron lesion that's affecting bladder control.

Palpating the kidneys

To palpate the right kidney, stand on the patient's right side. Place your left hand under the patient and your right hand on his abdomen, as shown.

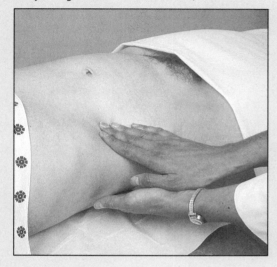

Instruct the patient to inhale deeply, so his kidney moves downward. As he inhales, press up with your left hand and down with your right hand.

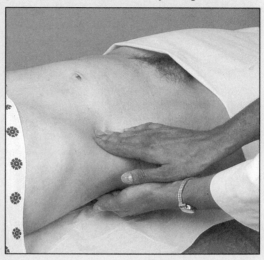

Urinary hesitancy
Difficulty starting a urine stream can occur with a UTI, a partial obstruction of the lower urinary tract, neuromuscular disorders, or the use of certain drugs. Hesitancy is most common in older men with prostatic enlargement.

Nocturia
Excessive urination at night, or nocturia, is a common sign of renal or lower urinary tract disorders. It can result from a disruption of the normal diurnal urine pattern or from overstimulation of the nerves and muscles that control urination. It may also be caused by cardiovascular, endocrine, or metabolic disorders and is a common adverse effect of diuretics.

Urinary incontinence
This common complaint may be transient or permanent, and the amount of urine may be small or large. Possible causes include stress incontinence; BPH; prostatic infection; tumor; bladder cancer or calculi; and neurologic disorders, such as Guillain-Barré syndrome, multiple sclerosis, and spinal cord injury. Urinary incontinence may also be the first sign of UTI.

Dysuria
This abnormality usually signals a lower UTI. The onset of pain suggests the cause of dysuria. Pain just before urination indicates bladder irritation or distention, whereas pain at the start of urination usually results from a bladder outlet obstruction. Pain at the end of urination can be a sign of bladder spasm. Pain throughout urination can indicate pyelonephritis, especially when accompanied by persistent high fever with chills, costovertebral angle tenderness, hematuria, and flank pain.

Pertinent diagnostic tests

After your assessment, certain diagnostic tests may be ordered to confirm a diagnosis of your patient's urinary problem. Urine tests commonly used to evaluate urinary problems include routine urinalysis and determination of creatinine clearance rate and creatinine level. Blood tests include those for blood urea nitrogen (BUN) and serum creatinine levels.

Tests that evaluate the structure and function of the urinary system may also be ordered. These tests include computed tomography (CT) scan, renal scan, intravenous pyelography (IVP), cystography, ultrasonography, renal angiography, and voiding cystourethrography.

Routine urinalysis. The simplest and perhaps most informative laboratory test, urinalysis measures urine pH, specific gravity, protein, glucose, blood ketones, and bacteria levels.

Creatinine clearance. This 24-hour urine test directly assesses kidney function. A low creatinine clearance rate may indicate reduced renal blood flow (associated with shock or renal artery obstruction), acute tubular necrosis, acute or chronic glomerulonephritis, bilateral renal lesions, or nephrosclerosis.

Blood urea nitrogen. Patients with renal disease and urinary tract obstruction will have an elevated BUN level. Because this test also reflects renal excretory capacity and protein intake, patients on high-protein diets will have an increased BUN level.

Serum creatinine. This test is a much more sensitive indicator of renal function than the BUN test because impaired renal function is usually the only cause of an elevated creatinine level.

CT scan. In a CT scan, a series of X-rays are taken at various angles to produce three-dimensional images. This test can be done with or without a contrast medium and helps in evaluating renal pelvic size, structural abnormalities, and parenchymal thickness.

Renal scan. In a renal scan, a contrast medium is used to show kidney size, blood flow, and excretion. Renal urinary stenosis and parenchy-

mal disease are commonly detected by this scan.

Intravenous pyelography. An IVP uses a contrast medium to view the renal parenchyma, ureters, and bladder. The test determines the size and shape of the kidneys as well as the presence of soft- or hard-tissue lesions.

Cystography. In this test, a contrast medium is used to determine the size and shape of a fluid-filled bladder. Cystography helps diagnose lower abdominal or pelvic trauma, bladder wall disorders, and some cases of pyuria or hematuria.

Ultrasonography. A noninvasive test, ultrasonography produces oscilloscopic, time-lapsed images by transmitting high-frequency sound waves into the abdomen. It helps determine the size and shape of the kidneys and the presence of calculi and differentiates between solid masses and fluid-filled cysts.

Renal angiography. After injection of a contrast medium, renal angiography shows renovascular pathways. It helps diagnose renal artery stenosis, renal vein thrombosis, and vascular damage from trauma. It also can differentiate vascular tumors from avascular cysts.

Voiding cystourethrography. In this test, a contrast medium is instilled through the urethra and into the bladder. Fluoroscopic films or overhead radiographs demonstrate bladder filling and then show excretion of the contrast medium while the patient voids. Voiding cystourethrography helps diagnose urethral obstructions or lesions.

Male reproductive system

Many common disorders of the male reproductive system may produce serious physiologic and psychological consequences. For instance, sexual and reproductive dysfunction, such as

ANATOMY

Reviewing the male reproductive system

Use this illustration to review the important structures of the male reproductive system.

Bladder
Symphysis pubis
Seminal vesicle
Common ejaculation duct
Prostate gland
Vas deferens
Corpus cavernosum
Penis
Urethra
Epididymis
Testicle
Scrotum
Glans penis
Prepuce
Urethral meatus

---

impotence and infertility, can dramatically reduce a patient's quality of life. Also, STDs, the most common communicable diseases in the United States, can cause serious complications unless they're detected and treated early.

Anatomy and physiology

The male reproductive system includes the penis, scrotum and testicles, epididymis and vas deferens, seminal vesicles, and prostate gland. An accurate assessment depends on understanding their structure and function. (See *Reviewing the male reproductive system.*)

Penis
The penis consists of the shaft, glans, corona, and urethral meatus. The shaft contains three

columns of vascular erectile tissue: two corpora cavernosa, which form the major part of the penis, and the corpus spongiosum, which encases the urethra. The skin of the penis is hairless and usually darker than the skin on other parts of the body.

The glans is located at the end of the penis. A slitlike opening, the urethral meatus is located ventrally at the tip of the glans. The corona is formed by the junction of the glans and the shaft. The prepuce (the loose skin covering the glans) is often surgically removed shortly after birth (circumcision).

When erect, the penis can discharge sperm. Erection occurs when the two corpora cavernosa become engorged with blood. During sexual activity, sperm is forcefully ejaculated from the urethral meatus along with secretions from the prostate gland, vas deferens, seminal vesicles, and epididymis.

Scrotum and testicles

A loose, wrinkled, deeply pigmented pouch, the scrotum is located at the base of the penis. It consists of a muscle layer covered by a layer of thin skin and is divided into two compartments, each containing a testicle and portions of the spermatic cord. The left side of the scrotum is usually lower than the right because the left spermatic cord is longer.

The testicles are oval, rubbery structures that are suspended vertically and slightly forward in the scrotum. The testicles produce both testosterone and sperm. Testosterone stimulates the changes that occur in puberty: the growth of genitalia and the appearance of secondary sex characteristics, such as facial and body hair, muscle development, and voice changes.

Epididymis and vas deferens

The epididymis curves over the posterolateral surface of each testicle, creating a visible bulge on the surface. (In a small number of men, the epididymis is located anteriorly.) The vas deferens begins at the lower end of the epididymis, climbs the spermatic cord, travels through the inguinal canal, and ends in the abdominal cavity where it lies on the fundus of the bladder.

The epididymis acts as a reservoir for sperm maturation; the vas deferens functions as the storage site for mature sperm and the pathway to the seminal vesicles.

Seminal vesicles

A pair of saclike glands, the seminal vesicles are found on the lower posterior surface of the bladder in front of the rectum. Secretions from the seminal vesicles help form seminal fluid, which mixes with sperm at ejaculation and is thought to protect the sperm until one of them reaches the ovum.

Prostate gland

A walnut-shaped gland about 2½" (6 cm) long, the prostate surrounds the urethra just below the bladder. It produces a thin, milky, alkaline fluid that mixes with seminal fluid during ejaculation. Prostatic fluid enhances sperm motility and the chance of fertilization by neutralizing the acidity of the urethra and the woman's vagina.

Health history

A male patient may be embarrassed to discuss his reproductive system. And you may be a bit uncomfortable yourself. But if you act professionally and use tact and sensitivity, you'll both be more at ease, and the patient will trust you and be less likely to withhold valuable information. Remember that sexual performance is an especially sensitive subject. Many men view sexual problems as a sign of diminished masculinity. An older man may see a normal decrease in sexual prowess as a sign of declining health.

Chief complaint

The most common reproductive system complaints expressed by men are penile discharge; impotence; infertility; and scrotal and inguinal masses, pain, and tenderness. To investigate these or any reproductive complaints, ask your patient relevant questions about such particulars as onset, duration, and severity. Also ask what precipitates the symptom, what makes it worse, and what makes it better. For more information on exploring chief complaints, see Chapter 3.

Medical history

Ask the patient if he's circumcised. If he's not, can he retract and replace the prepuce easily? An inability to retract the prepuce is called phimosis; an inability to replace it is called paraphimosis. Untreated, these conditions can impair local circulation and lead to edema and even gangrene.

Ask if the patient has ever had an STD or any other infection of the reproductive system. If so, how long did it last and how was it treated? Certain STDs or other infections can cause infertility and other reproductive system abnormalities.

Has the patient noticed any sores, lumps, or ulcers on his penis? If so, he may have an

STD or inflammatory disorder. Ask also if he's noticed any penile discharge or bleeding. Copious, thick, yellow discharge may indicate gonorrhea. Thin, watery discharge suggests nonspecific urethritis, prostatitis, or a chlamydial infection. Bloody discharge may indicate an infection or cancer in the urinary or reproductive tract. Has he noticed any scrotal swelling? Such swelling can indicate an inguinal hernia, a hematocele, epididymitis, or a testicular tumor.

Psychosocial history
Determine whether the patient is heterosexual, homosexual, or bisexual. Ask about his cultural and religious background and how it affects his sexual beliefs and practices. This information may help identify potential risk factors. For example, if the patient won't use a condom, he has an increased risk of contracting an STD.

If the patient is having sexual problems, find out if they're affecting his social relationships and emotional well-being. Feelings of emotional or social isolation can increase stress and exacerbate sexual dysfunction.

Activities of daily living
Ask if the patient takes any precautions to prevent contracting STDs. Also find out if he knows how to examine his testicles and if he does so periodically. Explain that testicular cancer, the most common cancer in men between ages 15 and 30, can be treated successfully when detected early.

Physical examination

First ask the patient to disrobe from the waist down and to cover himself with a drape. Then put on gloves and examine the patient's penis, scrotum and testicles, inguinal and femoral areas, and prostate gland.

Penis
Observe the penis. Its size will depend on the patient's age and overall development. The penile skin should be slightly wrinkled and pink to light brown in whites and light brown to dark brown in blacks. Check the penile shaft and glans for lesions, nodules, inflammation, and swelling. Also check the glans for smegma, a cheesy secretion. Then gently compress the glans to open the urethral meatus, and inspect it for discharge, lesions, inflammation and, specifically, genital warts. If you note any discharge, obtain a culture specimen.

Using your thumb and forefinger, palpate the entire penile shaft. It should be somewhat firm, and the skin should be smooth and movable. Note any swelling, nodules, or indurations.

Scrotum and testicles
Have the patient hold his penis away from his scrotum so that you can observe the scrotum's general size and appearance. The skin will be darker than the rest of the body. Spread the surface of the scrotum, and examine the skin for swelling, nodules, redness, ulceration, and distended veins. You'll probably notice some sebaceous cysts — firm, white to yellow, nontender cutaneous lesions. Also, check for pitting edema, a sign of cardiovascular disease. Spread the pubic hair and check the skin for lesions and parasites.

Gently palpate both testicles between your thumb and first two fingers. Assess their size, shape, and response to pressure (typically, a deep visceral pain). The testicles should be equal in size. They should feel firm, smooth, and rubbery, and should move freely in the scrotal sac. If you note any hard, irregular areas or lumps, transilluminate the area by darkening the room and pressing the head of a flashlight against the scrotum, behind the lump. The testicle will appear as an opaque shadow, as will any lumps, masses, warts, or blood-filled areas. Transilluminate the other testicle to compare your findings.

Next, palpate the epididymis, usually located in the posterolateral area of the testicle. It should be smooth, discrete, nontender, and free of swelling or induration.

Finally, palpate each spermatic cord, located above each testicle. Begin palpating at the base of the epididymis and continue to the inguinal canal. The vas deferens is a smooth, movable cord inside the spermatic cord. If you feel any swelling, irregularity, or nodules, transilluminate the problem area, as described above. If serous fluid is present, you'll see a

Palpating for an indirect inguinal hernia

To palpate for an indirect inguinal hernia in a man, place your gloved finger on the neck of the scrotum and insert it into the inguinal canal, as shown. Then ask the patient to bear down.

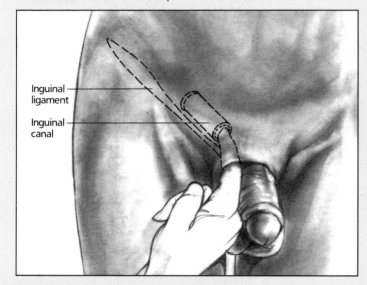

Inguinal ligament

Inguinal canal

red glow; if tissue and blood are present, you won't see this glow.

Inguinal and femoral areas

Have the patient stand. Then ask him to hold his breath and bear down while you inspect the inguinal and femoral areas for bulges.

To assess for a direct inguinal hernia, place two fingers over each external inguinal ring, and ask the patient to bear down. If he has a hernia, you'll feel a bulge.

To assess for an indirect inguinal hernia, examine the patient both standing and supine with his knee flexed on the side you're examining. Place your index finger on the neck of the patient's scrotum and gently push upward into the inguinal canal. When you've inserted your finger as far as possible, ask the patient to bear down or cough. A hernia will feel like a mass of tissue that withdraws when met by the finger. (See *Palpating for an indirect inguinal hernia*.)

Although you can't palpate the femoral canal, you can estimate its location to help detect a femoral hernia. Place your right index finger on the right femoral artery with your finger pointing toward the patient's head. Keep your other fingers close together. Your middle finger will then lie over the femoral vein; your ring finger, over the femoral canal. Note any tenderness or masses. Use your left hand to check the patient's left side.

Prostate gland

Before the examination, have the patient empty his bladder. Then have him stand and lean over the examination table. If he can't assume this position, have him lie on his left side with his right knee and hip flexed or with both knees drawn toward his chest. Inspect the skin of the perineal, anal, and posterior scrotal areas. It should be smooth and unbroken with no protruding masses.

Next, lubricate the gloved index finger of your dominant hand and insert it into the rectum. Tell the patient to relax to ease passage of the finger through the anal sphincter. With your finger pad, palpate the prostate gland on the anterior rectal wall just past the anorectal ring. The gland should feel smooth, rubbery, and about the size of a walnut. It shouldn't protrude into the rectal lumen; if it does, it's probably enlarged. An enlarged prostate gland is classified as Grade 1 (less than ³/₈″ [1 cm] into the rectal lumen) to Grade 4 (more than 1¼″ [3 cm] into the rectal lumen). Also note any tenderness or nodules. (See *Palpating the prostate gland*.)

Abnormal findings

During your assessment, you may detect certain abnormalities of the penis, scrotum and testicles, inguinal and femoral areas, or the prostate. This section will help you to interpret your findings.

Penile lesions

A hard, nontender nodule—especially on the glans or inner lip of the prepuce—may indicate carcinoma of the penis.

A syphilitic chancre is a hard, round papule usually found on the glans penis. Eventually, the papule erodes into an ulcer. You may also note swollen inguinal lymph nodes accompanying this finding.

A cluster of small, painful vesicles may indicate genital herpes. The lesions eventually disappear but tend to recur.

Genital warts appear as single or multiple, elongated or cauliflower-like lesions. They may be moist and malodorous or dry and firm.

Penile discharge

A profuse, yellow discharge suggests gonococcal urethritis. The patient may report urinary frequency, burning, and urgency. Without treatment, the prostate, epididymis, and periurethral glands will become inflamed.

A copious, watery, purulent urethral discharge may indicate chlamydial infection.

Other penile abnormalities

In paraphimosis, the prepuce is so tight that, when retracted, it gets caught behind the glans and can't be replaced. Edema can result.

Hypospadias is a ventral displacement of the urethral meatus on the penis. Epispadias is a dorsal displacement of the urethral meatus on the penis. Both conditions are congenital.

Scrotal and testicular abnormalities

A painless scrotal nodule that can't be transilluminated may be a testicular tumor. This disorder occurs most often in men ages 20 to 35.

Scrotal enlargement may be a sign of a hydrocele, or a collection of fluid, in the testicle. This condition is associated with poor fluid reabsorption, as occurs with cirrhosis, congestive heart failure, and a testicular tumor. A hydrocele can be transilluminated.

Inguinal or femoral abnormalities

A direct inguinal hernia emerges from behind the external inguinal ring and protrudes through it. It seldom descends into the scrotum and usually affects men over age 40.

An indirect inguinal hernia can be palpated in the internal inguinal canal with its tip in or beyond the canal. Or the hernia may descend

Palpating the prostate gland

First, insert your gloved, lubricated index finger into the rectum. Then palpate the prostate on the anterior rectal wall, just past the anorectal ring, as shown.

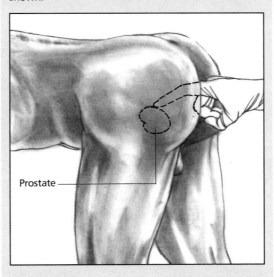

Prostate

into the scrotum. The most common type of hernia, it occurs in all age-groups.

A femoral hernia may be difficult to distinguish from a lymph node. It feels like a soft tumor below the inguinal ligament in the femoral area and is uncommon in men.

Prostate gland abnormalities

A smooth, firm, symmetrical enlargement of the prostate gland indicates BPH, which typically starts in the fifth decade of life. This finding may be associated with nocturia, urinary hesitancy and frequency, and recurring UTIs.

Hard, irregular, fixed lesions that make the prostate feel asymmetrical suggest prostate cancer. Palpation may or may not be painful. This condition also causes urinary dysfunction.

In acute prostatitis, the prostate gland is firm, warm, and extremely tender and swollen. Because this condition is caused by a bacterial infection, the patient usually will have a fever.

Pertinent diagnostic tests

Among the tests used to diagnose male reproductive system disorders are semen analysis; the Venereal Disease Research Laboratory (VDRL) test; measurement of serum alpha-fetoprotein, serum acid phosphatase, and prostate-specific antigen levels; and the divided urine test.

Semen analysis. This test measures the number of sperm in a semen sample. A below-normal level indicates infertility.

VDRL test. This blood test screens for or confirms a diagnosis of syphilis.

Serum alpha-fetoprotein test. By measuring the glycoprotein produced by tumors, this test helps detect testicular cancer and monitors the effectiveness of treatment. Above-normal levels suggest testicular cancer or inadequate treatment.

Serum acid phosphatase test. This test measures the phosphatase enzymes produced by prostatic tumors. Above-normal levels indicate prostate cancer.

Prostate-specific antigen test. In this blood test, elevated antigen levels suggest prostate cancer.

Divided urine test. By detecting bacteria in prostatic fluid or a urine sample, this test helps diagnose prostatitis.

Female reproductive system

Disorders of the female reproductive system may have wide-ranging effects on other body systems. Vaginitis, for example, can lead to a UTI because of the proximity of the vagina to the urethra. And ovarian dysfunction can alter a woman's endocrine balance.

But female reproductive system disorders may have psychosocial implications as well. A serious impairment in reproductive function can adversely affect a woman's self-image.

Anatomy and physiology

The female reproductive system is divided into external and internal genitalia. An accurate assessment depends on your understanding of the anatomy and function of this system. (See *Reviewing the female reproductive system*.)

The breasts are affected by ovarian production of estrogen and progesterone, especially during puberty, pregnancy, and lactation. So they'll also be discussed in this chapter.

External genitalia

Collectively called the vulva, the external genitalia include the mons pubis, labia majora, labia minora, clitoris, vaginal introitus, hymen, and Skene's and Bartholin's glands.

The mons pubis is the fat pad covering the symphysis pubis. After puberty, the mons pubis is covered by a patch of coarse, curly hair, which extends up to the lower abdomen in an inverted triangle.

The outer vulvar lips, or labia majora, are two rounded folds of adipose tissue that extend from the mons pubis to the perineum. After puberty, the outer surfaces of the labia majora are covered with hair, although the inner surfaces remain hairless.

The inner vulvar lips are called the labia minora. The anterolateral and medial parts join to form the prepuce and frenulum of the clitoris. The posterior union of the labia minora is called the fourchette.

Composed of erectile tissue similar to that of the corpora cavernosa of the penis, the clitoris lies between the labia minora at the top of the vestibule. The vestibule also contains the urethral and vaginal openings. The urethral orifice is an irregular slit posterior to the clitoris. The vaginal opening (or introitus) is posterior to the urethral orifice. It's a thin vertical slit in women with intact hymens and a large opening with irregular edges in women whose hymen has been perforated.

ANATOMY

Reviewing the female reproductive system

These two illustrations show you internal and external structures of the female reproductive system.

Fallopian tube

Ovary

Cervix

Fundus

Uterine cavity

External fornix

Vaginal vault

Mons pubis

Clitoris

Labia majora

Labia minora

Bartholin's glands

Skene's glands

Urethral orifice

Vaginal introitus

Perineum

Two kinds of glands have ducts that open into the vulva. Skene's glands are multiple, tiny structures located just below the urethra, each containing 6 to 31 ducts. Bartholin's glands are found posterior to the vaginal opening. Neither Skene's nor Bartholin's glands can be seen, but they can be palpated if enlarged.

Internal genitalia

The internal female reproductive system includes the vagina, cervix, uterus, ovaries, and fallopian tubes. A pink, hollow, collapsed tube, the vagina extends up between the urethra and the rectum and back to the uterus. Extremely dilatable, the vagina is about 6" (15 cm) long in adults. It acts as the route of passage for childbirth and menstruation.

The uterus is a hollow, muscular organ divided into the fundus and the cervix (the narrow, lower end that projects into the vaginal vault). The fundus and cervix are connected by the constricted isthmus. The position of the uterus may vary, depending on the fullness of the bladder. The only function of the uterus is to contain the developing embryo.

A pair of oval organs about 1¼" (3 cm) long, the ovaries are usually found near the lateral pelvic wall at the height of the anterosuperior iliac spine. The ovaries produce ova and release the hormones estrogen, progesterone, and testosterone. During puberty, they stimulate the growth of the uterus and its endometrial lining. They also stimulate the enlargement of the vagina and help thicken its epithelium as well as spur the development of secondary sex characteristics.

About 4" (10 cm) long, the two fallopian tubes extend from the ovaries into the upper portion of the uterus. Their funnel-shaped ends curve toward the ovaries, and during ovulation, they help guide the ova to the uterus after expulsion from the ovaries.

Breasts

The breasts are paired, modified sebaceous glands located on the anterior chest wall between the second and sixth ribs. They're composed mainly of subcutaneous and retromammary fat and contain many lymph nodes.

The upper lateral quadrant of each breast contains the largest amount of glandular tissue. This quadrant also contains the tail of Spence—a projection of breast tissue into the axilla. This is an important landmark because it's the site of most breast tumors.

The breasts are supported by a layer of subcutaneous connective tissue and by Cooper's ligaments. These ligaments are multiple fibrous bands that start at the subcutaneous connective tissue layer and run through the breasts, attaching to muscle fascia. Externally, each breast contains an areola and a nipple. (See *Reviewing the female breast*.)

The areolae are pigmented areas at the center of each breast. Their color varies from pink to brown; they also vary in size. The areolar surface contains sebaceous glands called Montgomery's tubercles or follicles. Located at the center of the areolae, the nipples are round, pigmented, protuberant structures. Their shape and size varies in adult women, and their color ranges from pink to dark brown.

Lymphatic drainage

Three types of lymphatic drainage occur in the breasts: cutaneous, areolar, and deep lymphatic drainage. Cutaneous lymph drainage comes from lymph nodes in the breast skin, except that of the areola and nipple. The lymph flows into the mammary, scapular, tracheal, and intermediate nodes. Formed in the areolar and nipple areas, areolar lymphatic drainage flows into the mammary nodes. Originating in the deep mammary tissues, deep lymphatic drainage flows into the anterior axillary nodes.

Health history

Conduct the interview before the patient is in the lithotomy position and, if possible, before she undresses. By doing so, you will help her feel more relaxed and less vulnerable.

Chief complaint

The most common reproductive system complaints expressed by women are pain, vaginal discharge, abnormal uterine bleeding, pruritus, breast lumps and masses, and breast changes,

Reviewing the female breast

Use this illustration to review the important structures of the female breast and associated nodes.

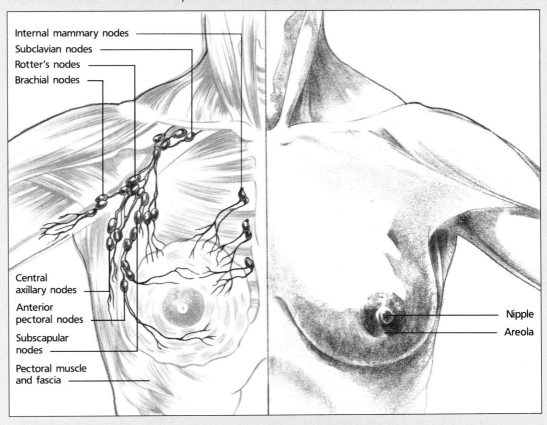

Internal mammary nodes
Subclavian nodes
Rotter's nodes
Brachial nodes
Central axillary nodes
Anterior pectoral nodes
Subscapular nodes
Pectoral muscle and fascia
Nipple
Areola

such as pain, nipple discharge, and nipple rash. To investigate these or any other reproductive complaints, ask your patient relevant questions about such particulars as onset, duration, and severity. Also ask what precipitates the symptom, what makes it worse, and what makes it better. For more information on exploring chief complaints, see Chapter 3.

Medical history

If appropriate, ask the patient when her last menstrual period started. The menstrual cycle—from the 1st day of one menses to the 1st day of the next—should be more than 21 days and less than 35 days. Deviations can indicate ovulatory problems, fibroid tumors, or cancer. Ask also how long the patient's periods usually last. The usual duration varies from 3 to 7 days. Extremely long or short periods may signal an abnormality, such as anovulation or anorexia nervosa. Ask the patient to describe her menstrual flow. An unusually heavy flow or clots can signal uterine fibroids. Women who use oral contraceptives or intrauterine devices (IUDs) report wide variations in menstrual flow.

Depending on the patient's age, ask if she's gone through menopause or is having symptoms of menopause. If she's experiencing symptoms, have her describe them. Also explore how she feels about going through menopause.

Ask the patient if she's sexually active. If not, is she a virgin? This information helps you assess her risk for some reproductive system disorders and provides clues for the physical assessment. If the patient has never had intercourse, use a small speculum during your examination.

Determine which method of contraception the patient uses. How long has she used it? If she uses an IUD or diaphragm, does she see her health care provider regularly to have it checked? If the patient uses a contraceptive device or spermicide, ask if she's ever had any adverse reactions to it. A diaphragm may cause urinary discomfort; a spermicide may cause vaginal irritation; and an IUD may increase the risk of pelvic inflammatory disease.

Has the patient had symptoms of an infection, such as vaginal discharge or itching, painful intercourse, sores or lesions, fever, chills, or swelling? These symptoms can result from an STD, candidiasis, vaginitis, or toxic shock syndrome. Ask if the patient has ever had vaginal bleeding after intercourse. Such bleeding can indicate a vaginal infection.

Determine if the patient has ever had an STD or another genital or reproductive system infection. Has it recurred? Recurring candidiasis infections can signal diabetes mellitus. Recurring STD infections may mean that the patient has an untreated partner or multiple partners.

Ask if the patient has ever been pregnant. If so, did she have any problems with her pregnancy or delivery? Did she deliver vaginally or by cesarean section?

Is the patient trying to get pregnant? How long has she been trying? If pregnancy doesn't occur after 1 year of trying, the patient may have a fertility problem.

Has the patient ever had reproductive system surgery, such as tubal ligation, dilatation and curettage, or a hysterectomy? If so, when and why?

Find out if the patient has ever had breast surgery. If so, when and why? Breast changes in a patient with previous breast cancer could indicate another malignant tumor. Has the patient ever had a mammogram? If so, when? Exposure to the excessive ionizing radiation from early mammography machines may increase the risk of breast cancer.

Family history
Ask if the patient's mother, maternal grandmother, or sisters ever had breast cancer. If so, was it in one breast or both? Did it occur before or after menopause? The patient's risk increases if the relative had cancer in both breasts, especially if it developed before menopause.

Psychosocial history
Has the patient experienced any changes in libido, the frequency of intercourse, or sexual function? Such changes may result from pain, infection, hormonal changes, depression, mental status changes, or role or relationship changes. Ask if the patient is having any other sexual problems. Physical problems of the reproductive system can affect sexuality.

Activities of daily living
Find out if the patient uses illicit drugs or drinks alcohol. If so, what kind and how much? Acquired immunodeficiency syndrome can be transmitted by sharing contaminated needles. Marijuana can produce a false-positive result on a urine test for pregnancy. Cocaine use during pregnancy can cause severe withdrawal symptoms and neurologic problems in neonates. Alcohol use during pregnancy can cause fetal alcohol syndrome.

Ask if the patient smokes. If so, how much and for how long? Smoking increases the risk of cardiovascular disease and occurrence of thrombi in women using oral contraceptives. Smoking during pregnancy is associated with fetal growth retardation and fetal and infant morbidity and mortality.

Does the patient eat a well-balanced diet? Eating patterns can affect the reproductive system at any age. For example, anorexia nervosa can cause menstrual irregularities.

Ask if the patient has had regular health checkups and gynecologic examinations. When was her last Papanicolaou (Pap) test? A Pap test can detect precancerous and cancerous cell changes in the cervix, human papillomavirus, *Chlamydia trachomatis,* and herpes simplex.

Does the patient perform a monthly breast self-examination? Make sure she knows the importance of the examination and the correct technique. Also, explain that breasts should be examined on the 5th to 7th day of the menstrual cycle when tenderness and lumpiness are reduced. Tell postmenopausal patients to choose a regular time each month. Tell those on estrogen replacement therapy to do the examination once a month on the day before they restart the drug.

Physical examination

Before starting the examination, ask the patient to urinate. Next, help her into the dorsal lithotomy position and drape her. After putting on gloves, examine the patient's external and internal genitalia and her breasts, as appropriate.

Inspecting the external genitalia
Observe the skin and hair distribution of the mons pubis. Spread the hair with your fingers to check for lesions and pediculosis.

Next, inspect the skin of the labia majora, spreading the hair to examine for lesions, parasites, and genital warts. The skin should be slightly darker than the rest of the body, and the labia majora should be round and full. Examine the labia minora, which should be dark pink and moist. In nulliparous women, the labia majora and minora are close together; in women who have experienced vaginal deliveries, they may gape open.

Closely observe each vulvar structure for syphilitic chancres and cancerous lesions. Examine the area of Bartholin's and Skene's glands and ducts for swelling, erythema, duct enlargement, or discharge. Next, inspect the urethral opening. It should be slitlike and the same color as the mucous membranes. Look for erythema, polyps, and discharge.

Palpating the external genitalia
Spread the labia open with one hand while you palpate the labia majora and labia minora with your other hand. The labia should feel soft. Note any swelling, hardness, or tenderness. If you detect a mass or lesion, palpate it to determine its size, shape, and consistency.

If you note labial swelling or tenderness, palpate the area of Bartholin's glands. Insert your gloved index finger into the patient's posterior introitus and place your thumb along the lateral edge of the swollen or tender labium. Then gently squeeze the labium. Obtain a culture specimen of any discharge. Usually, Bartholin's glands aren't palpable.

If you note urethral inflammation, milk the urethra and the area of Skene's glands. First, moisten the gloved index finger of your dominant hand with water. Separate the labia with your other gloved hand, and gently insert your index finger about $1\frac{1}{2}"$ (4 cm) into the anterior vagina. With your finger pad, gently press the anterior vaginal wall up into the urethra and pull outward. Continue palpating down to the introitus. This procedure shouldn't be painful. Obtain a culture specimen of any discharge.

Inspecting the internal genitalia
First, select a speculum that's appropriate for the patient. In most cases, you'll use a Graves speculum. However, if the patient is a virgin or nulliparous, or if she has a contracted introitus due to menopause, you should use a Pederson speculum.

Hold the speculum's blades under warm running water. This warms the blades and helps to lubricate them, making insertion easier and more comfortable for the patient. Don't use any commercial lubricants — they're bacteriostatic and will distort cells on Pap tests. Sit or stand at the foot of the examination table. Tell the patient that she'll feel some pressure; then insert the speculum. (See *How to insert a speculum,* page 240.)

While inserting and withdrawing the speculum, note the color, texture, and mucosal integrity of the vagina and any vaginal secretions. A white, odorless, thin discharge is normal.

How to insert a speculum

Place the index and middle fingers of your nondominant hand about 1″ (2.5 cm) into the vagina, and spread them to exert some pressure toward the posterior vagina.

Hold the speculum in your dominant hand, and insert the blades between your fingers, as shown.

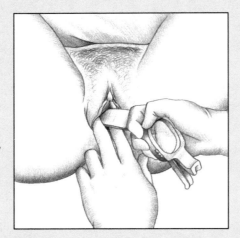

Ask the patient to bear down to open the introitus and relax the perineal muscles. Then point the speculum slightly downward, and insert the blades until the base of the speculum touches your fingertips inside the vagina.

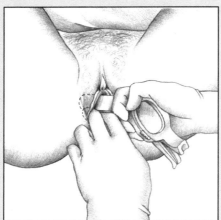

Then rotate the speculum to coincide with the plane of the vagina, and withdraw your fingers. Next, open the blades as far as possible and lock them. You should now be able to view the cervix.

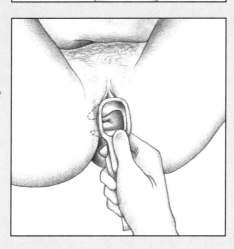

With the speculum in place, examine the cervix for color, position, size, shape, mucosal integrity, and discharge. The cervix should be smooth, round, rosy pink, and free of ulcerations and nodules. A clear, watery discharge is normal during ovulation; a slightly bloody discharge is normal just before menstruation. Obtain a culture specimen of any other discharge. After inspecting the cervix, obtain a specimen for a Pap test.

When you've completed your examination, unlock the speculum blades and close them slowly while you begin withdrawing the instrument. Close the blades completely before they reach the introitus. Then withdraw the speculum from the vagina.

Palpating the internal genitalia

With the patient still in the dorsal lithotomy position, palpate her vagina. To do so, lubricate your index and middle fingers and insert them into the vagina, exerting pressure posteriorly. Note any tenderness or nodularity in the vaginal wall. Also assess the support of the vaginal outlet by asking the patient to bear down, noting any bulging of the marginal walls that could indicate a cystocele or rectocele.

Next, palpate the cervix, which should be smooth and firm. If it feels nodular or irregular, cysts, tumors, or lesions may be present.

Then, place your other hand on the abdomen between the umbilicus and symphysis pubis. Elevate the cervix and uterus with the two fingers inside the vagina while you press down and in with the hand on the abdomen. Try to grasp the uterus between your hands. Then slide your fingers farther into the anterior fornix and palpate the body of the uterus between your hands. Note its size, shape, surface characteristics, consistency, and mobility. Note any tenderness of the uterine body and fundus. Also note the position of the uterus. (See *Bimanual palpation of the uterus.*)

The ovaries will usually be palpable in a premenopausal woman, unless she's obese. Palpable ovaries in a postmenopausal patient may mean an ovarian tumor. The ovaries should be flattened, ovoid, and 1¼″ to 1½″ (3 to 4 cm) in diameter. The fallopian tubes and supporting tissues usually aren't palpable unless an abnormal mass is present.

Rectovaginal palpation

A complete vaginal examination should include rectal palpation to assess the posterior portion of the uterus and pelvic cavity. This examination also confirms uterine position and allows you to assess the adnexal area (ovaries, fallopian tubes, and supporting tissues).

After completing the vaginal examination, change your gloves. Then lubricate your index and middle fingers, and insert them into the vagina and rectum respectively while the patient bears down. Insert them as far as possible. Place your other hand above the symphysis pubis and press down, palpating the posterior part of the uterus with your middle finger. The rectovaginal septum should feel firm, thin, smooth, and pliable.

Breast examination

Ask the patient to disrobe from the waist up and then to sit with her arms at her sides. Observe her breast skin, which should be smooth, undimpled, and the same color as the rest of her skin. Check for edema, which can accompany lymphatic obstruction and suggest cancer. Note breast size and symmetry. Inspect the nipples, noting their size and shape. If a nipple is inverted, ask the patient how long it's been that way. Also note any nipple discharge.

Have the patient hold her arms over her head and then put her hands on her hips while you examine her breasts. This helps you detect dimpling or retraction that wasn't obvious before. If the patient has large or pendulous breasts, have her stand with her hands on the back of a chair and lean forward. This helps reveal breast or nipple asymmetry that wasn't visible before.

Palpating the breasts

Ask the patient to lie supine so that you can palpate her breasts. Place a small pillow under her shoulder on the side you're examining. Ask her to put her hand behind her head, unless her breasts are very small. This spreads the breast more evenly across the chest and makes

Bimanual palpation of the uterus

To palpate the uterus bimanually, insert the index and middle fingers of one hand into the patient's vagina and place your other hand on the abdomen between the umbilicus and symphysis pubis. Press the abdomen in and down while you elevate the cervix and uterus with your two fingers, as shown. Try to grasp the uterus between your hands.

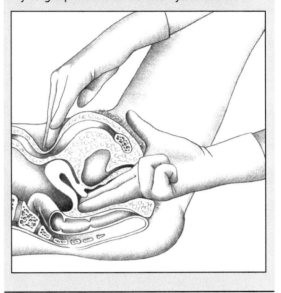

finding nodules easier. (See *Palpating the breasts and axillae,* page 242.)

Next, place your fingers flat on the breast and compress the tissues gently against the chest wall, palpating in concentric circles outward from the nipple. Cover the entire breast—periphery, tail of Spence, and areola. An alternative method, especially useful in patients with pendulous breasts, is palpating across or down the breast with the patient sitting up.

Note the consistency of the breast tissue. Normal consistency varies widely, depending in part on the proportions of fat and glandular tissue. Check for nodules and unusual tenderness. Nodularity may increase before menstruation; tenderness may result from premenstrual

Palpating the breasts and axillae

With the patient supine and her arm above her head, place a small pillow under the shoulder on the side you're examining. Using your finger pads, palpate the breast in concentric circles from the center to the periphery.

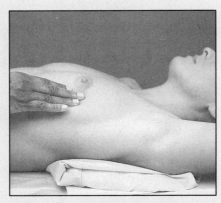

Palpate the areola and nipple, and compress the nipple between your thumb and index finger.

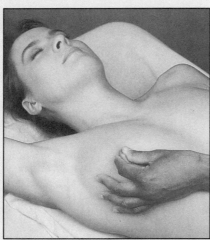

With the patient seated, palpate the axillae. Palpate the right axilla with the middle three fingers of one hand while supporting the patient's arm with your other hand.

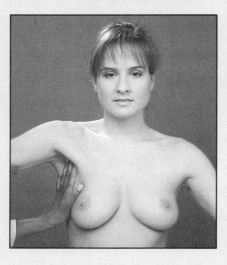

fullness, cysts, or cancer. Any lump or mass that feels different from the rest of the breast tissue may represent a pathologic change. If you detect a mass, note the following:
• location (centimeters from the nipple, using the quadrant or clock method)
• size (in centimeters)
• shape (round, discoid, regular, or irregular)
• consistency (soft, firm, hard)
• discreteness (borders in relation to surrounding tissue)
• mobility
• degree of tenderness.

Next, palpate the nipple, noting its elasticity. Then compress the nipple and areola to detect discharge. If you see any, note the color, consistency, and quantity.

Assessing the axillae

Have the patient sit up. Then inspect the skin of the axillae for rashes, infections, and any unusual pigmentation.

Next, palpate the axillae, starting with the right one. Ask the patient to relax her right arm while you use one hand to support her elbow or wrist. Cup the fingers of your other hand together, and reach high into the apex of the axilla. Your fingers should be directly behind the pectoral muscles, pointing toward the midclavicle. Press your fingers downward and in toward the chest wall to try to feel the central nodes. You can usually palpate one or more soft, small, nontender, central nodes. If the nodes feel large or hard or are tender, or if the patient has a suspicious-looking lesion, try to palpate the other groups of lymph nodes.

To palpate the pectoral or anterior nodes, grasp the anterior axillary fold between your thumb and fingers and palpate inside the borders of the pectoral muscle. To palpate the lateral nodes, press your fingers along the upper inner arm, trying to compress these nodes against the humerus. To palpate the subscapular or posterior nodes, stand behind the patient, and use your fingers to feel inside the muscle of the posterior axillary fold.

Abnormal findings

During your assessment, you may detect one of the following common abnormal findings: genital lesions, vaginal inflammation or discharge, vaginal prolapse, cervical lesions, cervical cyanosis, breast cysts or masses, prominent breast veins, breast inflammation, and nipple retraction or inversion.

Genital lesions
In the early stages, syphilitic chancre causes a painless, eroded lesion with a raised, indurated border. The lesion usually appears inside the vagina, but it may be on the external genitalia. You may also notice lymph node inflammation.

Genital herpes produces multiple shallow vesicles, lesions, or crusts inside the vagina and on the external genitalia, buttocks and, sometimes, the thighs. Dysuria, regional lymph node inflammation, pain, edema, and fever may be present. A Pap test reveals multinucleated giant cells with intranuclear inclusion bodies.

Vaginal inflammation and discharge
Vaginitis usually results from an overgrowth of infectious organisms. It causes redness, itching, dyspareunia, dysuria, and malodorous discharge.

Trichomonas vaginalis may cause gray or green, frothy or watery malodorous discharge. It may be transmitted sexually. Besides redness, you may note red papules on the cervix and vaginal walls.

Candida albicans causes a thick, white, curdlike discharge that appears in patches on the cervix and vaginal walls. The discharge has a yeastlike odor.

Chlamydia trachomatis produces a heavy, gray-white discharge.

Gonorrhea is often asymptomatic. Purulent green-yellow discharge and cystitis may appear.

Vaginal prolapse
Cystocele is the prolapse of the anterior vaginal wall and bladder into the vagina. During a speculum examination, you'll notice a pouch or bulging on the anterior wall as the patient bears down.

Rectocele is the herniation of the rectum through the posterior vaginal wall. On examination, you'll see a pouch or bulging on the posterior wall as the patient bears down.

Cervical lesions
During a speculum examination, you may detect late-stage cervical cancer as hard, granular, friable lesions; in the early stages, the cervix looks normal.

Cervical polyps are bright red, soft, and fragile. They're usually benign, but they may bleed. They usually arise from the endocervical canal.

Cervical cyanosis
This condition may accompany any disorder that causes systemic hypoxia or venous congestion in the cervix. It's also common during pregnancy.

Breast cysts or masses
In fibrocystic disease of the breast, you'll palpate one or more well-defined, movable lumps or cysts. This benign condition results from excess fibrous tissue formation and hyperplasia of the lining in the mammary ducts.

Fibroadenoma, a benign condition, produces a small, round, painless, well-defined, mobile lump that may be soft but is usually solid, firm, and rubbery.

Breast cancer usually appears in the upper outer quadrant as a hard, immobile, irregular lump. Nipple discharge may occur, and breast skin may become edematous with enlarged pores, discoloration, and an orange-peel appearance (peau d'orange). The skin feels thick, hard, and immobile.

Prominent breast veins
Prominent veins may be associated with cancer. However, they're normal in pregnancy and in some fair-skinned women.

Breast inflammation
Acute mastitis causes skin abrasions or cracking and reddened skin; fever and other signs of systemic infection may also occur. This condition is usually associated with lactation.

Erythema of the nipple and areola are early signs of Paget's disease, a cancer of the mammary ducts. Nipple thickening, scaling, and erosion occur later. Another common sign is a red, scaly, eczema-like rash over the affected nipple and areola.

Nipple retraction and inversion

Retracted (dimpled or creased) areas in breast skin or nipples result from fibrosis or scar tissue formation and may be a sign of cancer. The breast or nipple may also change contour. Retraction may be obvious during inspection, or it may not be evident until the patient changes position or you palpate her breast.

Inverted nipples may be normal if the patient has always had them. But suspect fibrosis or cancer if nipple inversion occurs suddenly, accompanied by a thickening and broadening of the skin.

Pertinent diagnostic tests

Depending on the patient's complaint and your findings, one or more of the following tests may be ordered: colposcopy, laparoscopy, endometrial biopsy, cytologic smear, Pap test, vaginal secretion culture, urinalysis, VDRL test, mammography, and transillumination. A description of the VDRL test appears in the section on the male reproductive system.

Colposcopy. In this test, a colposcope is inserted into the vagina to examine the cervix by means of a magnifying lens. Colposcopy can detect cervical cancer, a herpes virus infection, and other conditions of the cervix, vagina, and external genitalia.

Laparoscopy. A laparoscope inserted through an abdominal incision allows visualization of the pelvic organs to help pinpoint ovarian cysts and other problems. Surgical instruments can be passed through the laparoscope so that small lesions can be removed with a laser beam or cryosurgical or electrocautery device.

Endometrial biopsy. In this procedure, scrapings of endometrial tissue are obtained for culture. This test helps detect endometrial cancer.

Cytologic smear. In this test, a culture is made of abnormal nipple discharge to determine its cause.

Pap test. This test detects cervical cancer. Cervical and endocervical specimens are obtained during a speculum examination for a culture.

Vaginal secretion culture. With this test, a specimen is obtained and a culture performed to diagnose candidiasis, trichomoniasis, gonorrhea, chlamydial infection, and other vaginal infections and STDs.

Urinalysis. Used with a vaginal secretion culture, antibody titer urinalysis helps diagnose a chlamydial infection.

Mammography. This procedure uses low-dose radiation to view the breasts. It can detect lumps as small as 4 mm and calcium deposits as small as 1 mm.

Transillumination. Also called diaphanography or light scanning, this test projects infrared light through breast tissue. Then a video camera photographs the light, and a computer transforms it into images on a video screen. Lesions or areas of increased vascularity appear darker than the surrounding tissue. Because it emits no radiation, this test is useful for showing tumor changes.

Suggested readings and acknowledgments

Suggested readings

Alspach, J., ed. *Core Curriculum for Critical Care Nursing,* 4th ed. Philadelphia: W.B. Saunders Co., 1991.

Bates, B. *A Guide to Physical Examination and History Taking,* 5th ed. Philadelphia: J.B. Lippincott Co., 1991.

Bayley, E. "Wound Healing in the Patient with Burns," *Nursing Clinics of North America* 25(1):205-22, March 1990.

Braunwald, E. "The Physical Examination," in *Heart Disease: A Textbook of Cardiovascular Medicine,* 4th ed. Edited by Braunwald, E. Philadelphia: W.B. Saunders Co., 1992.

Bryant, G. "When the Bowel Is Blocked," *RN* 55(1):58-66, January 1992.

Danger Signs and Symptoms. Clinical Skillbuilders Series. Springhouse, Pa.: Springhouse Corp., 1990.

DeWitt, S. "Nursing Assessment of the Skin and Dermatologic Lesions," *Nursing Clinics of North America* 25(1):235-45, March 1990.

Dolan, J. *Critical Care Nursing: Clinical Management through the Nursing Process.* Philadelphia: F.A. Davis Co., 1991.

Goldberg, S., and Bronson, B. "Blistering Diseases: Diagnostic Help for Primary Care Physicians," *Postgraduate Medicine* 89(2):159-62, February 1991.

Guyton, A.C. *Textbook of Medical Physiology,* 8th ed. Philadelphia: W.B. Saunders Co., 1991.

Ignatavicius, D., and Bayne, M. *Medical Surgical Nursing: A Nursing Process Approach.* Philadelphia: W.B. Saunders Co., 1991.

Illustrated Manual of Nursing Practice. Springhouse, Pa.: Springhouse Corp., 1991.

Little, R., and Little, W. *Physiology of the Heart and Circulation,* 4th ed. Chicago: Year-book Medical Pubs., 1988.

Malasanos, L., et al. *Health Assessment,* 4th ed. St. Louis: C.V. Mosby Co., 1990.

Marshall, S.B., et al. *Neuroscience Critical Care: Pathophysiology and Patient Management.* Philadelphia: W.B. Saunders Co., 1990.

Pariser, R. "Allergic and Reactive Dermatoses: How to Identify and Treat Them," *Postgraduate Medicine* 89(8):75-80, 85, June 1991. Published errata appear in *Postgraduate Medicine* 90(2):54, August 1991.

Phillips, R., and Feeney, M. *The Cardiac Rhythms: A Systematic Approach to Interpretation,* 3rd ed. Philadelphia: W.B. Saunders Co., 1990.

Rapid Assessment. Clinical Skillbuilders Series. Springhouse, Pa.: Springhouse Corp., 1991.

Rodnitzky, R.L., ed. *Van Allen's Pictorial Manual of Neurologic Tests,* 3rd ed. Chicago: Year-book Medical Pubs., 1988.

Seidel, H., et al. *Mosby's Guide to Physical Examination,* 2nd ed. St. Louis: Mosby-Year Book, Inc., 1991.

Shapiro, B.A., et al. *Clinical Application of Respiratory Care,* 4th ed. St. Louis: Mosby-Year Book, Inc., 1991.

Sparks, S., and Taylor, C. *Nursing Diagnosis Reference Manual,* 2nd ed. Springhouse, Pa.: Springhouse Corp., 1993.

Traver, G.A., et al. *Respiratory Care: A Clinical Approach.* Rockville, Md.: Aspen Pubs., Inc., 1991.

Treseler, K.M. *Clinical Laboratory and Diagnostic Tests: Significance and Nursing Implications,* 2nd ed. East Norwalk, Conn.: Appleton & Lange, 1988.

Vonfrolio, L.G., and Bacon, K. "Abdominal Trauma," *RN* 54(6):30-34, June 1991.

Wardell, T. "Assessing and Managing a Gastric Ulcer," *Nursing91* 21(3):34-42, March 1991.

Wilson, J.D., et al. *Harrison's Principles of Internal Medicine,* 12th ed. New York: McGraw-Hill Book Co., 1991.

Acknowledgments

Carroll H. Weiss
Vitiligo, p. 89
Squamous cell carcinoma, p. 90
Cherry angioma, p. 90
Seborrheic keratosis, p. 89
Tinea corporis, p. 89
Scabies, p. 89
Telangiectasis, p. 87
Candidiasis (monilial), p. 88
Urticaria, p. 87
Basal cell carcinoma, p. 90
Kaposi's sarcoma, p. 90
Malignant melanoma, p. 90
Purpura, p. 87

Fran Heyl Associates
Contact dermatitis, p. 87

Biophoto Associates
Acne, p. 88

Photo Researchers, Inc.
Herpes simplex, St. Bartholomew's Hospital/ Science Photo Library, p. 88
Herpes zoster, p. 89
Eczema, St. Bartholomew's Hospital/Science Photo Library, p. 87
Cystic acne, J.F. Wilson, p. 88
Impetigo, Science Photo Library, p. 88
Psoriasis, John Radcliffe Infirmary/Science Photo Library, p. 87
Verruca, David Parker/Science Photo Library, p. 88
Spider nevus, Biophoto Associates, p. 90

PHOTOTAKE
Lupus erythematosus (discoid or systemic), p. 89

Advanced skilltest

This self-test presents case histories with related multiple-choice questions as well as general multiple-choice questions on advanced assessment. The questions begin on this page and continue to page 250. You'll find the answers along with rationales on pages 250 and 251.

Case history questions

Mrs. Baumann, age 45, is admitted to your unit with complaints of burning abdominal pain and nausea. She has had the pain for 2 weeks and gets relief only when her stomach is full. Because she eats to stop the pain, she has gained 5 lb over the last 2 weeks.

1. During the health history, Mrs. Baumann reports that she experiences pain 2 to 4 hours after eating. Which of the following causes would you suspect?

    a. Cholecystitis

    b. Appendicitis

    c. Duodenal ulcer

    d. Intestinal obstruction

2. When assessing Mrs. Baumann's abdomen, which technique would you use last?

    a. Palpation

    b. Auscultation

    c. Percussion

    d. Inspection

3. Which diagnostic test would confirm the diagnosis of a duodenal ulcer?

    a. Small-bowel series

    b. Upper GI series

    c. Endoscopy

    d. Ultrasound of the stomach

Mr. Klim, age 62, is admitted to your unit for hip surgery. During the history, he tells you that he has been smoking two packs of cigarettes a day for 45 years. He also reports that he becomes short of breath when he exerts himself and that he has a productive cough with white secretions.

4. You suspect that Mr. Klim has underlying chronic obstructive pulmonary disease (COPD). Given your suspicion, which inspection finding would you *not* expect to see?

    a. Barrel chest

    b. Mucous membrane cyanosis

    c. Clubbed fingers

    d. Abnormal expansion and collapse of an area of the chest wall

5. Upon auscultating Mr. Klim's lungs, which adventitious breath sounds would you expect to hear?

    a. Fine crackles and rhonchi that don't clear with coughing

    b. Wheezes

    c. Coarse crackles

    d. Pleural friction rubs

6. Which percussion and palpation findings would you expect?

    a. Dullness and increased fremitus

    b. Resonance and crepitus

    c. Hyperresonance and decreased fremitus

    d. Tympany and no fremitus

Mrs. Casalini, age 32, is admitted to your unit after a car accident. She complains of pain at the base of her head and down into her neck. In the accident, the right rear of her car was hit by a truck, and her head was thrown back against the headrest. Then she hit the steering wheel with the right side of her face and her right ear. Her eyes are swollen, irritated, and dry. She reports some hearing loss in her right ear as well as dizziness.

7. Mrs. Casalini's doctor diagnoses a basilar skull fracture. Which type of nasal drainage would you expect to see?

    a. Bloody

    b. Clear and thin

    c. Yellow and thick

    d. White and thick

8. Mrs. Casalini's complaints of dizziness and decreased hearing in her right ear would lead you to suspect damage to the:

    a. cochlea and vestibular and semicircular canals.

    b. auricle and auditory canal.

    c. malleus and stapes.

    d. tympanic membrane and incus.

9. You'd suspect that Mrs. Casalini's dry, irritated eyes may result from an obstruction of the:

    a. bulbar conjunctiva.

    b. lacrimal duct.

    c. fibrous tunic.

    d. choroid.

Mr. Tulliver, age 76, is admitted to your unit with balance and gait abnormalities. He tells you he used to lose his balance when he stood up from a sitting position, but now he loses his balance even when he sits down. He says he walks like a "drunken sailor."

10. Which area of the brain controls general balance and coordination?

    a. Brain stem

    b. Cerebrum

    c. Cerebellum

    d. Temporal lobes

11. When examining Mr. Tulliver, you'd be sure to assess the:

    a. vestibular branch of cranial nerve VIII.

    b. cranial nerve V.

    c. cranial nerve XII.

    d. cochlear branch of cranial nerve VIII.

12. Which gait abnormality would indicate cerebellar dysfunction?

    a. Ataxic gait

    b. Hemiparetic gait

    c. Steppage gait

    d. Parkinsonian gait

Mr. Wandowski, age 62, is admitted to your unit with a diagnosis of an inferior wall myocardial infarction. He has a history of unstable angina, which has been getting progressively worse over the last 2 days. When you examine him, he appears comfortable and says he's not having chest pain.

13. You note that Mr. Wandowski's heart rate alternates between 60 to 68 beats/minute (with a normal sinus rhythm) and 48 to 60 beats/minute. You can't detect any pattern to these changes. Which coronary artery would you expect to be affected?

    a. Left anterior descending artery

    b. Right coronary artery

    c. Left main artery

    d. Circumflex artery

14. When auscultating Mr. Wandowski's heart sounds, where would you expect S_2 to be the loudest?

    a. Pulmonary area

    b. Tricuspid area

    c. Mitral area

    d. Aortic area

15. Mr. Wandowski calls you into his room and complains that he's short of breath. He appears cyanotic, and he has all the other signs of congestive heart failure (CHF). Which abnormal heart sound would you expect to hear?

    a. S_3

    b. S_4

    c. Ejection click

    d. Summation gallop

General questions

16. Normal inspection findings for the nose include all of the following *except:*

    a. a moist, pinkish red mucosa.

    b. an absence of lesions and polyps.

    c. visible choana, cilia, and middle and inferior turbinates.

    d. thin mucus drainage and mild edema.

17. Which area of the brain contains the nuclei of cranial nerves III through XII and is a major sensory and motor pathway for impulses running to and from the cerebrum?

    a. Diencephalon

    b. Brain stem

    c. Pons

    d. Cerebellum

18. In a patient with chronic renal failure, you'd expect to see all of the following *except:*

    a. poor concentration, disorientation, and memory loss.

    b. red, flushed skin.

    c. dry skin, scratches, and dehydration.

    d. peripheral edema and pulmonary edema.

19. A 30-year-old woman complains of dyspnea on exertion and at rest, and of orthopnea. She also tells you she has a history of rheumatic fever. During your examination, you note a middiastolic or presystolic thrill at the apex; weak pulses; and a localized, delayed, rumbling, low-pitched murmur at or near the apex. You'd suspect:

    a. mitral stenosis.

    b. pulmonary stenosis.

    c. tricuspid stenosis.

    d. cardiomyopathy.

20. Urinary hesitancy, urinary frequency, and hematuria would suggest:

    a. diabetes mellitus.

    b. benign prostatic hyperplasia.

    c. urinary tract infection.

    d. renal and lower urinary tract disorders.

21. During your assessment of a man with congestive heart failure (CHF), you note scrotal enlargement. On transillumination, the scrotum transmits light. You'd suspect:

    a. a hydrocele.

    b. a testicular tumor.

    c. paraphimosis.

    d. hypospadias.

Answers

1. c. These are the classic symptoms of a duodenal ulcer. The pain associated with cholecystitis is usually in the right upper quadrant, shoulder, and scapular area. In appendicitis, pain is usually localized in the right lower quadrant. Diffuse abdominal pain as well as constipation and vomiting occur with intestinal obstruction.

2. a. Because palpation can alter auscultatory findings, you should follow this sequence when assessing the abdomen: inspection, auscultation, percussion, and palpation.

3. b. An upper GI series provides the most direct view of the duodenum and thus would be ordered to detect a duodenal ulcer. A small-bowel series detects problems in the small bowel, such as sprue, Hodgkin's lymphoma, and obstructions. Endoscopy is typically used to view the esophagus and stomach or the large bowel. Ultrasound isn't performed on the stomach because the air in the stomach prevents the sound wave transmission needed to produce an image.

4. d. You may see this abnormality in patients with chest wall injuries. In patients with COPD, barrel chest results from intercostal muscle hypertrophy due to chronic use. Cyanosis of the mucous membranes results from central hypoxia, usually associated with COPD. Patients with COPD also develop clubbed fingers as a result of chronic tissue hypoxia.

5. a. In patients with COPD, fine crackles and rhonchi that don't clear with coughing result from thick secretions in the bronchioles. Wheezes usually occur in patients with asthma or an airway obstruction caused by a tumor or foreign body. Coarse crackles usually occur in patients with increasing pulmonary congestion, such as pulmonary edema. Pleural friction rubs occur in patients who have inflamed visceral and parietal pleurae.

6. c. Hyperresonance results from air in the pleural space, and decreased fremitus indicates an increase of physiologic dead space — both of which occur in patients with COPD. Dullness and increased fremitus indicate fluid or tissue consolidation, as seen in pneumonia. You'll hear resonance over healthy lung tissue, and crepitus indicates air in the subcutaneous tissue. Normally, you'll hear tympany over the stomach, and you won't palpate fremitus in the lower chest.

7. b. Clear, thin secretions may indicate cerebrospinal fluid leakage from the basilar skull fracture. Epistaxis results from irritation or trauma. Thick yellow or white secretions indicate infection.

8. a. The cochlea is the organ of hearing, and the vestibular and semicircular canals help maintain equilibrium. The auricle and auditory canal collect auditory signals and direct them into the middle ear. The malleus, stapes, and incus are the bony structures of the middle ear that transmit sound vibrations to the inner ear. These structures aren't responsible for hearing. They protect the auditory apparatus from intense vibrations and equalize the air pressure on both sides of the tympanic membrane. The tympanic membrane separates the external ear from the middle ear.

9. b. The lacrimal duct allows tears to flow into the conjunctiva, keeping it moist. The bulbar conjunctiva lines the anterior surface of the eyeball up to the edge of the cornea. The fibrous tunic is the outer covering of the eyeball. The choroid lines most of the inner sclera, preventing light from being lost by reflection when it enters the eye.

10. c. The cerebellum controls general balance and coordination. The brain stem regulates respirations, vasomotor and cardiac functions, and relays messages between upper and lower levels of the nervous system. The cerebrum is responsible for mental status, including orientation, attention and concentration, general knowledge, memory and retention, reasoning, and mood and affect. The temporal lobes regulate speech, behavior, hearing, vestibular sense, and emotion.

11. a. The vestibular branch of cranial nerve VIII helps maintain equilibrium. Cranial nerve V innervates the muscles of the jaw and supplies pain and touch sensations to the face. Cranial nerve XII coordinates tongue movements. The cochlear branch of cranial nerve VIII is responsible for hearing.

12. a. Ataxia is characterized by a wide-based, reeling, "drunken" gait. Hemiparetic gait indicates damage to the upper motor neurons. Steppage gait is associated with lower motor neuron disease. Parkinsonian gait indicates Parkinson's disease.

13. b. The right coronary artery feeds the sinoatrial (SA) and atrioventricular (AV) nodes and the inferior muscles of the left ventricle. (An alteration in heart rate often indicates a problem with the SA and AV nodes.) The left anterior descending artery and the left main artery supply the left ventricle, and the circumflex artery supplies the left atria and the posterolateral surface of the left ventricle.

14. d. S_2 signals the beginning of ventricular diastole when the aortic valve snaps shut. S_1, heard best at the mitral area, signals the beginning of systole when the mitral valve is forced open by a surge of blood. S_3 may be heard at the tricuspid or mitral area during early to middiastole. And S_4 can be heard at the tricuspid or mitral area late in diastole, just before S_1.

15. a. S_3 results from vibrations during rapid ventricular filling and signals CHF. S_4 occurs in patients with hypertension, aortic stenosis, mitral regurgitation, and coronary artery disease. You may auscultate an ejection click in a patient with a stenotic aortic or pulmonary valve, hypertension, or a dilated aorta or pulmonary artery. A summation gallop occurs in patients with severe myocardial disease.

16. d. Drainage and edema are abnormal and may indicate an allergic reaction or an infection. The other findings are normal.

17. b. The brain stem includes the midbrain, the pons, and the medulla oblongata. The diencephalon divides the cerebrum and contains the thalamus, epithalamus, subthalamus, and hypothalamus. The cerebellum also contains major motor and sensory pathways.

18. b. The skin of a patient with chronic renal failure is usually pale because of decreased red blood cell production. Poor concentration, disorientation, and memory loss result from an inability to excrete toxins. Dry skin, scratches, and dehydration stem from the atrophy of sweat and oil glands. Peripheral edema and pulmonary edema may result from a buildup of fluid in the interstitial spaces and lungs.

19. a. These signs and symptoms indicate mitral stenosis. Pulmonary stenosis results in a split S_2 with a delayed or absent pulmonary component, a systolic murmur at the left sternal border, fatigue and, possibly, peripheral edema. Tricuspid stenosis causes a middiastolic thrill at the lower left sternal border, an apical impulse, and diastolic rumbling with a murmur along the lower left sternal border. Cardiomyopathy produces a systolic murmur, S_3, palpitations, basilar crackles, and a cardiac impulse displaced to the left.

20. b. These are classic signs and symptoms of benign prostatic hyperplasia. The most common sign of diabetes mellitus is polyuria. Urinary tract infections typically cause urinary urgency. Renal and lower urinary tract disorders may cause nocturia.

21. a. A hydrocele, a collection of fluid in the testicle, may be associated with systemic conditions of poor fluid reabsorption, such as CHF. A testicular tumor, a painless nodule palpable in the scrotum, wouldn't transmit light upon transillumination. Paraphimosis is a tight prepuce or foreskin. Hypospadias is a congenital displacement of the urethral meatus on the penis.

Index

i refers to illustration; t refers to table